Cancer Treatment and Research

Volume 191

This book series provides detailed updates on the state of the art in the treatment of different forms of cancer and also covers a wide spectrum of topics of current research interest. Clinicians will benefit from expert analysis of both standard treatment options and the latest therapeutic innovations and from provision of clear guidance on the management of clinical challenges in daily practice. The research-oriented volumes focus on aspects ranging from advances in basic science through to new treatment tools and evaluation of treatment safety and efficacy. Each volume is edited and authored by leading authorities in the topic under consideration. In providing cutting-edge information on cancer treatment and research, the series will appeal to a wide and interdisciplinary readership. The series is listed in PubMed/Index Medicus.

Rida Fatima Saeed · Sadr ul Shaheed
Editors

Nutrition and Dietary Interventions in Cancer

Springer

Editors
Rida Fatima Saeed
Department of Biological Sciences
National University of Medical Sciences
Rawalpindi, Pakistan

Sadr ul Shaheed
John Radcliffe Hospital
University of Oxford
Oxford, UK

ISSN 0927-3042 ISSN 2509-8497 (electronic)
Cancer Treatment and Research
ISBN 978-3-031-55621-0 ISBN 978-3-031-55622-7 (eBook)
https://doi.org/10.1007/978-3-031-55622-7

This Springer imprint is published by the registered company Springer Nature Switzerland AG
The registered company address is: Gewerbestrasse 11, 6330 Cham, Switzerland

Paper in this product is recyclable.

Contents

Introduction to Nutrition and Cancer

1

Hanadi Talal Ahmedah, Haneen Adel Basheer, Inas Almazari, and Kawther Faisal Amawi

Contents

Abbreviations

ATCC	American Type Culture Collection
BMI	Body mass index

H. T. Ahmedah (✉)
Department of Medical Laboratory Technology, Faculty of Applied Medical Sciences, King Abdulaziz University, Rabigh 25732, Saudi Arabia
e-mail: hehmedouh@kau.edu.sa

H. A. Basheer
Faculty of Pharmacy, Zarqa University, PO Box 132222, Zarqa 13132, Jordan
e-mail: hbasheer@zu.edu.jo

I. Almazari
Department of Clinical Pharmacy, Faculty of Pharmacy, Zarqa University, Zarqa, Jordan
e-mail: ialmazari@zu.edu.jo

K. F. Amawi
Department of Medical Laboratory Science, Faculty of Allied Medical Science, Zarqa University, PO Box 132222, Zarqa 13132, Jordan
e-mail: kamawi@zu.edu.jo

R. F. Saeed and S. ul. Shaheed (eds.), *Nutrition and Dietary Interventions in Cancer*, Cancer Treatment and Research 191, https://doi.org/10.1007/978-3-031-55622-7_1

CNS	Central nervous system
COVID	Coronavirus disease
CVD	Cardiovascular disease
DNA	Deoxyribonucleic acid
DNP	Dictionary of natural products
DRI	Dietary reference intakes
EBV	Epstein–Barr virus
ER	Estrogen receptor
GI	Glycemic index
GL	Glycemic load
HDI	Human Development Index
HPV	Human papillomavirus
IF	Intrinsic factor
MCV	Microcytic volume
NOC	*N*-nitroso carcinogenic compounds
PAH	Polycyclic aromatic hydrocarbons
PEITC	Phenethyl isothiocyanate
RAE	Retinol activity equivalents
RNA	Ribonucleic acid
ROS	Reactive oxygen species
UV	Ultraviolet
VKOR	Vitamin K epoxide reductase
WHO	World Health Organization

1.1 Introduction

1.1.1 What is Cancer?

The human body consists of cells that grow and divide to create new cells. Consequently, as old and damaged cells die, they are replaced by these new cells. Gene defects resulting in either loss or gain of gene functions can promote cells to grow and divide rapidly and uncontrollably. This creates abnormal masses of tissue known as tumors, which are classified according to their behavior or histogenetic. In histogenetic classification, the tumor is named according to the cells or tissue type from which the tumor originates. For example, cancers that occur in epithelial, mesoderm, and glandular tissues are classified as carcinomas, sarcomas, and adenocarcinomas, respectively. This classification is very important when selecting the best treatment option for the patient. Tumors can also be classified as benign or malignant, according to their behavior. Benign tumors are those that stay localized, grow slowly, and are unable to invade surrounding tissues or spread to other sites in the body. By contrast, malignant tumors are cancerous; they grow rapidly and have the ability to invade and destroy adjacent tissue and spread to distant sites via the bloodstream or the lymphatic system in the process known as metastasis [1].

The term cancer describes a group of diseases that progress by undergoing specific steps known as the hallmarks of cancer. In 2000, Hanahan and Weinberg defined six hallmarks of cancer: sustaining proliferative signaling, evading growth inhibitory signals, resisting cell apoptosis, enabling immortality, inducing angiogenesis, and activating invasion and metastasis. Later, they add two further hallmarks: reprogramming cellular metabolism and avoiding immune destruction.

1.1.2 Epidemiology of Cancer

Cancer is a major human health problem and one of the reasons for decreasing life expectancy in every country of the world. The World Health Organization (WHO) data show that cancer ranked as the first or second cause of death in 112 of 183 countries in 2019 [2]. According to the GLOBOCAN 2020 survey, cancer cases were estimated at 19.3 million and cancer deaths were about 10.0 million in 2020 globally [3]. The most prevalent cancer type is carcinoma, which arises from epithelial cells. Four carcinomas, namely cancers of the lung, large intestine (colon and rectum), prostate, and breast, are particularly important concerning incidence as well as mortality. Sung et al. reported that breast, lung, colorectal, prostate, and stomach cancers are the most common human cancers, accounting for 11.7, 11.4, 10.0, 7.3, and 5.6%, of the estimated 2.3 million new cases worldwide in 2020. Lung cancer remained the leading cause of cancer death, accounting for 18% of all cancer deaths. Other common causes of cancer death were colorectal (9.4%), liver (8.3%), stomach (7.7%), and female breast (6.9%) cancers [3].

The cancer incidence rates are higher in the High/Very High Human Development Index (HDI) countries than in the Low/Medium HDI countries. The cancer incidence was 104.3 and 128.0 cases per 100,000 persons for men and women, respectively, in low HDI countries and 335.3 and 267.6 per 100,000 persons for men and women, respectively, in very high HDI countries. The mortality rates in men were about twofold higher in high HDI countries, at 122.9–141.1 per 100,000 persons than in low HDI countries, at 76.7–78.0 per 100,000 persons. By contrast, in women, the mortality rates were nearly the same across HDI levels, at 67.0–88.4 per 100,000 persons [3].

The causes underlying these geographical differences are now being addressed by molecular biology research on human cancers, and the understanding these studies bring about can help in cancer prevention. The prevention of cancer is brightest for those cancers that show large geographical differences. For example, the incidence of lung cancer is threefold lower in low HDI countries than in very high HDI countries. Knowing the cause of this difference would therefore be very helpful in preventing lung cancer. Studies have shown that people who migrate to other countries often develop the types of cancer common in the countries to which they immigrated rather than the types of cancer prevalent in their home countries. This shows that the causes of most cancers are lifestyle factors rather than inherited genetic factors [4].

Lifestyle factors, population growth, and aging all lead to increases in cancer incidence rates. The coronavirus disease of the 2019 pandemic period (COVID-19) is expected to have an impact on cancer statistics in different world regions. A short-term drop in cancer incidence, followed by a slight increase in advanced-stage disease and a subsequent increase in mortality, is predicted due to delays in patient diagnosis and treatment, health system closures (including suspension of screening programs), and reduced availability of and access to care.

1.1.3 What Causes Cancer?

Scientists believe that some types of cancer can be prevented if the causes are known. As mentioned before, cancer is a group of diseases whose only common feature is uncontrolled cell growth and proliferation. The fundamental cause of all cancers is genetic damage, which is usually acquired due to exposure to environmental factors or behavioral influences, although it is sometimes congenital and occurs naturally when deoxyribonucleic acid (DNA) is replicated during the process of cell division. Some genetic changes that increase the risk of cancer are also inherited and passed from parent to child. The following sections will cover the hereditary factors and major carcinogens and their roles in the etiology of cancers.

1.1.3.1 Congenital and Hereditary Cancers

The genome is the entire set of genetic material in an organism. The agents that cause cancer are termed carcinogens, and when they cause alterations and mutations to the DNA sequence, they are known as mutagens. DNA mutations lead to diseases, including cancer. Studies have confirmed that the DNA of cancer cells contains mutations. These can be very small DNA changes that affect a single base pair (termed point mutations) or they can be very large and cause major changes in the structure of chromosomes (termed deletion or translocations).

Cancers arise from the accumulation of mutations that eliminate the normal constraints that prevent proliferation and assure the genetic integrity of cells. In general, several types of genes, if inherited in a faulty state, can cause genetic dysregulation that gives rise to uncontrolled cell proliferation and the development of cancer. These genes are classified as proto-oncogenes, tumor suppressor genes, genes that regulate programmed cell death (apoptosis), and genes involved in DNA repair [5, 6].

Two types of DNA mutations can occur, somatic mutations and germline mutations. Somatic mutations are the most frequently occurring genetic mutations in cancer cells, and they arise due to damage to the DNA of a somatic cell (body cell) due to exposure to environmental mutagens, such as cigarette smoke, and ultraviolet irradiation, and others. Mutations of this type are not passed on to the next generation of offspring and cannot be inherited. Cancers that occur because of somatic mutations are referred to as sporadic cancers and account for the majority of cancer patients (90%). By contrast, the alterations in the DNA of egg or sperm cells (germline mutations) are passed on to offspring. A small proportion of many cancers are due to inherited germline mutations, which result in a high risk of developing specific cancers in the individual with the mutation [7].

A congenital defect is one of the strongest known risk factors for cancer in children. For example, studies have shown associations between chromosomal anomalies and cancer in children with trisomy 21, who have a 20-fold increased risk of developing acute lymphoblastic leukemia. Other studies have indicated that children with nonchromosomal birth defects may also be at an increased risk of developing cancer. The risk of cancer increases with the number of defects and decreases with age for both nonchromosomal and chromosomal anomalies [8].

1.1.3.2 Infection

Infection is another of the main contributors to cancer development. Many infectious agents, including viruses, parasites, fungus, and bacteria, are carcinogenic. Several DNA and ribonucleic acid (RNA) viruses are known to cause cancer. For example, human papilloma (HPV) viruses, especially both strains HPV16 and HPV18, are responsible for cervical and other genital cancers [9, 10], as well as the development of skin, head and neck, and other cancers [11]. Specific strains of herpes viruses, such as Kaposi sarcoma herpes virus (KSHV) and Epstein–Barr virus (EBV), have also been shown to be carcinogens or co-carcinogens. KSHV is the causative agent of Kaposi sarcoma (KS) [12], while EBV has been implicated in the pathogenesis of many types of cancer, such as Burkitt's lymphoma, Hodgkin's disease, non-Hodgkin's lymphoma, nasopharyngeal carcinoma, and lymphomas [13, 14]. Chronic infections by hepatitis B or hepatitis C viruses are known to increase the risk of hepatocellular carcinoma [15]. In addition, some retroviruses, such as human immunodeficiency virus (HIV), cause cancer by interfering with the immune system, while others, such as human T-cell leukemia virus (HTLV1), cause cancer by direct growth stimulation [16, 17].

Some studies have also proven that bacterial infections can play an important role in cancer development [18]. For example, *Helicobacter pylori* infection is associated with stomach cancer, while infections by *Chlamydia trachomatis* and *C. pneumonia* are associated with cervical carcinoma and lung cancer, respectively [19, 20]. Similarly, parasitic infection with *Schistosoma* trematodes is implicated in the development of urinary bladder cancer [21].

1.1.3.3 Sunlight and Ionizing Radiation

Radiation is a form of energy propagated from a propagating source through the material in space. It consists of ionizing radiation or nonionizing radiation. Nonionizing radiation is a type of low-energy radiation, such as sunlight, that does not have enough energy to remove an electron from an atom or molecule [22].

Sunlight is divided into three types: visible (color), infrared (heat), and ultraviolet (UV) light [23]. UV radiation is probably responsible for all the carcinogenic effects of sunlight. UV radiation is subdivided into UVA (315–400 nm), UVB (280–315 nm), and UVC (100–280 nm) [24]. Exposure to UV light can cause skin damage, such as benign changes, pigmentation, discoloration, freckles, sunburn, cancer (basal cell carcinoma, squamous carcinoma, and melanoma), and destruction of elastin and collagen proteins [23, 25, 26]. Moreover, UV exposure increases the risk of ocular surface squamous neoplasia (OSSN), which includes dysplasia, carcinoma in situ, and squamous cell carcinoma of the conjunctiva or cornea [27, 28]. Long sleeves, long pants, a hat, and sunglasses with lenses that absorb UV must be worn and sunscreen must be used to protect against UV radiation and prevent skin cancer.

Ionizing radiation is propagated through space and has enough energy to interact with an atom and ionize it; that is, it can remove tightly bound electrons from the orbit around an atom [22]. Ionizing radiation has always been present everywhere at low doses, but our bodies are adapted to it. Ionizing radiation falls into two categories: natural and manmade. The natural sources of ionizing radiation are cosmic radiation (e.g., fallout), terrestrial radiation (e.g., radon gas), and radiation from building materials (e.g., sandstone and concrete). The manmade sources of radiation include medical procedures, such as diagnostic X-rays, nuclear medicine, and radiation therapy [23]. Ionizing radiation has many forms, including alpha, beta, gamma, and X-rays. These radiation types can be classified as either electromagnetic or particulate energy. Gamma and X-rays are classified as electromagnetic and can penetrate human tissues and cause serious damage to organs. Alpha and beta rays are classified as particulate energy and can penetrate only a few millimeters of skin. These particles do not cause significant damage to organisms due to their weak penetrating power, but they may induce cancer or have other adverse health effects when injected or inhaled [22, 29]. Exposure to ionizing radiation at low doses induces rapid repair of damage by the cells. At moderate and high doses, the cells become able to repair radiation damage and may choose to die (apoptosis) or to become changed permanently. These altered cells may become cancerous or produce other abnormalities (e.g., birth defects) [23]. Highly proliferative and sufficiently oxygenated cells are the most radiosensitive cells in the body. Consequently, bone marrow, reproductive and gastrointestinal systems, skin, muscle, and the brain are the most radiosensitive organs in the body [30].

Knowledge of the role of radiation exposure in human cancer began fifty years ago. Studies have linked leukemia and lung, skin, and bone cancers with external radiation exposure among Japanese atomic bomb survivors, with radon exposure in underground miners, radiation exposure in radiologists, and exposure in luminous dial painters, respectively. Knowledge of the role of radiation exposure in the risk of cancer has increased in the last half-century, with most evidence coming from studies of atomic bomb survivors in Hiroshima and Nagasaki, who have now been observed for more than 50 years. The remaining evidence comes from studies conducted on people exposed to radiation for medical, occupational, or environmental reasons [31]. Studies have confirmed that populations exposed to high to moderate doses of ionizing radiation have an increased risk of several types of cancers [32–35].

1.1.3.4 Environment

Several chemical substances (carcinogens) are known to induce cancer when they are used at high concentrations. In our environment, only 30,000 of 100,000 chemical elements have been analyzed. Of those, only 275 proved to be carcinogenic [23]. Some people, such as painters, construction workers, and pesticide and petroleum workers, are at a higher risk of cancer than others due to their jobs [23]. Epidemiologic studies have shown associations between several chemical agents and elevated risks of various cancers. For example, asbestos, which occurs naturally in the environment as bundles of fibers that are used in commercial and industrial applications, is known to lodge in the small airways of the lungs, causing tissue damage and leading to lung cancer, as well as mesothelioma [36]. Other agents, including heavy metals such as arsenic, cadmium, chromium, and nickel, are also involved in lung cancer. Soot, shale oil, and coal tar are now implicated in scrotal cancer. Certain substances, such as aromatic amines (e.g., naphthylamine and benzidine), aflatoxin, and vinyl chloride, are associated with increased risks of bladder and liver cancer [6]. Presenting the long list of chemicals that increase the risk of cancer section is beyond the scope of this text, but awareness of the broad range is important when obtaining the occupational and social history of patients with newly diagnosed cancers.

1.1.3.5 Lifestyle (Diet, Alcohol Consumption, Smoking, and Physical Inactivity)

The incidence of cancer is predicted to increase substantially over the next few decades [3], largely due to an increase in lifestyle-related cancers arising from economic and demographic transitions worldwide. Lifestyle factors, such as diet, alcohol consumption, smoking, and physical inactivity, are increasing the risk of cancer and are therefore important targets for primary prevention. Epidemiologic evidence suggests that physical activity decreases the risk of cancer of the liver, lung, kidney, gastric cardia, esophagus, endometrium, colon, rectum, head and neck, bladder, and breast, as well as myeloid leukemia and myeloma [37]. The latest data show that 40% of all cancer deaths are due to smoking, making this the strongest lifestyle-related risk factor overall. Moreover, alcohol consumption increases the risk of cancer of the mouth, oesophagus, breast and liver. Smoking and alcohol consumption have been known to have a synergistic effect that means the risk of cancer from both alcohol and smoking together is more than the effect of each risk alone [1]. The role of smoking, alcohol and diet will be discussed later in this chapter.

1.1.4 Principles of Conventional Therapies

This section provides the general principles of cancer conventional therapies including surgical therapeutic options, radiotherapy, and antineoplastic therapeutic strategies.

1.1.4.1 Surgery

Recent considerations imply that cancer is a localized disease that can spread later, so removing the tumor also means removing the disease. Surgery is the accepted primary treatment for cancer once a solid tumor is diagnosed, according to this paradigm. Before this paradigm's acceptance, cancer was thought to be a systemic disease. Surgery has been accepted as the primary cancer treatment for more than 130 years [38].

There is little doubt about surgery's efficacy because it has been the accepted cancer treatment for over a century. Most people would have no reason to doubt its efficacy because they believe cancer begins as a localized disease that spreads later, and surgery is capable of removing the tumor. As a result, "clinicians know that almost every type of cancer can be treated more successfully if detected at an early stage" [39]. According to the study of Wei et al. [42], the tumour can be removed surgically, which also provides instant relief from the obstruction that was preventing the patient from breathing and swallowing normally. Careful planning of surgery is vital to ensure the optimal outcome of therapy and prevent complications, some of which may be fatal. The hypopharynx has a wide diameter above, which is in continuity with the oropharynx, and a small circumference below, which is where it meets with the cervical oesophagus. This gives it the appearance of a funnel. Because of this, while the removal of a portion of the hypopharynx is necessary for the treatment of small tumours, a total, circumferential pharyngectomy is required for the treatment of large tumours, particularly those that involve the post-cricoid region [42].

Surgery is still the sole cure for pancreatic cancer patients, although only around 20% of them are candidates for surgery [40, 41]. The major goal of surgery is to completely resect the tumor such that no cancer cells can be observed at the initial tumor location under a microscope. R0 refers to a successful resection. A resection is referred to as R1 when cancer cells may be seen microscopically at the primary tumor location. Unfortunately, even in specialized surgical centers, the frequency of R1 resection reaches 75%, according to a recent study. Pancreatoduodenectomy, which includes removal of the pancreatic head, duodenum, distal common bile, and sometimes gastric antrum, is followed by pancreatoenterostomy, hepaticojejunostomy, and gastrojejunostomy in the Whipple surgery for resection of pancreatic head cancer. A substantial morbidity rate of up to 45% is associated with this surgery. When a tumor is discovered in the tail or body of the pancreas, a distal pancreatectomy is performed, in which the tail and maybe a portion of the body of the pancreas are excised [41].

For resectable gastric cancers, surgery is suggested. Each guideline advocated for perioperative care. Gastrectomy with sufficient margins, perigastric and extragastric lymph node dissection, and subsequent gut reconstruction are the usual procedures for gastric cancer. The goal of surgical treatment is complete resection with no residual disease; however, there is disagreement over the type of gastric resection, the extent of lymph node dissection, and repair [42].

Sarcomatous tumor cells linked with the development of osteoid matrix or bone characterize bone sarcomas, which are primary malignant bone tumors. They are further divided into three categories based on cytologic features: osteosarcomas (up to 40%), chondrosarcomas (20–27%), and Ewing sarcomas (up to 15%). Another quarter of a percent of all bone cancers is unspecified.

1.1.4.2 Radiotherapy

Significant advancements have been made in recent years in our understanding of potential cancer development and treatment indicators. Cancer clinical care is still a challenge in the twenty-first century due to the disease's increased prevalence. Some of the treatment choices include hormone therapy, chemotherapy, immunotherapy, radiation therapy, and surgery. Nearly half of all cancer patients receive radiation therapy at some time during their treatment, making it a crucial component of cancer care today [42, 43]. 40% of curable cancer treatments include it. The fundamental goal of radiation therapy is to prevent cancer cells from proliferating (cell division). The United Kingdom has proclaimed 2011 as the Year of Radiation Therapy to commemorate a century of advancement since Marie Curie won her second Nobel Prize for radium research. Over the past century, studies into the biology of cancer cell responses to radiation and ongoing advancements in radiation treatment methods have sought to increase cancer patient survival and reduce the adverse effects of treatment [43].

X-rays were initially recognized for their clinical utility as a cancer treatment strategy after Wilhelm Conrad Röntgen of Germany discovered them in 1895. One hundred years ago, Marie Curie received her second Nobel Prize for radium research, confirming her status as a forerunner in the field of radiation therapy. In commemoration of a century of advancement, the United Kingdom has proclaimed 2011 as the Year of Radiation Therapy. Since then, radiation therapy has developed into a recognized medical speciality, with Radiation Oncology functioning as a field where scientists and medical experts from several fields work together [43].

Radiation therapy, also known as radiotherapy, is a very cost-effective single modality treatment that accounts for just approximately 5% of the entire cost of cancer care. It is used in conjunction with surgery and chemotherapy. Furthermore, roughly half of all cancer patients will undergo radiation therapy at some point during their disease [45, 46], with radiation therapy contributing around 40% to curative treatment [47].

One kind of physical agent that can be used to kill cancer cells is radiation. The radiation is referred to as ionizing radiation because it produces ions (electrically charged particles) and deposits energy in the cells of the tissues it passes through.

This accumulated energy may harm cancer cells or result in genetic changes that cause cell death. High-energy radiation deteriorates the genetic material (DNA) of cells, preventing them from further multiplying and dividing [48]. Radiation kills both healthy and cancerous cells, but the goal of radiation therapy is to expose abnormal cancer cells to more radiation while sparing healthy cells that are nearby or in the radiation's path. As opposed to cancer cells, normal cells can typically repair themselves more quickly and continue to function normally. Differential cancer cell mortality results from cancer cells' inferior ability to repair radiation damage compared to healthy ones [46]. Radiation can be provided to cure cancer, or it can be used as a very effective palliative treatment to relieve cancer-related symptoms.

1.1.4.3 Antineoplastic Therapy

Cytotoxic systemic chemotherapy and targeted biological therapy are two types of antineoplastic therapies. Cytotoxic chemotherapy is "targeted" in many ways against specific components that drive cell cycle development; nevertheless, these targets are rarely unique to tumor cells. Because systemic cytotoxic chemotherapy targets all rapidly dividing cells, it also targets hair follicles, gastrointestinal mucosa, and hematopoietic cells, causing alopecia, nausea, diarrhea, mucositis, and bone marrow suppression, among other side effects. The newer generation of targeted biological therapies is still given systemically as traditional chemotherapy; however, these medications are distinct in that they are designed to target specific molecular components in tumor cell biology with the hopes of reducing damage to non-cancerous cells [49].

Alkylating and Alkylating-Like Agents

Alkylating agents are a type of antineoplastic or anticancer medicine that works by preventing protein synthesis by reducing the transcription of DNA into RNA. Alkylating chemicals replace hydrogen atoms on DNA with alkyl groups, resulting in the development of cross-links within the DNA chain and hence cytotoxic, mutagenic, and carcinogenic consequences. Although this activity occurs in all cells, alkylating chemicals have the greatest impact on quickly dividing cells that lack the opportunity to repair their DNA. Because cancer cells divide at such a high rate, they are among the most vulnerable. Anemia, pancytopenia, amenorrhea, poor spermatogenesis, intestinal mucosal injury, baldness, and an increased risk of cancer are some of the major side effects of alkylating drugs. As a result of the alkylation process, the DNA code is misread, DNA, RNA, and protein synthesis are inhibited, and programmed cell death (apoptosis) is triggered in rapidly reproducing tumor cells. The alkylating agents are divided into six categories:

(1) Mechlorethamine, cyclophosphamide, ifosfamide, melphalan, and chlorambucil are nitrogen mustards.
(2) Altretamine, thiotepa, and other ethylenamine and methylenamine compounds.
(3) Alkyl sulfonates [busulfan] are a type of alkyl sulfonate.

(4) Nitrosoureas [carmustine, lomustine].
(5) Dacarbazine, procarbazine, and temozolomide triazenes.
(6) Platinum coordination complexes, which are platinum-containing antineoplastic drugs [cisplatin, carboplatin, oxaliplatin] [50].

Antimetabolites

Antimetabolites are referred to as "cytotoxic" medications because they cause cell death. They function by imitating the chemical processes necessary for cell development. Instead of the usual genetic material's RNA and DNA, antimetabolites are employed to trick cells into absorbing the drugs. Antimetabolites, which are widely used to treat cancer, are antimetabolites. Examples include fludarabine, gemcitabine, cytarabine, pemetrexed, 6-mercaptopurine, and 5-fluorouracil [51].

Antitumor Antibiotics

Antibiotics and anticancer chemicals produced by Streptomyces bacteria have piqued the interest of pharmaceutical and biotech businesses. The xylem sap from grapevines has a good influence on the manufacture of various antibiotics by numerous Streptomyces species, including S. ambofaciens, American Type Culture Collection (ATCC 23,877) and S. argillaceous ATCC 12,596, according to this study. Actinomycin D, chromomycin A3, fungichromin B, mithramycin A, and other well-known compounds were synthesized, as well as four compounds with molecular formulae not found in the Dictionary of Natural Products (DNP v28.2) [52].

Streptomyces bacteria are common soil bacteria that assist in the degradation of complex carbohydrates, lipids, and proteins with a variety of hydrolytic enzymes [53]. These bacteria also create a variety of antibiotics and anticancer chemicals, which are their primary source of revenue [54–56]. Doxorubicin is used to treat severe lymphoma, childhood solid tumors, bone and soft tissue sarcomas, and breast cancer, with new indications being discovered all the time. Daunorubicin, on the other hand, has risen to the forefront of research in the treatment of acute leukemia. Epirubicin has a similar range to doxorubicin but is less hazardous. The potential of ICRF-187 to protect against cardiotoxicity piques clinical interest in using changes in doze intensity for therapeutic purposes. In leukemia, idarubicin is as least as effective as daunorubicin and doxorubicin. Introduction of new anthracycline antibiotic analogs, insight into mechanisms of resistance, the reversal of multidrug resistance in vitro, the protection of cardiac toxicity, and the study of other important biochemical reactions relevant to cytotoxicity are all new areas of research concerning anthracycline antibiotics. Orally active anthracyclines, such as idarubicin, are being developed, as are molecules that lack cross-resistance to the parent medicines or have different mechanisms of cytotoxicity. These changes are anticipated to broaden the therapeutic range of these already commonly used medications [57].

Hormonal Agents

The most common therapies for severe and recurrent gynecological cancers are hormone therapy and chemotherapy, and responsiveness to therapy is a key component in prognosis and survival [58]. Hormone therapy has been more popular in recent years as a result of chemotherapy's terrible side effects. Hormone treatment for cancer is taking drugs that prevent or slow cancer growth by inhibiting biological activity or lowering hormone levels. Hormone therapy either stops hormones from allowing cancer cells to proliferate and divide or suppresses hormone production. It is not, however, effective against all tumors types [59]. In recent years, the treatment of individuals with gynecological malignancies has advanced dramatically [60].

Hormone therapy has recently been proven to be an effective cancer treatment approach. Hormone treatment for gynecological cancers is taking drugs that lower hormone levels or impede their biological activity, halting or slowing cancer progression. Hormone therapy works by preventing cancer cells from multiplying due to hormones. Vulvar cancer, cervical cancer, vaginal cancer, uterine cancer, and ovarian cancer can all be treated with aromatase inhibitors, anti-estrogens, progestin, estrogen receptor antagonists, gonadotropin-releasing hormone agonists, and progestogen. Hormone replacement therapy is quite effective. In women infected with the human papillomavirus, progestogen and estrogen replacement are linked to a lower risk of gynecological malignancies. Gene products of HPV may either stimulate or inhibit estrogen activation via the transcriptional activity of estrogen receptor. Patients with hormone-sensitive recurrent or metastatic gynecologic cancers are often treated with hormones, while response rates and therapeutic outcomes are variable. As a result, this review examines the use of hormone therapy in the treatment of gynecological malignancies and identifies information gaps [58].

1.1.5 Role of Nutrition in Cancer

Nutrition and nutritional status are crucial in the management of cancer patients, as malnutrition is common due to a variety of factors, including poor intake and dietary habits. The most common cause of malnutrition in those patients is that cancer causes anorexia and cachexia which leads to loss of appetite [61, 62].

1.1.5.1 Definition of Nutrition

The simple definition of nutrition is the essential requirement for a certain amount of raw materials for the ideal and potential generation of all biological products and the maintenance of the biochemical processes. The good nutrition concept focuses on the dietary requirements to sustain life in addition to physical, physiological, and structural integrity. Three classes of nutrients provide all energy (calories): fats, carbohydrates, and protein, which are needed in large amounts, hence called macronutrients. Other nutrients needed in lesser amounts (mg or μg) are called micronutrients, which are vitamins and minerals. Thus, it is necessary to focus on their nature, types, and the effects of these nutrients on human health [62, 63].

A well-balanced diet provides all of the essential elements, such as energy, proteins, fats, vitamins, minerals, and others, for the body's proper function for the maintenance of life. Organic substances such as amino acids, proteins, carbohydrates, lipids, and vitamins are the primary sources of nutrients that are vital for living things. Minerals, primarily calcium, phosphorus, and magnesium, make up the skeletal system. Other minerals, including iron, copper, zinc, cobalt, manganese, and fluorine, are required in trace amounts for numerous bodily activities [62, 63].

Proteins

Although all cells are capable of synthesizing proteins, there is a significant variation between plant and animal cells. Plants can synthesize proteins from inorganic nitrogen, carbon dioxide, and water in the chlorophyll via photosynthesis, which uses sunlight as the primary source of energy [63].

Protein is an essential part of our diets. Nitrogen, carbon, hydrogen, and oxygen are the four main necessary components of proteins. Aside from nitrogen, the other three elements are also necessary components of carbohydrates and lipids. Proteins are large, complex macromolecules made up of smaller monomers of amino acids. Protein architectures are influenced by a variety of parameters such as the number of amino acids, their sequence, and the inclusion of nonprotein components and chemicals. Only 20 distinct amino acids are used to construct the hundreds of proteins that make up our body. Nine of the 20 amino acids can't be manufactured in human bodies, thus they're deemed "essential" and must be taken from the diet. The remaining 11 are "nonessential" amino acids because our bodies can make them in adequate amounts. Our bodies must produce and store enormous amounts of protein during periods of development. As a result, the need for protein in our diets increases as we develop [62, 64].

The finest sources of protein include lean meats and dairy products, fish, lentils, and grains. Protein is present in almost all foods with varying quality. The proteins that include all of the necessary amino acids needed for development, pregnancy, breastfeeding, and overall health are called "complete" proteins. Lean meats and poultry, fish, low-fat dairy products, and eggs are the finest sources of complete protein. Although grains and cereals are high in protein, they are referred to as "incomplete" proteins because they frequently lack one or more essential amino acids. However, this does not imply that humans must consume meat, eggs, and dairy products (items derived from animals) to obtain all of the essential amino acids. These amino acids can be obtained by eating a variety of grains and legumes even if they are consumed at different times throughout the day [65].

Excess protein is not stored in our systems, thus consuming more than the appropriate quantity will not result in greater muscles. Instead, it is converted to carbohydrates or fat and stored. Excess protein (amino acids) consumption is counterproductive, as it adds to the metabolic burden and wastes energy through excess nitrogen excretion in the form of urea in the urine. Also, excess protein is deaminated and used in the gluconeogenesis process to produce glucose, and the excess amino acids are converted to fat, which is then stored. On the other hand, eating too little protein results in some health hazards as the body begins to break down muscle protein into its constituent amino acids [66, 67].

Lipids

Lipids are water-insoluble compounds that are either structural or storage, whether their source is plant or animal. Structural lipids are fats found in the layer that covers the surface of plants or membrane components present in animal tissues, while plant storage lipids are primarily oils stored in seeds and fruits, and animal body storage lipids are usually found in fat depots [68].

Dietary fats, often known as triglycerides, are fats found in the diet that comprise three fatty acids (chain-like molecules of carbon, hydrogen, and oxygen) connected to a glycerol backbone. Dietary fats also allow fat-soluble vitamins (A, D, E, and K) to be absorbed from meals during digestion. The quantity of hydrogen atoms connected to a carbon chain determines whether a fatty acid is saturated or unsaturated. Because our bodies require small amounts of several fatty acids from foods (known as essential fatty acids) to build cell membranes and produce several essential hormones, such as the steroid hormones testosterone, progesterone, and estrogen, as well as the hormone-like prostaglandins, fat is considered an essential nutrient. Additionally, the essential fatty acids, linoleic and linolenic acids, are polyunsaturated fats. Omega-3 fatty acids are a kind of polyunsaturated fatty acid found in fish (particularly tuna, mackerel, and salmon) and plant oils like canola (rapeseed) oil. Polyunsaturated fats, like monounsaturated fats, reduce blood cholesterol and can be used to replace saturated fats in the diet [69, 70].

Cholesterol is a waxy, fat-like molecule found in cell membranes that serve as a precursor for bile acids (needed for digestion), vitamin D, and a set of hormones (the steroid hormones). The liver is capable of producing nearly all of the cholesterol required for these vital processes. Cholesterol is found in only animal-based foods, such as meat, poultry, milk, butter, cheese, and eggs. On the other hand, cholesterol is absent in plant-based foods, such as fruits, vegetables, nuts, seeds, legumes, grains, and the oils obtained from them [69].

Carbohydrates

Carbohydrates (saccharides) are a diverse group of nutrients and the most abundant organic molecules in nature that are found in most foods. Their name is taken from French terminology "hydrate de Carbone" which means the natural products containing carbon, hydrogen, and oxygen. Because of their single (mono) ring structure, sugars like fructose and glucose are known as monosaccharides, whereas two-ringed carbohydrates like sucrose are known as disaccharides. Foods are sweetened using simple sugars, which are tiny molecules that may be found in a variety of foods and various forms. Sweeteners such as hexoses and disaccharides are the most frequent in human diets. Fructose, for example, is the sugar that gives some fruits their sweet flavor. The most common simple sugar is table sugar, commonly known as sucrose, which is made from sugar cane or sugar beets.

Sucrose is made up of a molecule of fructose chemically bonded to another simple sugar called glucose. Lactose, the sugar that gives milk its somewhat sweet taste, is another disaccharide made up of glucose coupled with another simple sugar called galactose. The most common polysaccharides, which are glucose polymers linked via glycosidic linkages include branched glycogen (from animal sources) and branched starch, and unbranched cellulose (from plant sources) [71–74].

Glucose in the bloodstream and glycogen (animal starch) in other tissues are two types of carbohydrates found in modest amounts in the animal body. These come from plant sources in diets. Starch and fibre are two types of complex carbohydrates found in plant-based meals. Grain, various fruits and vegetables, legumes, nuts, and seeds all contain starch as a type of carbohydrate. Fibrous polysaccharides, particularly cellulose molecules, are more numerous in plants than all other types of carbohydrates. Fibre is the harder substance that makes up a seed's coat and other plant structural components. While starches are metabolized by our bodies for energy, fibre is not degraded or metabolized [73].

The majority of human diets are made up of various types of carbs, as is widely known. Carbohydrates are not required for the provision of blood glucose, which is required for the body's fundamental processes. The process of gluconeogenesis can provide blood glucose by supplying it from the metabolism of lipids and proteins. Carbohydrates are still the cheapest source of nutritional energy for animals in the current world. For the brain, glucose is required to satisfy its energy needs, whereas the muscles use it for temporary short periods of activity. The liver and muscles also convert small amounts of the dietary sugar into glycogen, the storage form. Muscle glycogen stores must be replenished after a long workout [75].

Carbohydrates are known for their protein-sparing impact in which a sufficient supply of metabolizable carbs saves proteins (amino acids) for bodily tissue development and repair instead of being used for providing energy (glucose) in the body. In the lack of sufficient glucose, the rate of fat and protein metabolism is accelerated to produce glucose, which is required for energy supply. This oxidation process is frequently imperfect, resulting in the buildup of ketone molecules (acetoacetic acid, β-hydroxybutyric acid, and the release of acetone as a byproduct). Ketosis is caused by a high buildup of ketone bodies over the threshold [62].

Foods high in added sugar are frequently deficient in vital elements like vitamins and minerals. Unfortunately, these foodstuffs are frequently substituted for more nutrient-dense meals like fruits, vegetables, and low-fat whole-grain goods, and they may deprive us of critical nutrients while also contributing to weight gain. Sugar is often used to compensate for the flavor lost when fat is reduced; hence, these meals have a high sugar level. Foods heavy in sugar, or sugar and fat, with few other nutrients, appear at the top of the Food Guide Pyramid (Fig. 1.1) because they should be consumed in moderation. Choosing naturally containing fructose fresh fruits, or low-fat yogurt naturally containing lactose, on the other hand, allows us to obtain the vitamins and minerals found in those foods as well as other food components that contribute to health [72].

Fiber (a material found in bran, fruits, vegetables, and legumes) is a form of complex carbohydrate that is necessary for our health even though it is not digested

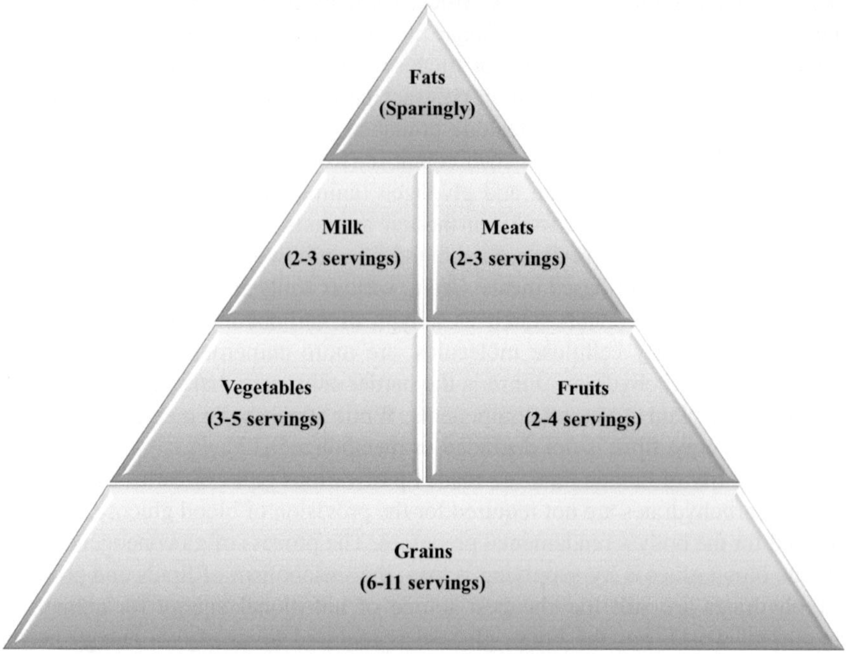

Fig. 1.1 The food guide pyramid

by our systems. Insoluble fiber, also known as roughage, is found in vegetables, nuts, and some cereal grains and is made up of cellulose, hemicellulose, and lignin. Pectin, found in fruits, and gums, and present in certain grains and legumes, are a good example of soluble fibers. Diets high in fiber, such as whole grains, legumes, and fresh vegetables and fruits, have been associated with a decreased risk of a variety of ailments. Fiber also gives us a feeling of fullness, which can help in avoiding overeating and weight gain. Fiber and complex carbohydrate-rich diets have been linked to reduced serum cholesterol, as well as a lower risk of high blood pressure, coronary artery disease, and some forms of cancer. Although studies show that our consumption of carbs is growing, whole-grain meals continue to play a minor role, largely due to the difficulty in finding whole-grain items. Studies that have proved the benefits of a high fiber diet (containing 25–30 g of fiber per day) have used dietary fiber from fruits, vegetables, whole grains, and cereals as the source of dietary fiber. These and other studies imply that the health-promoting effects of these foods are due not just to the fiber, but also to the vitamins, minerals, and other chemicals they contain [76].

Vitamins and Dietary Minerals:
Vitamins and minerals are required by every process in your body in lesser amounts than the macronutrients (carbohydrate, protein, and lipid), this explains why vitamins and minerals are termed micronutrients. Vitamins and minerals

do not carry energy on their own, unlike macronutrients. Instead, they cooperate with the body to release, utilize, and store the energy from the energy-rich macronutrients (carbohydrates, protein, and fats) and with one another.

For each vitamin, dietary reference intakes (DRIs) specify the vitamin intake plus a small bit of additional to help most people avoid deficient symptoms. Today, those who are extremely undernourished or who have specific medical problems are more likely to get illnesses caused by vitamin deficiencies. Instead, in what could be considered a nutrition revolution, research has advanced beyond the detection and treatment of simple nutrient deficiencies to the realization that some vitamins (or foods that contain them) may help maintain health by preventing the onset of chronic diseases like cancer and heart disease in otherwise well-nourished individuals. The theory that some vitamins, particularly those referred to as antioxidants, may give even more benefit if consumed in levels somewhat larger than the recommended doses has also started to gain support in nutrition research. Essential vitamins can be divided into two categories: water-soluble and fat-soluble vitamins [77, 78].

Water-Soluble Vitamins

Nine vitamins are categorized as water-soluble because they dissolve in water, including folic acid, cobalamin, ascorbic acid, pyridoxine, thiamine, niacin, riboflavin, biotin, and pantothenic acid. Toxicity with these is uncommon since they are easily eliminated in the urine. Water-soluble vitamins need to be supplied nearly every day, ideally by consuming meals high in these nutrients. Excellent sources of water-soluble vitamins include fruits, vegetables, cereals, and legumes (except vitamin B12, which is found only in foods of animal origin). Deficiencies can, however, emerge fast since they are not significantly stored in the body [79].

Fat-Soluble Vitamins

A, D, E, and K are fat-soluble vitamins that are taken from food, absorbed into the circulation, and transported (in chylomicrons) with dietary fat. They are not easily eliminated, and they are kept in large quantities in the liver and adipose tissue. Fat-soluble vitamins do not need to be supplied regularly since they are stored in the body. Vitamins A and D are stored in the liver, and reserves can last up to six months. Vitamin K reserves, on the other hand, may last only a few weeks, while vitamin E supplies might last anywhere from a few days to many months. Fat-soluble vitamins can build up in the body if taken in excess, generally as a supplement. Vitamin A and D intakes that exceed the DRI can be detrimental. Fortunately, obtaining toxic levels of fat-soluble vitamins from meals is difficult [80].

Minerals

Minerals are elements that may be found on the earth, and like vitamins, serve a variety of roles in our systems. Some minerals, such as calcium and phosphorus, have a structural role, unlike vitamins. Our bones and teeth are made up of these minerals. Calcium, like several other key minerals such as sodium, chlorine, potassium, and magnesium, is a cell function regulator. The minerals salt, chloride, and potassium (commonly known as electrolytes) are in charge of maintaining the equilibrium of fluids within and outside of cells, as well as managing nerve impulse movement, together with calcium. Trace minerals are minerals that your body needs in little quantities, generally less than 20 mg per day. Iron, chromium, cobalt, copper, fluoride, iodine, manganese, molybdenum, selenium, and zinc are among these elements. The mineral iron is a component of hemoglobin, a protein in your blood that transports oxygen and collects carbon dioxide. Although DRIs have been established for certain trace minerals, those for which there is insufficient information to determine specific DRIs have an adequate intake recommendation [71].

Vitamins and Minerals as Antioxidants

Antioxidants include a variety of vitamins and minerals. Vitamins E and C, beta-carotene and other carotenoids, as well as the minerals selenium, copper, zinc, and manganese, are among them. When cells consume oxygen to utilize the nutrients that food offers, however, free radicals are produced as a byproduct. These free radicals can harm tissues, cells, and deoxyribonucleic acid if they are allowed to build up. The generation of free radicals in our bodies is also aided by environmental contaminants such as cigarette smoke and UV rays from the sun. Excess free radical production has been linked to an increased risk of cancer, heart disease, cataracts, and other forms of cell degeneration related to age, according to research (DNA, the genetic material of cells) [81].

Antioxidants in our bodies scavenge and counteract the effects of free radicals. Each antioxidant has a different impact. Water-soluble vitamin C eliminates free radicals from physiological fluids and cell structures. Vitamin E and beta-carotene are fat-soluble. They appear to be most active in adipose tissues and cell membranes throughout the body. Selenium is an antioxidant that aids in the absorption of vitamin E. Food is the best source of antioxidants, except for vitamin E. Fruits, vegetables, and grains include a wide range of antioxidants [81].

1.1.5.2 Nutrition and Risk of Cancer Development

Although the association between diet and cancer risk is complex due to the varieties of nutrients and food included in different types of diets, many epidemiological and animal studies have gathered profound evidence on the correlation between cancer and certain unhealthy dietary habits. For instance, many have reported an increased risk of cancer incidence related to higher consumption of carbohydrates, saturated fat, meat, and iron. On the other hand, vegetables, fruits, calcium, vitamin D, and folic acid have a protective role against cancer. Here we provide an overview of the role of nutrition, obesity, and alcohol consumption on cancer risk, and highlight the role of diet/nutrition in cancer prevention and treatment.

Diet and Cancer Risk

There is convincing evidence that associates the Western diet with cancer risk. The Western diet is known for high consumption of simple carbohydrates (refined sugar), meats (especially red meat), and animal fats (high amounts of saturated and trans fats), with low consumption of whole grains, fruits, vegetables, nuts, and seeds. On the other hand, diets based on regular consumption of vegetables, fruits, fibers, vitamins, and antioxidants with low consumption of meat, fat, refined sugars, and alcohol, such as the Mediterranean diet, play an important role in protecting against cancer development by counteracting the inflammatory effect of many carcinogens [82]. Here in this section, we represent the most reported harmful dietary patterns associated with cancer risk.

Meat

Meat is an important part of a balanced diet as it provides vital nutrients such as proteins, essential amino acids, vitamins, and other micronutrients. Meat can be fresh or processed by different procedures such as salting and curing, and it is usually classified as a white or red subtype.

It has been observed in many studies that the increased consumption of meat has been involved with a range of diseases, including diabetes, cardiovascular, gout, arthritis, and cancer. Regarding cancer risk, this was mainly reported for red, processed, and meat cooked at high temperatures but not with white meat. This risk has been documented in many types of cancers such as colorectal, breast, gastric, esophagus, prostate, and lung. On the other hand, the association between meat consumption and cancer risk in other types of cancer such as bladder cancer is still unclear and therefore needs further investigation. Of note, the consumption of white meat has not been associated with an increased risk of cancer development in cancers such as gastric, oral cavity, and pharynx cancers. This could be related to the fact that amount of iron is relatively less in white meat compared to red and therefore the generation of carcinogens is lower [83, 84].

Red meat is known to have great quantities of iron, which can cause direct DNA damage and the formation of *N*-nitroso carcinogenic compounds (NOCs). The formation of NOCs is also reported in the making of processed meat. Furthermore, meat cooked at high temperatures can lead to the formation of carcinogens such as heterocyclic amines and polycyclic aromatic hydrocarbons (PAHs). These carcinogens can cause mutations in our DNA leading to an increased risk of cancer. Nonetheless, some studies have shown that the increase in colorectal cancer risk is related to red meat consumption, despite its carcinogenic content. Meat consumption can elevate bile acid production which can promote mitosis leading to colorectal adenomas and carcinomas. In the breast, studies have shown that meat consumption can cause an increase in NOCs, PAHs, estrogen, insulin-like growth factor-1, and pro-inflammatory cytokines which can lead to breast cancer. Furthermore, in prostate cancer, it was shown that meat consumption can lead to infiltration of mast cells and macrophages, which leads to inflammation that can contribute to increased cancer risk. For prostate cancer risk specifically, it is noteworthy that the effects of diet on cancer risk are more likely to be observed with advanced rather than total prostate cancers [83, 85].

Currently, there is no conclusive evidence about meat consumption, particularly red meat and cancer risk. Therefore, the current recommendation is not to completely avoid meat, because of its valuable nutrients, but to limit consumption of red meat to no more than 350–500 g cooked in three portions per week.

Carbohydrates

Carbohydrates can be categorized as good or bad carbohydrates based on their glycemic index (GI), glycemic load (GL), and fiber content. GI classifies foods by their ability to cause a quick rise in blood glucose and insulin responses following food ingestion and GL describes as the amount of carbohydrate in each type of food multiplied by GI [86].

It has been hypothesized that our Westernized lifestyle which includes a high level of refined sugars high GI and GL types of food, such as cakes, cookies, sweetened products, and soft drinks, can contribute to an increased risk of cancer. However, for most types of cancers, there are scarce data with mixed findings on the association between carbohydrate consumption and increased cancer risk [87].

The most convincing evidence was shown in colorectal and breast cancers. It has been reported that refined sugars, high GI and GL types of food are associated with increased colon cancer risk. There are also some specific studies on the association of increased colon cancer risk with high quantities of sucrose intake. Furthermore, breast cancer risk was increased with higher GI and GL types of foods and this risk was stronger in postmenopausal women. This increased cancer risk might be related to the fact that high GI foods lead to an immediate rise in blood glucose, which triggers the secretion of insulin and insulin-like growth factors that can cause DNA alteration and mutations leading to cancer. However, since research on carbohydrates is too sparse, further research is needed to draw any conclusions and recommendations [88].

Fat

The role of dietary fat consumption in the risk of cancer has been a source of dispute. Nonetheless, epidemiologic studies on the increased consumption of fat as a huge part of the Westernized type of diet have shown an increased cancer risk. The risk was highly associated with animal diet, mostly the saturated and trans fats, especially in colorectal, prostate, breast, skin, pancreas, and lung cancers [89]. Although the research in this area is still emerging, great attention has been drawn toward saturated fats, most particularly palmitic fatty acids. It has been reported that the increased consumption of palm oil, butter, olive oil, corn oil and lard is linked to cancer development, due to their high content of palmitic acid [90, 91].

A high-fat diet can lead to a higher level of palmitic acid production that has a stimulatory effect on β2-adrenergic receptor expression [92]. The β2-adrenergic receptor is known to enhance tumor growth by increasing cell proliferation as seen in colorectal cancer. In addition, it has been established that the increased consumption of fat can promote the synthesis of hepatic bile acids, which undergoes biotransformation to generate higher amounts of reactive nitrogen and oxygen species. These reactive species can cause various mutations that lead to cancer [93, 94].

It is noteworthy that despite the evident link between fat consumption in cancer development, the complete cut-off on fat consumption does not reduce cancer risk [91]. Therefore, it is currently recommended to consume fat in moderation, increase the level of unsaturated fats, which are known to have a protective role against inflammation and cancer, and avoid the high consumption of saturated and trans fats.

Obesity and Cancer Risk

Obesity is a serious problem that occurs when energy intake is higher than energy expenditure leading to excessive accumulation of fat in adipose tissue. The percentage of individuals suffering from obesity with a body mass index (BMI) of greater than or equal to 30 kg/m^2, is increasing in the modern world, reaching a pandemic level in countries, known to highly depend on the Westernized diet. Obesity intensifies the risk of several chronic diseases, including diabetes mellitus type 2, hypertension, dyslipidemia, nonalcoholic fatty liver disease, Alzheimer's disease, osteoarthritis, kidney failure, liver disease, and many types of cancer [95].

Recently, the association between obesity and increased cancer risk or cancer-related mortality has been confirmed in many studies. It has been reported that obesity can cause 14% of cancer deaths in men and 20% in women [95]. This risk is strongest in cancers of the gastrointestinal origin, endometrium, kidneys, liver, and breast cancer in women. The development of cancer may take up to 10 years in the presence of obesity. However, in hormonal-related cancers occurring in postmenopausal women, such as breast and endometrial cancer, this lag time may be shorter. Also, it has been shown that the risk of colon cancer death in adulthood is doubled when patients have suffered from obesity in their teenage years. On the other hand, there have been several studies that showed that weight loss can lower the risk of colon, breast, and endometrial cancers. For instance, weight loss of higher than 10 kilos in postmenopausal women can lower the risk of breast cancer by 50% [96]. All of this can confirm the link between obesity and cancer development and cancer-related deaths [97].

The mechanism by which obesity triggers cancer development is complex and can be tissue-specific; however, there have been reports on the most significant biological mechanisms mediating the increased risk of cancer including insulin production, insulin resistance, sex hormones, oxidative stress, inflammation, alterations in adipose tissue production of adipokines and vascular growth factors, and alterations in immune function. All of these mechanisms caused by obesity can contribute to cell mutations and thus increase the risk of cancer development. Of note, inflammation is particularly important as it could be a major factor in all types of obesity-related cancers. It has been established that during tumor development, there is an increase of inflammatory cytokines, that are associated with promoting cancer development by causing an increase in cell proliferation, apoptosis, angiogenesis, and metastasis, Also, inflammation can cause a major change in the macrophages present in the microenvironment of adipose tissue, from an M1-like protective phenotype against tumorigenesis to a more tumor-promoting M2-like phenotype [97].

It is also noteworthy that in many epidemiological studies, obesity can contribute to cancer development through low-serum levels of vitamin D. The biological mechanisms linking obesity, low vitamin D, and cancer risk are not completely confirmed, but the majority of research is pointing toward that the obesity can lead to increased levels of vitamin D in adipose tissue, which can activate vitamin D receptor, leading to a higher state of chronic inflammation. Therefore, further research specifically addressing the biological mechanism underlying the relationship between obesity and vitamin D leading to increased cancer risk is needed [98].

It is confirmed that obesity can lead to 20% of cancer development, and therefore weight loss might play a significant role in reducing the risk of cancer in obese individuals [95]. Therefore, the current guidelines from the Public Health Goals of the World Cancer Research Fund advise that the BMI in adults should be between 21 and 23 kg/m^2, to reduce the risk of disease development including cancer.

Alcohol and Cancer Risk

It is well known that a high intake of alcohol is linked to an increased risk of cancer. It is estimated that 5.5% of cancers are due to alcohol consumption [99]. The association between cancer risk and alcohol has been highly approved in many epidemiological studies on breast, oral cavity, pharynx, larynx, esophagus, stomach, colon, rectum, pancreas, and liver cancer. However, for other types of cancers such as lung and prostate, there might be a minimal risk that requires further research. It has been observed that in certain types of cancers such as pancreatic cancer, the amount of heavy alcohol intake is more important than the type of alcohol in increasing the cancer risk. On the other hand, a light or moderate alcohol intake can increase the risk of cancer of the oral cavity and pharynx [100].

There are multiple proposed biological mechanisms through which alcohol can cause cancer. One of the major mechanisms is the metabolism of alcohol which can lead to the formation of acetaldehyde, a very toxic metabolic that can cause direct DNA damage and mutations. Another important mechanism can be related to the formation of oxidative stress species leading also to DNA damage. Alcohol metabolites can also inhibit the activity of DNA methylation enzymes, such as methionine synthase, and methionine adenosyl transferase, which can cause DNA hypomethylation that results in the activation of oncogenes that promotes tumor development and growth. For breast cancer, alcohol consumption may lead to increased hormonal receptor levels and estrogen concentrations, leading to a higher risk of developing breast cancer [101].

In addition, other studies have shown that alcohol might not be a causative factor of cancer by itself; however, it might act as a solvent that modifies the cells in a way that eases the penetration of carcinogens. For instance, there is a synergistic effect of alcohol and smoking in increasing the risk of upper gastrointestinal cancers. It has been shown that smokers, who consume the same amount of alcohol, have double the amount of acetaldehyde in their saliva compared to non-smokers [101].

Since alcohol consumption has been identified as a leading risk factor for the development of cancer, it is highly recommended to limit its intake to up to one drink per day for women and up to two drinks per day for men. Accordingly, interventional health programs are highly warranted for individuals who drink at a heavy level. Furthermore, as this risk of cancer onset has been observed at even low to moderate levels for some types of cancer, it is not recommended for individuals who do not drink to not start drinking for any reason as more research is needed in this area.

1.1.5.3 Nutrition and Cancer Prevention

The three stages of carcinogenesis are initiation, promotion, and progression. After exposure to a carcinogenic substance, a normal cell undergoes a fast and irreversible transformation into a cancer cell known as initiation. Tumor promotion is thought to be a somewhat prolonged and reversible process, in contrast to tumor initiation, where preneoplastic cells that are actively multiplying increase. The development of a tumor with the ability to invade and spread throughout the body is considered progression, the last stage of neoplastic transformation. The burden of cancer is significant and rising worldwide. In many regions of the world, cancer has surpassed cardiovascular disease as the main cause of mortality, accounting for one in eight of all fatalities. Still, preventing cancer is the best course of action. More than 33% of cancer-related fatalities can be prevented by changing one's lifestyle and eating habits, along with taking the right nutritional supplements. As a result, diet plays a crucial part in cancer prevention [102].

Chemoprevention is the term for the prolonged use of artificial, organic, or biological chemicals to prevent or postpone the manifestation of cancer. Blocking agents and suppressing agents are the two primary types of chemopreventive agents. Blocking drugs halt carcinogens from entering the target areas, activating their metabolism, or interacting with significant cellular macromolecules (DNA, RNA, and proteins). Conversely, suppressing drugs prevent initiated cells from transforming into malignant cells at either the promotion or the progression stage. The premalignant stage (initiation and promotion) of multistep carcinogenesis can be stopped or reversed by chemopreventive phytochemicals. They can also slow down the transformation of precancerous cells into malignant ones, if not completely stop it [103].

A material undergoes oxidation when it transfers electrons or hydrogen to an oxidizing agent. This chemical reaction can result in the production of free radicals, which can cause oxidative damage to lipids, proteins, and DNA, which promotes the pathogenesis of cancer. These free radicals are either nitrogen oxide reactive species, which include nitric oxide, peroxynitrite, and nitrous anhydride, or reactive oxygen species (ROS), which include hydroxyl and superoxide radicals. Antioxidants are reducing substances that are present in foods, especially those with a vegetable origin, and are believed to act as chemoprotective agents [104].

The prevention of cancer is greatly influenced by diet. In humans, vitamin E is the primary lipid-soluble antioxidant while vitamin C is the primary water-soluble antioxidant. For malignancies of the stomach, mouth, esophagus, lung, pancreas, and uterine cervix, in particular, epidemiologic studies of dietary vitamin C demonstrate an inverse correlation. Carotenoids and flavonoids, among other plant dietary components, have antioxidant effects (in addition to other anticarcinogenic properties). Additionally, eating fruits high in polyphenols has been shown to lower the chance of developing cancer. Because each antioxidant has distinct properties and a different distribution inside the body, different antioxidants presumably do not have the same effects across the body. In this context, dietary phytochemicals with potential antioxidant activities have great relevance as chemopreventive agents to prevent oxidative stress [104].

Previous studies have shown that these dietary phytochemicals' biological action is caused by their strong free radical scavenging and antioxidant activity, which in turn regulates the expression of oncogenes and tumor suppressor genes. Additionally, numerous dietary chemopreventive phytochemicals have been found to inhibit a particular regulatory step throughout the carcinogenic process. Dietary phytochemicals control the proliferation and differentiation of cancer cells, the arrest of the cell cycle at various stages, and the initiation of cell death pathways including apoptosis and autophagy [105].

It appears that numerous phytochemicals have anti-inflammatory effects. Many studies confirmed the profound relationship between inflammation and cancer. Food varieties, food preparation techniques, portion sizes, food diversity, and total calorie balance are some of the dietary variables that might influence cancer risk. A general dietary pattern with a high proportion of vegetal foods (fruits, vegetables, grains, and legumes), less meat, dairy, and other high-fat foods, and a balance between calorie consumption and physical exercise can lower the risk of cancer. Strong data suggests that increasing a fruit and vegetable diet lowers the risk of colon cancer. For malignancies deemed hormonal, including breast and prostate cancer, the evidence is less compelling. The vast majority of the numerous scientific researches on this topic demonstrates that consuming fruits and vegetables, particularly those that are green, dark yellow, and in the cabbage family, as well as soy products and legumes, protects against colon cancer [105].

A decreased risk of lung cancer has also been linked to increased consumption of fruits, vegetables, or both. Tobacco use is the main cause of lung cancer risk, although diet can interfere with the risk. Fruits and vegetables lower cancer risk regardless of whether a person smokes, despite studies showing that smokers tend to eat less healthfully than nonsmokers. Scientists have proposed that beta-carotene itself may lower the incidence of lung cancer since several studies show that meals high in beta-carotene protect against lung cancer. But according to recent studies on beta-carotene supplements, smokers who took them were more likely to get lung cancer than those who took a placebo. These results provide credence to the hypothesis that beta-carotene in meals may serve as a stand-in for other protective nutrients or compounds, either alone or in combination. They also imply that consuming one nutrient in excess might have negative effects [104].

Despite the strong evidence linking eating fruits and vegetables with a lower risk of developing cancer, few adults and kids regularly consume these items. The National 5 A Day for Better Health Program aims to improve fruit and vegetable intake to five or more servings per day due to the concerns about low intake levels. Although particular nutrients or other compounds that may be derived from foods are not included in this advice, it nevertheless applies to foods in their fresh, frozen, canned, dried, or juice forms. The main candidates are certain vitamins and minerals, fiber, and phytochemicals found in meals with a plant origin, such as carotenoids, flavonoids, terpenes, sterols, indoles, and phenols [104].

The foundation of a healthy diet, as shown by the Food Guide Pyramid, is made up of grains like wheat, rice, oats, and barley, as well as the meals created from them. Six to eleven standard portions of these items are included daily in healthy diets. Numerous vitamins and minerals, including folate, calcium, and selenium, which have all been linked to a decreased risk of colon cancer, are abundant in grains. In comparison to items made with refined flour, whole grains are richer in fiber and several vitamins and minerals. It is recommended to receive fiber from fruits, vegetables, and whole grains rather than from fiber supplements since the advantages of grain foods may come from both their other nutrients and their fiber content [77].

Beans are a great source of fiber, protein, and a variety of vitamins and minerals. The family of plants that includes dry beans, pinto beans, lentils, and soybeans among many others is referred to scientifically as legumes, or simply as beans. Beans are a good low-fat but high-protein substitute for meat since they are particularly rich in elements that may prevent cancer. Protein, fat, and carbohydrates all give energy to the diet, therefore consuming too much of one or more of these macronutrients may increase your chance of developing cancer. However, there is an ongoing debate about whether certain macronutrients might raise risk without affecting energy balance. For instance, calories from fat are substituted by calories from carbohydrates and/or proteins in intervention trials of low-fat diets under isocaloric settings. Other nutrients may also vary. It is therefore challenging to distinguish between the impact of lower fat consumption and these other modifications. Similarly, merely increasing fat in the diet cannot be distinguished from increasing energy (or the consequent weight gain). Therefore, total energy and other nutrients that include energy must be carefully considered in epidemiologic investigations of macronutrients [78].

According to a fundamental epidemiological study, getting more sun exposure that boosts the endogenous synthesis of vitamin D3, leads to a decrease in the risk of colorectal cancer. This gave rise to the hypothesis that a lack of vitamin D may increase the chance of developing cancer. Trials including vitamin D interventions supported this idea. Observational epidemiologic research has shown that having insufficient vitamin D levels increases the chance of developing many cancers, such as colorectal, prostate, and breast cancer, and that taking enough vitamin D3 supplements helps prevent cancer. However, for the general population, randomized control trials were unable to corroborate these findings, pointing to the need for segmentation into more sensitive subpopulations [77].

It has been discovered that indoles and sulforaphane are more effective against breast cancer. Additionally, they have had a big impact on how the skin is protected from UV radiation damage. The prostate tumorigenesis process has been significantly inhibited by sulforaphane. For its chemopreventive effect against breast, lung, cervical, prostate, and numerous myeloma cell lines, phenethyl isothiocyanate (PEITC) has been extensively researched. PEITC has shown extremely strong inhibitory efficacy against melanoma [102].

1.1.5.4 Nutrition and Cancer Treatment

Currently, studies on the role of nutrition in cancer treatment are limited to very few studies that only explored the role of nutrition supplementation in improving cancer therapy. For instance, the use of vitamins and antioxidants can in breast cancer can either enhance or diminish the efficacy of conventional treatments including chemotherapy and radiotherapy. For instance, one can argue that the use of vitamins C, D, and E can enhance cancer treatment response as they exert anti-inflammatory and antioxidant effects. However, it is well known that radiotherapy and chemotherapeutic agents exert their anticancer effects through the production of ROS and damaging cancer cells; therefore these vitamins may interfere with the anticancer actions of these agents and reduce their efficacy [82, 102].

Dietary phytochemicals demonstrate improved anticancer efficacy due to the modulation of various cell death mechanisms, including apoptosis and autophagy, in close interaction with cell cycle regulation, suppression of cellular proliferation, invasion, and migration. In numerous tumor and cancer cell lines, quercetin triggers both apoptosis and autophagy. Skin and gastrointestinal tract tumors have been successfully decreased by resveratrol's anticarcinogenic properties. Breast, lung, colon, and brain tumors can all be effectively treated with curcumin, an extract of turmeric, thanks to its chemopreventive properties. Green tea's phytonutrient epigallocatechin gallate is effective in treating prostate, bladder, cervical, and brain malignancies. Similar to this, Kaempferol has been linked to a decrease in pancreatic and lung cancer. Another potent phytochemical extracted from fresh ginger, gingerol, is useful in treating cancers with origins in the colon, breast, ovary, and pancreas [41, 104].

The abundance of non-nutritive disease-preventing bioactive substances present in everyday dietary supplements, such as polyphenols, carotenoids, glucosinolates, organo-sulfides, nitrogen-containing chemicals, and terpenoids, has enormous potential as chemotherapeutic agents. These bioactive dietary phytochemicals operate as solo medication candidates or in combination with other traditional chemotherapy medicines to produce nontoxic, target-specific chemotherapeutic effects with effective bioactivity and increased bioavailability [104].

There have been several studies on the relationship between cancer and vitamins, and vitamin supplements are frequently used by cancer patients. Unfortunately, vitamin supplements might not be a smart idea; using multivitamins was associated with an increase in cancer-related mortality in male smokers. Additionally, second research on prostate cancer patients revealed a higher death rate among those using multivitamins. Vitamin supplements are only one aspect of food's significance in the treatment of cancer. Therefore, at the moment due to sparse research in this area, it is advisable to have a healthy diet such as the Mediterranean diet, instead of taking supplements that might negatively impact treatment response.

1.2 Concluding Remarks

- Cancer is a group of diseases in which some of the body's cells grow uncontrollably and spread to other parts of the body.
- Cancer is an important cause of morbidity and mortality worldwide, in developing and developed countries.
- Hereditary, lifestyle, and environment are factors that play an important role in carcinogenesis.
- There are different treatments for cancers based on conventional strategies. Surgical treatment is the most common conventional treatment for cancer. Other conventional cancer treatments include radiation and chemotherapy.
- Without a doubt, cancer could be prevented, and in some circumstances, it may even be reversed.
- Cancer survivors should be concerned about their food as well to maintain good health and prevent cachexia.
- There are certain guidelines to promote overall health and prevent chronic illnesses like cancer that are linked to nutrition.
- The general guidelines that apply to both cancer prevention and treatment include:
  - Eating a varied and balanced diet that gives your body all the nutrients it needs. Protein, carbs, lipids, vitamins, and minerals.
  - The diet should include more fruits and vegetables, a balance of omega-3 and-6 fats, vitamin D, and fewer sugars.
  - Include other plant-based foods in your diet regularly, such as bread, cereals, grain products, rice, pasta, and beans.
  - Include wholegrain carbs in each meal. Instead of processed (refined) grains, use whole grains.
  - Limit red meat to two servings per week and avoid processed meats.
  - Including protein in at least 2–3 of daily meals.

– Include two to three pieces of dairy or dairy substitutes every day in the diet. Select substitutes that are enriched with vitamin D and calcium.
– Reduce the number of fats and fatty meals.

References

1. Pecorino L (2021) Molecular biology of cancer: mechanisms, targets, and therapeutics. Oxford University Press
2. Hanahan D, Weinberg RA (2000) The hallmarks of cancer. Cell 100(1):57–70
3. Hanahan D, Weinberg RA (2011) Hallmarks of cancer: the next generation. Cell 144(5):646–674
4. (WHO) W.H.O. Global health estimates: leading causes of death. Cited 6 June 2022. Available from: https://www.who.int/data/gho/data/themes/mortality-and-global-health-estimates/ghe-leading-causes-of-death
5. Sung H et al (2021) Global cancer statistics 2020: GLOBOCAN estimates of incidence and mortality worldwide for 36 cancers in 185 countries. CA Can J Clin 71(3):209–249
6. Blackadar CB (2016) Historical review of the causes of cancer. World J Clin Oncol 7(1):54
7. Hill BT (2019) Etiology of cancer. Clinical ophthalmic oncology. Springer, pp 11–17
8. Modiano J, Breen M (2007) The etiology of cancer. In: Withrow and MacEwen's small animal clinical oncology
9. Hodgson S (2008) Mechanisms of inherited cancer susceptibility. J Zhejiang Univ Sci B 9(1):1–4
10. Lupo PJ et al (2019) Association between birth defects and cancer risk among children and adolescents in a population-based assessment of 10 million live births. JAMA Oncol 5(8):1150–1158
11. Monsonego J et al (2015) Prevalence of high-risk human papilloma virus genotypes and associated risk of cervical precancerous lesions in a large US screening population: data from the ATHENA trial. Gynecol Oncol 137(1):47–54
12. Pfister H (1987) Human papillomaviruses and genital cancer. Adv Cancer Res 48:113–147
13. Haedicke J, Iftner T (2013) Human papillomaviruses and cancer. Radiother Oncol 108(3):397–402
14. Goncalves PH et al (2017) Kaposi-Sarcoma herpesvirus associated cancers and related diseases. Curr Opin HIV AIDS 12(1):47
15. Thompson MP, Kurzrock R (2004) Epstein-Barr virus and cancer. Clin Cancer Res 10(3):803–821
16. Kanda T, Yajima M, Ikuta K (2019) Epstein-Barr virus strain variation and cancer. Cancer Sci 110(4):1132–1139
17. Ringehan M, McKeating JA, Protzer U (2017) Viral hepatitis and liver cancer. Philos Trans R Soc B Biol Sci 372(1732):20160274
18. Clifford GM et al (2005) Cancer risk in the Swiss HIV Cohort study: associations with immunodeficiency, smoking, and highly active antiretroviral therapy. J Natl Cancer Inst 97(6):425–432
19. Zhang L-L et al (2017) Human T-cell lymphotropic virus type 1 and its oncogenesis. Acta Pharmacol Sin 38(8):1093–1103
20. Parsonnet J et al (1991) Helicobacter pylori infection and the risk of gastric carcinoma. N Engl J Med 325(16):1127–1131
21. Koskela P et al (2000) Chlamydia trachomatis infection as a risk factor for invasive cervical cancer. Int J Cancer 85(1):35–39

22. Littman AJ, Jackson LA, Vaughan TL (2005) Chlamydia pneumoniae and lung cancer: epidemiologic evidence. Cancer Epidemiol Biomark Prev 14(4):773–778
23. Dematei A et al (2017) Angiogenesis in Schistosoma haematobium-associated urinary bladder cancer. APMIS 125(12):1056–1062
24. Mu H et al (2018) Ionizing radiation exposure: hazards, prevention, and biomarker screening. Environ Sci Pollut Res 25(16):15294–15306
25. Parsa N (2012) Environmental factors inducing human cancers. Iran J Public Health 41(11):1
26. World Health Organization, Ultraviolet radiation and health. Cited 20 June 2022. Available from: https://www.who.int/health-topics/ultraviolet-radiation#tab=tab_1
27. Cleaver JE, Crowley E (2002) UV damage, DNA repair and skin carcinogenesis. Front Biosci Landmark 7(4):1024–1043
28. Singh AD et al (2004) Sunlight exposure and pathogenesis of uveal melanoma. Surv Ophthalmol 49(4):419–428
29. Gichuhi S et al (2014) Pathophysiology of ocular surface squamous neoplasia. Exp Eye Res 129:172–182
30. Ng J et al (2008) Ultraviolet radiation and the role of matrix metalloproteinases in the pathogenesis of ocular surface squamous neoplasia. Invest Ophthalmol Vis Sci 49(12):5295–5306
31. Wolbarst AB et al (2010) Medical response to a major radiologic emergency: a primer for medical and public health practitioners. Radiology 254(3):660–677
32. Cox JD, Ang KK (2009) Radiation oncology E-book: rationale, technique, results. Elsevier Health Sciences
33. Doll R (1995) Hazards of ionising radiation: 100 years of observations on man. Br J Cancer 72(6):1339–1349
34. Gilbert ES (2009) Ionising radiation and cancer risks: what have we learned from epidemiology? Int J Radiat Biol 85(6):467–482
35. Preston DL et al (1994) Cancer incidence in atomic bomb survivors. Part III: Leukemia, lymphoma and multiple myeloma, 1950–1987. Radiat Res 137(2s):S68–S97
36. Folley JH, Borges W, Yamawaki T (1952) Incidence of leukemia in survivors of the atomic bomb in Hiroshima and Nagasaki, Japan. Am J Med 13(3):311–321
37. Ozasa K et al (2012) Studies of the mortality of atomic bomb survivors, report 14, 1950–2003: an overview of cancer and noncancer diseases. Radiat Res 177(3):229–243
38. Wakeford R (2013) The risk of childhood leukaemia following exposure to ionising radiation—a review. J Radiol Prot 33(1):1
39. Mossman BT, Gee JBL (1989) Asbestos-related diseases. N Engl J Med 320(26):1721–1730
40. Lynch BM, Leitzmann MF (2017) An evaluation of the evidence relating to physical inactivity, sedentary behavior, and cancer incidence and mortality. Current Epidemiol Rep 4(3):221–231
41. Barnett GC et al (2009) Normal tissue reactions to radiotherapy: towards tailoring treatment dose by genotype. Nat Rev Cancer 9(2):134–142
42. Baskar R et al (2012) Cancer and radiation therapy: current advances and future directions. Int J Med Sci 9(3):193–199
43. Begg AC, Stewart FA, Vens C (2011) Strategies to improve radiotherapy with targeted drugs. Nat Rev Cancer 11(4):239–253
44. Blasius F et al (2022) Surgical treatment of bone sarcoma. Cancers (Basel) 14(11)
45. Bethesda (2012) Clinical course and diagnosis of drug induced liver disease. In: LiverTox: clinical and research information on drug-induced liver injury, Bethesda
46. Cutler DM (2008) Are we finally winning the war on cancer? J Econ Perspect 22(4):3–26
47. Chaudhry P, Asselin E (2009) Resistance to chemotherapy and hormone therapy in endometrial cancer. Endocr Relat Cancer 16(2):363–380
48. Benjamin DJ (2014) The efficacy of surgical treatment of cancer—20 years later. Med Hypotheses 82(4):412–420
49. Delaney G et al (2005) The role of radiotherapy in cancer treatment: estimating optimal utilization from a review of evidence-based clinical guidelines. Cancer 104(6):1129–1137

50. Esposito I et al (2008) Most pancreatic cancer resections are R1 resections. Ann Surg Oncol 15(6):1651–1660
51. Guideline Committee of the Korean Gastric Cancer Association, Development Working Group and Review Panel (2019) Korean practice guideline for gastric cancer 2018: an evidence-based, multi-disciplinary approach. J Gastric Cancer 19(1):1–48
52. Guidozzi F (2013) Estrogen therapy in gynecological cancer survivors. Climacteric 16(6):611–617
53. Hopwood DA (2019) Highlights of streptomyces genetics. Heredity (Edinb) 123(1):23–32
54. Tiwari M (2012) Antimetabolites: established cancer therapy. J Cancer Res Ther 8(4):510–519
55. Jackson SP, Bartek J (2009) The DNA-damage response in human biology and disease. Nature 461(7267):1071–1078
56. Kemung HM et al (2018) Streptomyces as a prominent resource of future anti-MRSA drugs. Front Microbiol 9:2221
57. Mitra S et al (2022) Hormonal therapy for gynecological cancers: how far has science progressed toward clinical applications? Cancers (Basel) 14(3)
58. Muggia FM, Green MD (1991) New anthracycline antitumor antibiotics. Crit Rev Oncol Hematol 11(1):43–64
59. Ajani JA et al (2022) Gastric cancer, version 2.2022, NCCN clinical practice guidelines in oncology. J Natl Compr Canc Netw 20(2):167–192
60. Ringborg U et al (2003) The Swedish council on technology assessment in health care (SBU) systematic overview of radiotherapy for cancer including a prospective survey of radiotherapy practice in Sweden 2001–summary and conclusions. Acta Oncol 42(5–6):357–365
61. Robatel S, Schenk M (2022) Current limitations and novel perspectives in pancreatic cancer treatment. Cancers (Basel) 14(4)
62. Rojas GA et al (2021) International trends in incidence of osteosarcoma (1988–2012). Int J Cancer 149(5):1044–1053
63. Santamaria RI et al (2022) Grapevine xylem sap is a potent elicitor of antibiotic production in *Streptomyces* spp. Antibiotics (Basel) 11(5)
64. Spasic J et al (2018) *Streptomyces* spp. in the biocatalysis toolbox. Appl Microbiol Biotechnol 102(8):3513–3536
65. Takahashi Y, Nakashima T (2018) Actinomycetes, an inexhaustible source of naturally occurring antibiotics. Antibiotics (Basel) 7(2)
66. Haddad T, Yee D (2011) Basic principles of antineoplastic therapies. In: Breast surgical techniques and interdisciplinary management, pp 707–715
67. Carrato A et al (2022) Clinical nutrition as part of the treatment pathway of pancreatic cancer patients: an expert consensus. Clin Transl Oncol 24(1):112–126
68. Cembranel F et al (2017) Relationship between dietary consumption of vitamins and minerals, body mass index, and waist circumference: a population-based study of adults in southern Brazil. Cad Saude Publ 33(12):e00136616
69. Corino C, Rossi R (2021) Antioxidants in animal nutrition. Antioxidants (Basel) 10(12)
70. de Carvalho C, Caramujo MJ (2018) The various roles of fatty acids. Molecules 23(10)
71. Ebbeling CB et al (2020) Effects of sugar-sweetened, artificially sweetened, and unsweetened beverages on cardiometabolic risk factors, body composition, and sweet taste preference: a randomized controlled trial. J Am Heart Assoc 9(15):e015668
72. Fernandez-Lazaro CI et al (2021) Dietary antioxidant vitamins and minerals and breast cancer risk: prospective results from the SUN Cohort. Antioxidants (Basel) 10(3)
73. Kerr BJ, Kellner TA, Shurson GC (2015) Characteristics of lipids and their feeding value in swine diets. J Animal Sci Biotechnol 6(30)
74. Koom WS et al (2012) Nutritional status of patients treated with radiotherapy as determined by subjective global assessment. Radiat Oncol J 30(3):132–139
75. Lee T, Suh HS (2019) Associations between dietary fiber intake and bone mineral density in adult Korean population: analysis of national health and nutrition examination survey in 2011. J Bone Metab 26(3):151–160

76. Li P, Wu G (2020) Composition of amino acids and related nitrogenous nutrients in feedstuffs for animal diets. Amino Acids 52(4):523–542
77. Li S et al (2021) Advances on monosaccharides and oligosaccharides: structural modifications and bioactivities. Mini Rev Med Chem 21(17):2551–2566
78. Lykstad J, Sharma S (2022) Biochemistry, water soluble vitamins, in StatPearls. Treasure Island
79. Morris AL, Mohiuddin SS (2022) Biochemistry, nutrients, in StatPearls. Treasure Island
80. Qi X, Tester RF (2020) Lactose, maltose, and sucrose in health and disease. Mol Nutr Food Res 64(8):e1901082
81. Reddy P, Jialal I (2022) Biochemistry, fat soluble vitamins, in StatPearls. Treasure Island
82. Reszczynska E, Hanaka A (2020) Lipids composition in plant membranes. Cell Biochem Biophys 78(4):401–414
83. Saha SK, Pathak NN (2021) Fundamentals of animal nutrition
84. Saha SK et al (2017) Correlation between oxidative stress, nutrition, and cancer initiation. Int J Mol Sci 18(7)
85. Carlberg C, Velleuer E (2022) Vitamin D and the risk for cancer: a molecular analysis. Biochem Pharmacol 196:114735
86. Kamal N et al (2022) Genesis and mechanism of some cancer types and an overview on the role of diet and nutrition in cancer prevention. Molecules 27(6)
87. Donaldson MS (2004) Nutrition and cancer: a review of the evidence for an anti-cancer diet. Nutr J 3:19
88. Logan J, Bourassa MW (2018) The rationale for a role for diet and nutrition in the prevention and treatment of cancer. Eur J Cancer Prev 27(4):406–410
89. Patra S et al (2021) Chemical diversity of dietary phytochemicals and their mode of chemoprevention. Biotechnol Rep (Amst) 30:e00633
90. Azeem S et al (2015) Diet and colorectal cancer risk in Asia—a systematic review. Asian Pac J Cancer Prev 16(13):5389–5396
91. De Cicco P et al (2019) Nutrition and breast cancer: a literature review on prevention, treatment and recurrence. Nutrients 11(7)
92. Kim SR et al (2019) Effect of red, processed, and white meat consumption on the risk of gastric cancer: an overall and dose-response meta-analysis. Nutrients 11(4)
93. Lippi G, Mattiuzzi C, Cervellin G (2016) Meat consumption and cancer risk: a critical review of published meta-analyses. Crit Rev Oncol Hematol 97:1–14
94. Matsushita M, Fujita K, Nonomura N (2020) Influence of diet and nutrition on prostate cancer. Int J Mol Sci 21(4):1447
95. Key TJ, Spencer EA (2007) Carbohydrates and cancer: an overview of the epidemiological evidence. Eur J Clin Nutr 61(Suppl 1):S112–S121
96. Maino Vieytes CA et al (2019) Carbohydrate nutrition and the risk of cancer. Curr Nutr Rep 8(3):230–239
97. Dydjow-Bendek D, Zagożdżon P (2019) Selected dietary factors and breast cancer risk. Przegl Epidemiol 73(3):361–368
98. Ocvirk S, O'Keefe SJD (2021) Dietary fat, bile acid metabolism and colorectal cancer. Semin Cancer Biol 73:347–355
99. Kesteloot H, Lesaffre E, Joossens JV (1991) Dairy fat, saturated animal fat, and cancer risk. Prev Med 20(2):226–236
100. Karunanithi S, Levi L (2018) High-fat diet and colorectal cancer: myths and facts. Future Oncol 14(6):493–495
101. Bojková B, Winklewski PJ, Wszedybyl-Winklewska M (2020) Dietary fat and cancer-which is good, which is bad, and the body of evidence. Int J Mol Sci 21(11)
102. De Pergola G, Silvestris F (2013) Obesity as a major risk factor for cancer. J Obesity 2013:291546–291546
103. Kolb R, Sutterwala FS, Zhang W (2016) Obesity and cancer: inflammation bridges the two. Curr Opin Pharmacol 29:77–89

104. Shanmugalingam T et al (2014) Obesity and cancer: the role of vitamin D. BMC Cancer 14:712–712
105. Rumgay H et al (2021) Alcohol and cancer: epidemiology and biological mechanisms. Nutrients 13(9):3173
106. Cao Y, Giovannucci EL (2016) Alcohol as a risk factor for cancer. Semin Oncol Nurs 32(3):325–331

Metabolic Carcinogenesis

2

Mahwish Ali, Syeda Mehpara Farhat, and Abdul Haleem

Contents

M. Ali (✉) · S. M. Farhat
National University of Medical Sciences, Rawalpindi, Pakistan
e-mail: mahwishmalik67@gmail.com

A. Haleem
Quaid-I-Azam University, Islamabad, Pakistan

R. F. Saeed and S. ul. Shaheed (eds.), *Nutrition and Dietary Interventions in Cancer*,
Cancer Treatment and Research 191, https://doi.org/10.1007/978-3-031-55622-7_2

Abbreviations

ATG5	Autophagy related 5
BMI	Body mass index
BRCA1	Breast cancer gene 1
CAA	Chloroacetaldehyde
CEO	Chloroethylene oxide
Cr	Chromium
CT	Computed tomography
CYP	Cytochrome P450 mono-oxygenase
CYP2E1	Cytochrome P450 2E1
Cys	Cysteine
EPA	Environmental Protection Agency
GSH	Glutathione
HMGB1	High mobility group box 1
IARC	International agency for research on cancer
LD50	Lethal dose
MAPK	Mitogen-activated protein kinase
NNK	4-(*N*-nitrosomethylamino)-1-(3-pyridyl)-1-butanone
NNN	*N′*-nitrosonornicotine
PET	Positron emission tomography
POB	Pyridyloxobutyl

2.1 Chemical Carcinogens, Fate, Causes and Associated Risks

Various different types of chemical compounds are used every day for the benefit of mankind in different ways. For example, the use of pesticides helps the production of foodstuff in ample quantities which is enough to fulfill the needs of millions of people. It has consequently lead to an increase in the life expectancy and helped in providing better living for mankind [1]. But at times, the toxic effects caused by these chemical compounds offset their benefits. The cancer-causing ability, i.e., carcinogenesis, of certain chemicals, called carcinogens, is a matter of great concern in the modern era. In 1997, Gomes-Carneiro defined carcinogen as a compound that has the capacity to act on several tissues and organs and initiate the process of cancer development in humans and animals under appropriate conditions [2]. This definition was considered incomplete after the various mechanisms involved in carcinogenesis were discovered [3]. Later in 2001, the carcinogen was defined from an experimental point of view. It states that a carcinogen is a compound that when administered in experimental animals causes statistically significant rise in the histological changes related to cancer development as compared to those animals which are not exposed to that chemical [4].

2.1.1 Historical Perspective for Identification of Chemical Carcinogens

According to Hayes, the relationship between the cancer development and exposure to different environmental factors was first identified by an English surgeon Percivall Pott in 1775 [5]. Percivall Pott observed that the children called "chimney sweeps" who used to clean chimneys by climbing them up frequently developed skin cancer of the scrotum due to repeated localized contamination with soot. On the basis of these observations, the Danish chimney sweeps were recommended to take daily bath so that the cancer occurrence can be avoided. In the eighteenth century, a high incidence of cancer in nasal mucosa was reported by John Hill that was traced to be caused by long-term exposure to snuff. A high proportion of bladder cancer was also reported across Europe in 1890 in the workers of rubber and chemical industry [1]. It had become evident by the end of the nineteenth century that occupational exposure to certain chemicals or chemical mixtures can lead to the development of cancer.

2.1.2 Experimental Evidence of Chemical Carcinogenesis

The first experimental proof of chemical carcinogenesis was provided in 1915 by Yamagiwa and Ichikawa [6]. In their experiment, they observed the development of papillomas and carcinomas in rabbit on rubbing their ear with coal tar. This provided a mechanistic base for the observed skin cancer by Percivall Pott. Later Beremblum and Shubik demonstrated that polycyclic aromatic hydrocarbons and croton oil can lead to the skin cancer development in mice [7]. Many other scientists proved the carcinogenic activity of different chemicals in bladder, liver, kidney, lungs and pancreas of animals. After successful translation of carcinogenic activity in animals, the foundation was laid for the use of animal models for different human diseases [8].

2.1.3 Hazard Identification of Chemical Carcinogens

The chemical carcinogens may act in a genotoxic or a non-genotoxic manner, i.e., exerting their effects via interacting with the genetic material. If the chemical is proved to have non-genotoxic potential, then its safe dose may be calculated which is the dose at which the chemical does not pose a harm to induce cancer. But if the compound is genotoxic, then it is difficult to identify its safe dose; however, it can be inferred that high doses of the chemical may pose a greater threat of inducing cancer while the lower doses have a lower risk [9].

According to the Environmental protection agency (EPA) of USA, the data for the carcinogenic potential of a compound can be obtained from three sources:

(1) Epidemiological data from humans.
(2) Results from long-term exposure to the animals. (However, it should be investigated that the tumor causing mechanism in animals is relevant to that in humans.)
(3) Supporting data including various small experiments for metabolic and pharmacokinetic studies, short-term tests for genotoxicity and other properties.

A combination of all three above-mentioned evidences is used to characterize the weight of evidence regarding the carcinogenic potential of the chemical in humans. Based on this characterization, the EPA has categorized chemical carcinogens as follows [10].

- Carcinogenic to humans
- Likely to be carcinogenic to humans
- Suggestive evidence of carcinogenic potential
- Inadequate information to assess carcinogenic potential
- Not likely to be carcinogenic to humans.

2.1.4 Mechanism of Chemical Carcinogenicity

In 1977, Jerina [11] demonstrated the mechanism of action of chemical carcinogens through their ground breaking discovery which revealed that the polycyclic aromatic hydrocarbons are unable to cause cancer directly but need to be metabolically activated by the action of certain enzymes termed as cytochrome P450 mono-oxygenase (CYP). Their discovery was further confirmed by Elizabeth and Millar [12] and others [13]. The CYP enzymes are located in the endoplasmic reticulum of different cells and are able to catalyze a large spectrum of chemical reactions the most prominent of which is insertion of oxygen atom to the organic substrates. The biological functions of the CYP enzymes are the detoxification of various exogenous and endogenous compounds through modification of their structure which makes them more hydrophilic or prepares them for further conjugation reactions [14]. However, some carcinogenic chemicals such as polycyclic aromatic hydrocarbons are converted to highly reactive unstable forms by the action of CYP enzymes. Due to the high hydrophilic nature, the modified polycyclic aromatic hydrocarbons have the ability to react with the nucleophilic targets including different proteins and DNA. The covalent modification of the DNA results in a permanent change, i.e., mutation, which may put them on the track toward becoming malignant [9]. Such cells become more vulnerable to accumulating further genetic alterations. It is important to understand that a single change is highly unlikely to cause malignancy, in any cell, but cumulative effect of various genetic alterations may result in a malignant cancer cell. This cancer cell may lead to the development a full-blown cancer through clonal expansion [15].

The mechanism of non-genotoxic carcinogens is more complex and includes various different modes of action including receptor mediated carcinogenesis, histone acetylation that leads to epigenetic alterations, oxidative stress, disruption of DNA repair mechanisms [16] and many others [17]. There are also some indirect genotoxic compounds that affect DNA by creating reactive oxygen species or other metabolites that react with DNA and alter the structure of DNA and consequently compromising its integrity [18].

2.1.5 Heavy Metals Carcinogenicity

Heavy metals are those metallic compounds which have at least five times higher density than water [19]. The heavy metals have various technological, industrial, domestic and agricultural utilities due to which their exposure to the humans has exponentially increased in the recent years. Therefore, there is an increasing public health concern, globally, in association with the contamination of environment with these heavy metals [20]. Although the heavy metals are naturally present in the environment due to different geological processes, most human exposure to these metals occurs due to anthropogenic activities such as industrial production, domestic effluents, and agricultural and pharmacological waste. In addition, the individuals working in smelters, foundries, mines and other industrial operations based on metallic process have very high exposure to the heavy metals [20]. This occupational exposure puts these individuals at higher risk of being affected by the toxic effects of the heavy metals.

Some of the heavy metals are micronutrients and are involved in various biochemical processes and physiological functions. While some heavy metals are considered non-essential because no biological function is known to be regulated by these heavy metals. The toxic effects of the non-essential heavy metals are known at various concentrations. The essential micronutrients have a narrow range of concentration between essential and toxic range and tissue and cellular damage is caused by the excessive amount of these essential heavy metals [21, 22]. The arsenic, cadmium, chromium, lead and mercury are ranked among top priority metals of public health concern due to their ability to produce reactive oxygen species and oxidative stress, (Fig. 2.1) which plays a key role in the toxicity and carcinogenicity of these metals [19].

2.1.5.1 Arsenic

Occurrence in Environment and Human Exposure

Arsenic is ubiquitously present in almost all environmental matrices [23]. The arsenic exists either as trivalent arsenite and pentavalent arsenate. In experiments conducted on rats, it was observed that the trivalent arsenite is more cytotoxic as compared to the pentavalent arsenite with LD50 of 36 and 220 μM respectively [24]. In addition to the natural processes such as volcanic eruption and soil erosion, the anthropogenic activities also contribute to the environmental pollution

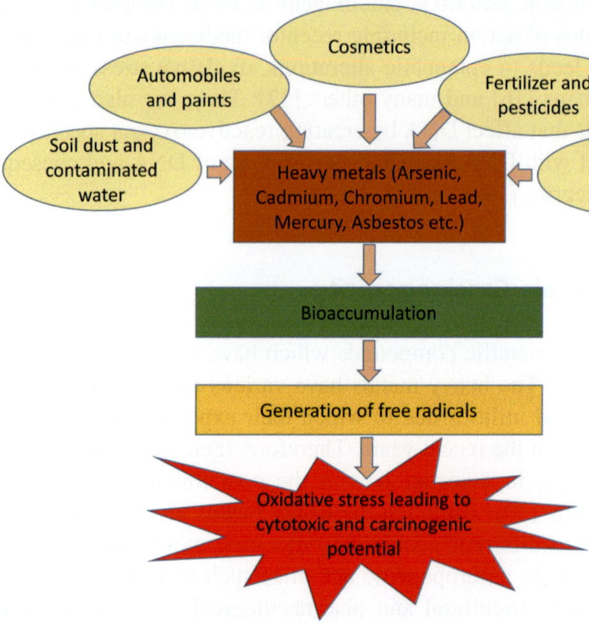

Fig. 2.1 Summary of the sources and carcinogenic potential of various heavy metals

by arsenic [23]. Various industrial products such as insecticides, fungicides, herbicides, dye-stuff and wood preservatives contained arsenic in 1980s. But the toxic effects of arsenic caused severe poisoning in humans resulting in headache, dizziness, vomiting diarrhea and fall in blood pressure due to which the use of arsenic in these products was inhibited by US EPA in 2004 [25]. In addition, arsenic is also component of various medicines were used from 1940 to 1970, for a variety of disorders in humans and veterinary ailments including diabetes, psoriasis, syphilis and trypanosomiasis [26]. The advancement of science and the requirement of extensive clinical trials for marketing and use of drugs has resulted in discontinuation of arsenic in drugs [27].

The oral ingestion, via intake from water and foods, of arsenic is the major contributor of human exposure to this metal. Other routes of exposure including inhalation, parenteral route and dermal exposure have a lesser contribution to the human exposure to this metal. Although the exposure from soil, air and water is much smaller however in the areas where these sources are contaminated with arsenic the exposure may become significant [28].

Carcinogenic Potential of Arsenic

High incidence of carcinoma and various other diseases, such as cardiovascular disease, peripheral neuropathy and diabetes [29], were reported in the population of Bangladesh, Taiwan, Thailand, West Bengal, Mexico, Finland, Chile, Argentina and Hungary due to contamination of drinking water with arsenic in these areas

[30]. Arsenic affects all organ systems, and high mortality rate due to cancer of skin, kidney, liver and bladder is reported in areas of high arsenic pollution. However, the adverse health effects are related to the arsenic dose, time duration and form of exposure [31]. Although there is strong evidence for carcinogenic potential of arsenic in humans, its underlying mechanism is not completely understood.

Mechanism of Carcinogenicity

In addition to being influenced by various intrinsic and extrinsic factors, the toxicity of arsenic greatly depends on its oxidation state and solubility which makes it toxicity analysis more complicated [32]. Epidemiological studies also support the carcinogenicity resulting from long-term exposure to arsenic in which different mechanisms have been proposed. Although arsenic has weak mutagenic properties, it might act as a clastogenic agent [33]. The DNA damage induced by arsenic trioxide was identified almost 3 decades ago in human lymphocytes [34]. The genotoxic studies of arsenic in human and rodent cell cultures have shown that arsenic can cause DNA repair inhibition, chromosomal aberrations, exchange between sister chromatids (due to its ability to cause a break in DNA strand) and formation of micronuclei [35, 36]. Arsenic compounds can also cause cell arrest in mitosis, induces expression of *c-fos* gene, and heme oxygenase protein [36]. Zhao et al. reported that arsenic may cause DNA hypomethylation through which it can cause aberrant gene expression. Moreover, arsenic stimulates the transactivational activity of Erk-1 and AP-1, which are extracellular signal transduction proteins, which in turn induces *c-fos* and *c-jun* gene expression [37]. In addition, the arsenic also affects the activity of P53 gene, which is involved in various cellular functions including DNA repair, cell cycle control, apoptosis and many others. The altered expression of P53 gene due to long-term exposure with arsenic can substantially contribute to its carcinogenicity [38]. Collectively arsenic has the ability to interfere with the cell signaling pathways that are frequently found associated with cancer promotion and progression in experimental animal models.

Due to the adverse health effects of arsenic the methods are being sought out to reduce its toxic effects on human body. The diet and nutrition have been observed to affect the metabolism and bio-accessibility of arsenic. It has been reported that the deficiency of micronutrients such as betaine, choline, folic acid vitamin B2, B12, B6 and zinc may impair the arsenic metabolism and can exacerbate its toxic effects. In addition, the dietary polyphenols and flavonoids contained in jiggery and honey can be helpful to combat the arsenic-induced toxicity [39].

The arsenic is known to produce reactive oxygen species, the use of exogenous dietary supplementation of antioxidants may help to remove the reactive oxygen species and repair the oxidized membranes of the cell caused by arsenic toxicity. Moreover, the proper diet and nutrition has a prophylactic effect rather than therapeutic effect on arsenic-induced toxicity. Therefore, the natural compounds and adequate nutrition can help to prevent any adverse effects caused by arsenic toxicity. Furthermore, the nutrition combination therapy may prove to be more useful for managing the arsenic toxicity as compared to the chelation therapy [40].

2.1.5.2 Cadmium

Occurrence in Environment and Human Exposure

Cadmium is a heavy metal with wide distribution in the environment. It occurs in the form of chloride, carbonate, sulfate, sulfide and hydroxide salts. It also has various industrial applications and is used in the production of pigments, alloys, electroplating industries, glass production and batteries. The people working in these industries have high exposure to this metal. The industrial activities may result in contamination of air, water and soil with cadmium which leads to extensive human exposure to this metal. Ingestion of the cadmium contaminated food and smoking have the capability to elevate cadmium concentration in blood and urine [41, 42]. After ingestion of the food contaminated with cadmium small portion of it is absorbed across gastrointestinal tract. However, the cadmium inhaled through industrial dust is efficiently absorbed via lungs [38].

Cadmium is currently used in various industries, e.g., as an alloy in electroplating, as a pigment in paints, stabilizer for polyvinyl plastics and in batteries. The release of cadmium from these industries may be a great source of cadmium exposure to humans [43]. The anthropogenic activities may result in the entry of cadmium in the soil–plant environment, and its presence in agricultural soil is a matter of great concern. As cadmium is more soluble in water than other heavy metals therefore it is readily available to the plats and accumulates in different plant parts and consequently enters the food chain [44]. For example, in Iran the farmers tried to increase the yield of rice, the biggest staple food in Iran, by using enormous amount of phosphate fertilizers and sludge waste, which contain high concentration of cadmium. This practice resulted in high cadmium concentration in rice and ultimately high human exposure to this metal [43]. Similarly, in a study conducted in USA about the sources of dietary intake of cadmium it was observed that the food groups that contributed most to the cadmium intake are cereal and bread, leafy vegetables, potato and greatest of all, lettuce [45].

Long-term exposure to cadmium results in toxicity to various organ systems including skeletal, reproductive, urinary, central and peripheral nervous system, cardiovascular and respiratory system. The measurement of cadmium levels in the body can be done through samples from hair, saliva, blood, nail and urine [43]. The chelation therapy as a mitigation strategy for cadmium toxicity is not very effective due to various safety and efficacy issues. Therefore, dietary supplements may play a better role in protecting against cadmium toxicity. Zhai et al. reported that tomatoes, berries, onion, garlic and grapes are very effective natural antagonists for cadmium toxicity and should be consumed regularly [46].

Carcinogenic Potential

The international agency for research on cancer has classified cadmium as carcinogenic in humans [47]. This classification of cadmium as carcinogenic is based on repeated observation of lung cancer occurrence in the individuals having occupational exposure to cadmium. Moreover, the animal studies have also strongly suggested the pulmonary effects of cadmium. After being absorbed in the blood stream, the cadmium may occur as free form or bound with other chemicals such as GSH and Cys in the body. The free forms are taken up via metal transporters and conjugated forms are transported to cells via receptor mediated pathways. Inside the cell the cadmium may cause various toxic effects including carcinogenicity [38]. It was observed that chronic inhalation of cadmium resulted in the pulmonary adenocarcinomas in the rodents [48]. The mechanism of cadmium induced carcinogenicity is poorly known, but it is speculated that it results from the generation of reactive oxygen species [49]. As a result of this oxidative stress, the nucleic acid and protein synthesis are disrupted and cause single-stranded DNA [50]. Previous studies have demonstrated that various stress responses such as heat shock, cold shock, stringent response, oxidative stress are elicited as a result of cadmium toxicity in the cell [50].

Mechanism of Carcinogenicity

Cadmium is reported to have a toxic effect on cellular proliferation, differentiation and apoptosis. The binding of cadmium to mitochondria results in inhibition of oxidative phosphorylation and cellular respiration. This results in chromosomal aberration, DNA strand breaks and sister chromatid exchange which may potentially result in chromosomal deletions. As a result of cadmium toxicity, the reduced glutathione (GSH) may be depleted resulting in increased production of reactive oxygen species. Furthermore, the activity of antioxidant enzymes is also inhibited further augmenting the cadmium-induced cellular damage. Similarly, metallothionine, a zinc concentrating protein, consists of 33% cysteine acts as cadmium scavenger as the cells being able to produce this protein are resistant to cadmium toxicity. Cadmium can also modulate the cellular levels of calcium, caspase and MAPK, where these processes cause indirect apoptosis [43].

2.1.5.3 Chromium

Occurrence in Environment and Human Exposure

Chromium (Cr) occurs in the environment in the oxidation states ranging from Cr (-2 to $+6$) of which trivalent and hexavalent are most common stable forms. The trivalent state is more stable and is found in ores, whereas the hexavalent state is a second most stable form. The chromium enters into the environment due to various natural and anthropogenic activities. The discharge from industrial units is a major contributor of chromium release into the environment [51]. The chromium released from the industrial effluents is in the hexavalent form which is considered to be the most carcinogenic [19]. Previously, all hexavalent chromium compounds were considered to be manmade and only trivalent chromium was considered natural which is an essential nutrient in humans. Inhalation is the principal route of human exposure to chromium, but contact through significant also presents a significant route of exposure. The exposure through skin leads to dermatitis in individuals having occupational exposure to chromium [52]. The inhalation from a person's occupational exposure and ingestion, a non-occupational exposure leads to multiorgan toxicity including renal damage, asthma, allergy and cancer of the respiratory tract.

Mechanism of Carcinogenicity

The toxicity of chromium depends on its oxidation state. The hexavalent chromium is more toxic, due to being a powerful oxidizing agent, as compared to similar amounts of trivalent chromium [53]. The high toxicity might be because of the reason that the hexavalent chromium can easily cross the cell membrane, as compared to trivalent chromium, and reduce to reactive intermediates inside the cell. The reduction of hexavalent chromium by hydrogen peroxide, glutathione peroxidase and ascorbic acid produces reactive intermediates which includes hydroxyl radicals and other oxidation states of chromium such as Cr(IV), Cr(V) and even Cr(III) [54]. The Cr(III) produced as a result of this intracellular chromium reduction gets trapped in the cell, due to its poor permeability across cell membrane. The products produced from reduction of hexavalent chromium may have genotoxic and mutagenic effects. These products may form DNA adducts DNA strand breaks, DNA protein cross links, oxidized bases, DNA inter- and intrastrand cross links and ultimately genome unstability. The damage induced by Cr(VI) can lead to dysregulation in DNA replication and transcription, non-functional DNA repair mechanism, dysregulated cell cycle checkpoints and disruption of gene networks that regulate the balance of cell survival and cell death. All of these mechanisms play an important role in chromium-induced carcinogenicity [55]. The ease of permeability of hexavalent chromium is evident from high penetration through the respiratory tract, gastrointestinal tract and even the intact skin [56] which in turn results in the reported high incidence of lung cancer in the individuals professionally exposed to high chromium levels [57]. Moreover, the carcinogenicity of chromium in humans is also supported by the presence of DNA breaks in peripheral lymphocytes in the urine of workers occupationally exposed to chromium [58]. The DNA damaging effects such as fragmentation of DNA due to breaks in the DNA strand that result in chromosomal abnormalities were observed in Sprague–Dawley rats and carcinoma cells of human liver [59, 60].

Although the excessive amounts of chromium can be damaging for the body, still it is an essential micronutrient and its dietary requirements are fulfilled by the foods such as broccoli, potatoes, whole grain products, beef, poultry, milk, dairy products and fruits like apple, banana and grape juice. Although the chromium deficiency is very rare (only in the individuals who have overall poor nutrition), still some people take chromium pills. The chromium pills have shown beneficial effects, in some studies, for type 2 diabetes, insulin resistance, heart disease risk and Parkinson's disease. But the use of these pills is highly controversial and is not recommended, due to toxic effects of excess chromium (https://www.webmd.com/diet/supplement-guide-chromium).

2.1.5.4 Lead

Occurrence in Environment and Human Exposure

The lead is naturally occurring in the environment, but burning of fossil fuel, mining and use of lead in manufacturing of various industrial goods leads to its further addition into the environment. Lead has various domestic and industrial applications. Its use in paints and lead acid batteries is the highest contributor of its total exposure to humans [61]. Although the use of lead has been greatly reduced in different countries, it is still used in various developing and underdeveloped countries in paints, smelting and batteries. The measurement of lead concentration from the blood samples is the most common method to determine the lead levels in the body. In addition the lead absorbed in the bones can be measured through X-ray fluoroscopy [62]. The lead has toxic effects on all body systems, but the nervous system is more susceptible to its toxic effects which are of high concern in children. The infants and children are prone to being affected by even low levels of lead [63] as their absorption capacity for lead present in water is more than 50%, whereas adults absorb 35–50% of the lead through drinking water [19]. After entry into the body, the lead is taken up by bones and various soft tissues including kidney, liver, heart and brain. The brain is the most vulnerable target causing headache, loss of memory and poor attention span [64].

The lead is a non-essential metal which is not used by our body. Although some of the people's favorite foods such as chocolate contain high levels of lead. High lead concentration in the body can interfere with the absorption of iron and calcium. The iron deficiency in the body may also lead to increased absorption of lead in the body. Therefore, reducing the use of lead rich foods and increasing the uptake of foods containing calcium iron and vitamin C may be a mitigation strategy for the lead toxicity. Moreover, the consumption of foods rich in antioxidants, Vitamin B6, B1 and flavonoids may also be helpful in combating the toxic effects produced by lead [62].

Mechanism of Carcinogenicity

The experimental evidence shows that lead has the ability to induce renal tumors in rats and mouse and therefore considered a probable carcinogen in humans [65]. The carcinogenic potential of lead is attributed to its ability to cause genetic damage via various indirect mechanisms including inhibition of DNA damage repair, oxidative stress and interact with tumor suppressor proteins [19]. Lead also has the ability to mimic calcium and interact with proteins that results in retardation of their function. It may also replace calcium in the skeleton which leads to the lead deposition in the bones and its release into the blood vessels during bone resorption that elevates lead level in the blood [64]. Moreover, lead binds to amide and sulfhydryl group of enzymes leading to alteration in the transportation of essential cations. In addition, the lead also causes cellular damage via production of reactive oxygen species [65]. This lead-induced carcinogenicity results from various cellular and molecular mechanisms including induction of oxidative stress, DNA damage, upregulation of stress gene transcription, caspase-3 activation and externalization of phosphatidylserine [19].

2.1.5.5 Mercury

Occurrence in Environment and Human Exposure

Mercury (Hg) is a heavy metal that exists in three forms, i.e., elemental, inorganic and organic either as mercurous (+ 1) or mercuric (+ 2) state. Although mercury is a naturally occurring chemical, anthropogenic mercury is a matter of great international concern and a priority toxic pollutant [66].

The humans are exposed to mercury mainly through dental amalgam and fish consumption. The natural process of off-gassing results in the release of mercury from earth crust into the water reservoirs [67]. Moreover, the polluted water from industries also causes an elevation of mercury concentration in the water bodies. The mercury in waterways is converted to methyl mercury through methylation by algae and bacteria. The methyl mercury, which is the most absorbed form of mercury, becomes part of the food chain into the fish and eventually to humans [68]. The mercury from fish is absorbed through the gastrointestinal tract, and due to its lipophilic nature, it easily gains entry through the placenta and blood brain barrier.

The second most absorbed form of mercury, elemental mercury, is mainly absorbed from dental amalgam that contains over 50% of elemental mercury. The elemental form of mercury is highly lipophilic and effectively absorbed through the tissue lining the mouth [66]. Once inside the cell, the mercury Hg^0 is oxidized to Hg^{+2} which is a very reactive form. Moreover, the rate of clearance of mercury is very slow and therefore it gets accumulated in kidney, liver and brain where it produces its toxic effects [19].

Mechanism of Carcinogenicity

The toxicity of mercury is observed to be resulting from its ability to induce oxidative stress through the sulfhydryl reactivity mechanism [69]. The + 2 state of mercury and methyl mercury have the ability to bond with the cysteine group of proteins and deplete the antioxidant enzymes. This depletion of antioxidant enzymes, induced by mercury, causes a hindrance in the removal of oxidative stress species resulting in their build-up in the cell [70]. The carcinogenic effects of mercury are quite controversial. Some studies report a genotoxic potential of mercury which is attributed to its ability to induce production of the reactive oxygen species. These reactive oxygen species may cause DNA damage and initiate the carcinogenic process. While other studies report no association between mercury and cancer development [19].

2.1.5.6 Asbestos

Occurrence in Environment and Human Exposure

Asbestos is a group of minerals that forms bundles of long thin fibers. The asbestos are silicate compounds and contain silica and oxygen in their structure. Their ability to resist heat, fire and being nonconductors of electricity makes them a widely used material in various industries including building and construction where it is used to strengthen the cement and plastic. Moreover, these are also used as insulators in the buildings for fire and sound proofing. In addition to being manmade the asbestos minerals are also naturally occurring. These are released into the environment when asbestos containing materials are disturbed. The natural activities such as weathering, land sliding and anthropogenic activities like gardening, construction and demolition in asbestos-bearing land may result in the release of asbestos Fibers into the air. These tiny asbestos fibers when inhaled by the exposed individuals may get trapped in the lungs and may remain there for a long time. If a person is continuously exposed to asbestos fibers, for example through occupational exposure, then their inhalation for longer duration may cause them to buildup in the lungs resulting in scarring and inflammation in the lungs called asbestosis [71].

Mechanism of Carcinogenicity

Asbestos is classified as a known carcinogen by the International Agency for Research on Cancer (IARC), US Environment Protection Agency (EPA) and US department of health and human services. The asbestos has also been implicated in the development of intrahepatic cholangiocarcinoma [72], lung cancer [73, 74], laryngeal cancer [75], ovarian cancer [76, 77] and prostate cancer [78].

The asbestosis, i.e., inflammation caused in the lung by asbestos deposition, causes the dysregulation of autoimmunity. The asbestos fibers present in the alveoli elicit local immune response in lungs against these foreign bodies. The macrophages phagocytize these asbestos fibers, and fibroblasts are stimulated to deposit connective tissue. The asbestos fibers are resistant to digestion and therefore causes the death of the macrophages which cause release of cytokines and recruiting further macrophages. The involvement of further fibroblastic cells to lay down fibrous tissue causes buildup of fibrous masses resulting in interstitial fibrosis [79]. The immunocompetent cells are altered as a result of progression of fibrosis, as a result of which the tumor immunity is declined. Moreover, the production of reactive oxygen species in the regional lymph nodes and pleural cavity, due to the presence of asbestos fibers, causes a chronic inflammation. Due to repeated encounter with the asbestos fibers and presence of surrounding inflammation the cellular and molecular features of immunocompetent cells are altered which further reduces the decreased tumor immunity [80].

Asbestos are reported to be associated with the development of mesothelioma, a rare cancer of the mesothelium, which is the thin membrane lining the chest and abdomen [81]. Usually with exposure to asbestos the cell death occurs, but there are some human mesothelial cells that escape this death resulting in accumulation of DNA damage in these calls and consequently the transformation into malignant cells. The cells that have the ability to escape cell death are reported to express high levels of high mobility group box 1 (HMGB1) protein which activates ATG5, an autophagy marker, which helps a large fraction of human mesothelial cells to survive asbestos exposure and become malignant [82].

2.1.5.7 Tobacco and Vinyl Chloride

Tobacco contains more than 70 carcinogenic chemicals. The tobacco-specific *N*-nitrosamines are considered to be most associated with carcinogenesis. The 4-(*N*-nitrosomethylamino)-1-[3-pyridyl]-1-butanone **5** (NNK) and *N'*-nitrosonornicotine (NNN) are the major contributors of tobacco associated carcinogenesis and are particularly reported to be associated with lung, esophagus and oral cavity cancer [83]. Therefore, both these nitrosamines are categorized as group I carcinogens by the IARC [84]. The NNK and NNN are bioactivated via several metabolic pathways. The α-hydroxylation is considered to be their primary bioactivation mechanism. The initial oxidation of tobacco-specific nitrosamines is catalyzed by P450. Various intermediate steps catalyzed by different enzymes lead to the formation of pyridyloxobutyl (POB), which is a highly reactive specie and makes DNA adducts [83] which is an essential step toward tumor formation [85].

Vinyl chloride is an industrially produced colorless gas which is used in the production of poly vinyl chloride. Vinyl chloride is also produced as a combustion product of tobacco. The polyvinyl chloride has vast industrial applications and is used for the production of pipes, cables, wires and packaging material. The individuals having occupational exposure to polyvinyl chloride are reported to have a high incidence of hepatobiliary cancer [86]. After inhalation the vinyl chloride is metabolized to chloroethylene oxide (CEO) by CYP2E1. The CEO rapidly rearranges to chloroacetaldehyde (CAA). Both CEO and CAA are reported to be genotoxic and result in DNA mutation. Moreover, the various adducts formation has also been reported to be formed from vinyl chloride [87].

2.2 Environmental Carcinogens, Fate, Causes and Associated Risks

Changes in the certain genes altering the function of the cell which may cause cancer. These variations can occur naturally or it can be the result of environmental factors that damage the DNA. The environmental factors include exposure to harmful chemicals such as metallic compounds or on the other side the tobacco smoke. Moreover, the other environmental factors take into account in this section are Alcohol, Diet, Radiation, Sunlight and Obesity. All these factors are discussed in detail in this section, about how such exposures contributes toward the development of cancer, where they are found and how may help people to avoid them.

2.2.1 Alcohol and Cancer

Many studies have revealed the impact of consumption of alcohol on the development of cancer in the human body. The strongest association was found between the risks of cancer development in the people consuming alcohol regularly compared to the persons who do not drink alcohol [88]. Alcohol when consumed can cause head and neck cancer, esophageal, liver, breast and colorectal cancer.

Alcohol increases the risk of developing cancer by converting the ethanol present in the alcohol to acetaldehyde, which is a probable toxic carcinogen for human body which can damage both DNA and proteins. Moreover, in the process of oxidation of alcohol reactive oxygen species are generated which can also damage DNA and proteins in the human body. Furthermore, last but not the least, consumption of alcohol impaired the human body in the break down and absorption of the vital nutrients such as Vitamin A, Vitamin B complex and Vitamin C, D and E, which become the associated risks of cancer development [89].

2.2.2 Obesity and Cancer

Obesity is one of the major risk factors in developing cancer. People with obesity are at higher risk of developing different type of cancers which include breast cancer, endometrium and colon cancer and cancers of colon, kidney, pancreas, gallbladder and esophagus.

Conversely, people having ideal weight and having healthy eating habits are less prone to developing cancer. In this regard, medical doctors suggest to maintain the ideal body mass index (BMI) (18.5–24.9) to reduce the risk of cancer. Moreover, taking healthy diet, keep body weight healthy and staying physically active help to reduce this risk of cancer.

2.2.3 Radiation and Cancer

Some radiation with certain wavelength which is called ionizing radiations can be the major inducer of cancer. These radiations include radon, X-rays and other high-energy radiations. Other forms of radiations include radiation from cell phones and visible light which are not harmful and did not cause cancer in living bodies.

2.2.3.1 Radon

Radon is an ionizing gas produced from the rocks and soil. Radon gas is produced from the breakdown of radium element which is formed when uranium and barium is the breakdown. The persons who are exposed to the radon gas very often are at high risk of developing lung cancer. Keeping a distance from such areas or wearing a mask while traveling through such areas to minimize the risk of its toxicity.

2.2.3.2 X-Rays

Many high-energy radiations such as alpha, beta, gamma radiations and X-rays can may cause damage to gene and DNA, which may lead to develop cancer.

Such types of radiations emit from the atomic bomb testing and accidental escape from nuclear power plant. Many other radiations use in the medical care such as CT scans, chest X-ray and PET scan can lead to cell damage which may lead to develop cancer. But the risk associated with medical imaging technologies to develop cancer is very rare as compared to the human benefits.

2.2.4 Sunlight and Cancer

Sunlight and tanning beds are the main source of UV radiations which can be a cause of skin cancer. Exposure to UV's cause early aging of the skin which may lead to develop skin cancer. The best way to reduce the risk is to avoid going outside in the mid-morning and late-afternoon, if necessary, try to wear sunscreen while going out. Although skin cancer is more common in light skin color, but people with all skin colors can develop cancer.

2.2.5 Tobacco and Cancer

Tobacco is the most leading cause of many types of cancer such as lung, mouth, larynx, mouth, liver, kidney, bladder, esophagus, rectum, colon, pancreas and cervix. The people who smoke regularly and the persons who inhaled cigarette smoke are mostly termed as "secondary smokers" are both at the higher risk of developing cancer at any stage of their lives. Quit smoking is the only way to lower the risk of developing cancer or the person who already developed cancer can increase his life expectancy.

2.3 Metabolic Carcinogens, Fate, Causes and Associated Risks

2.3.1 Diet and Cancer

Diet is an important part of our daily routine. Healthy diet not only reduce the risks of cancer but also contribute toward the better living. It is evident from the studies that diet does not directly involve in causing cancer; however, it may change the risk pattern to develop cancer [90]. Many observational studies have revealed that excessive intake of certain foods may increase the likelihood of developing cancer. For this reason, scientists have studied many dietary compounds, food additives to evaluate their possible connection with the risk of cancer development. Some of the potential compounds are discussed below in this section.

2.3.2 Sugar and Refined Carbs

Processed foods that are low in nutrients and fiber and have high sugar content may increase the risk of developing cancer. Moreover, it has also been found in many scientific studies that a diet that can elevate the blood glucose level is also associated with the increased risks of developing breast, stomach and colorectal cancers [91]. In addition to the blood glucose increase level of insulin is also contributing toward the cancer risks by stimulating the cell division and supporting the cell growth and proliferation of cancer cells [92]. This is the reason that people suffering with diabetes are at high risk of developing cancer [93].

2.3.3 Processed Meat and Over-Cooked Food

Processed meat mainly refers to the meat that has been preserved by curing, salting or smoking. Such type of food includes bacon, hot dogs, salami, ham and deli meats. The IARC categorized processed meat as a carcinogen [94]. Furthermore, observational studies had also revealed the close association of processed meat with colorectal cancer [95]. Furthermore, harmful compounds such as glycation end-products and heterocyclic amines are produced by cooking food at elevated temperatures which includes frying, grilling, broiling and barbecue [96]. Building-up of these compounds in excess causes inflammation in the body which may become a reason for the development of cancer and other fatal diseases.

2.3.4 Dairy

Many observational studies linked the consumption of dairy products with prostate cancer. In one study, they followed the 4000 men suffering with the prostate cancer to find the link between the prostate cancer and dairy products [97]. The study resulted that high intake of whole milk could become the risk of prostate cancer, due to the increase amount of insulin like growth factor and elevated levels of calcium in the milk from pregnant cows. These findings need in depth study as these reasons are very weakly linked with the progression of prostate cancer [98].

2.3.5 Other Risk Factors

Other risk factors associated with the diet that can cause cancer include acrylamide, antioxidants, tobacco smoke, artificial sweeteners, calcium, Vitamin D and tea [89]. But the mechanism of their association with developing cancer is still unclear. In-depth studies are needed to evaluate their relationship with developing cancer.

2.3.6 Genetics and Cancer

It is proved from the studies that cancer is not transferred genetically from one generation to another. However, if a genetic change is present in parents and transferred to the egg or sperm cells than the off-spring inherited that genetic change may be at a greater risk of developing cancer. For instance, if parents transfer BRCA1 gene to their kid than that child is at higher risk of developing cancer in his/her life [85].

2.4 Necessary Preventive Measures Against Carcinogens

It has been estimated that by changing the dietary habits and lifestyles almost 30–40% of the cancers can be cured. Many factors such as concentrated sugars, refined flour products, increased consumption of red meat, low intake of Fiber, imbalance of omega 6 and 3 contribute to increase risk of cancer. Cruciferous vegetables, flax seeds, broccoli sprouts and the very rich source of sulforophane which can lower the risk of cancer. Moreover, folic acid, Vitamin B-12 & D, and carotenoids are enlisted as protective elements in cancer prevention diet. Furthermore, probiotics and oral digestive enzymes are also considering good in anticancer diet measures. Such types of diets are not only very conducive to prevent cancer but also favors recovery from cancer. Along with the diet physical health is also a good preventive measure from developing cancer. By doing exercise daily and maintaining ideal body weight and BMI can also reduce the risks of developing cancers.

2.5 General Relevance of Carcinogen Metabolism to Cancer

Major factors that contribute to human carcinogenesis are (i) cigarette smoking, (ii) infection and (iii) diet and nutrition. The dietary and nutritional components can be either genotoxic or constituents having tumor promotion. Some microcomponents present in food or produced during cooking food are important genotoxic agents. For example, heterocyclic amines produced during cooking of meat and fish may cause breast, prostate and colon cancer. Similarly, the food contaminated with mycotoxins such as aflatoxin B_1 is reported to cause the development of hepatic carcinoma in various experimental animals. Furthermore, pyrrolizidine alkaloids present in various edible plants, cycasin present in cycad nuts, hydrazine in mushrooms and various flavonoids present in fruits and vegetables are among some other dietary components that may cause carcinogenesis (for a detailed description of these dietary carcinogens, please see the review [99]).

Once inside the body the chemicals are either able to produce their carcinogenic potential in the form they are taken in or their pre-carcinogenic form is metabolized to become active carcinogen inside the body. The pre-carcinogenic chemical metabolism can take one of the two routes, it is either detoxicated and excreted out of the body or is converted into reactive (carcinogenic) product which causes mutations by reacting with the genome and ultimately resulting in development of cancer [100].

2.6 Conclusion

It is necessary to raise awareness among the general population about adopting healthy lifestyle and especially to those who have high exposure to carcinogens about having precautionary measures to reduce cancer perils.

References

1. Oliveira PA, Colaço A, Chaves R, Guedes-Pinto H, De-La-Cruz P, Luis F et al (2007) Chemical carcinogenesis. An Acad Bras Ciênc 79:593–616
2. Gomes-Carneiro MR, Ribeiro-Pinto LF, Paumgartten FJR (1997) Environmental risk factors for gastric cancer: the toxicologist's standpoint. Cad Saude Publica 13:S27–S38
3. Butterworth BE, Bogdanffy MS (1999) A comprehensive approach for integration of toxicity and cancer risk assessments. Regul Toxicol Pharmacol 29(1):23–36
4. Bello Gutiérrez J, López de Cerain Salsamendi A (2001) Fundamentos de ciencia toxicológica. Ediciones Díaz de Santos
5. Hayes R (1995) Genetic susceptibility and occupational cancer. Med Lav 86(3):206–213
6. Yamagiwa K, Ichikawa K (1918) Experimental study of the pathogenesis of carcinoma. J Cancer Res 3(1):1–29
7. Berenblum I, Shubik P (1947) The role of croton oil applications, associated with a single painting of a carcinogen, in tumour induction of the mouse's skin. Br J Cancer 1(4):379
8. Toth B (2001) Species susceptibilities to chemical carcinogenes: a critical appraisal of the roles of genetic and viral agents. In Vivo (Athens, Greece) 15(6):467–478
9. Schrenk D (2018) What is the meaning of 'a compound is carcinogenic'? Toxicol Rep 5:504–511
10. EPA (2005) US. Guidelines for carcinogen risk assessment. 70 FR 17765–17817
11. Lehr RE, Jerina DM (1977) Metabolic activations of polycyclic hydrocarbons. Structure-activity relationships. Arch Toxicol 39(1–2):1–6
12. Miller EC, Miller JA (1981) Mechanisms of chemical carcinogenesis. Cancer 47(5 Suppl):1055–1064
13. Conney AH, Chang RL, Jerina DM, Wei SJ (1994) Studies on the metabolism of benzo[a]pyrene and dose-dependent differences in the mutagenic profile of its ultimate carcinogenic metabolite. Drug Metab Rev 26(1–2):125–163
14. Nebert DW, Russell DW (2002) Clinical importance of the cytochromes P450. Lancet 360(9340):1155–1162
15. Brouwer AF, Meza R, Eisenberg MC (2017) Parameter estimation for multistage clonal expansion models from cancer incidence data: a practical identifiability analysis. PLoS Comput Biol 13(3):e1005431
16. Fenga C, Gangemi S, Giambo F, Tsitsimpikou C, Golokhvast K, Tsatsakis A et al (2016) Low-dose occupational exposure to benzene and signal transduction pathways involved in the regulation of cellular response to oxidative stress. Life Sci 147:67–70
17. Hernandez AF, Parron T, Tsatsakis AM, Requena M, Alarcon R, Lopez-Guarnido O (2013) Toxic effects of pesticide mixtures at a molecular level: their relevance to human health. Toxicology 307:136–145

18. Barnes JL, Zubair M, John K, Poirier MC, Martin FL (2018) Carcinogens and DNA damage. Biochem Soc Trans 46(5):1213–1224
19. Tchounwou PB, Yedjou CG, Patlolla AK, Sutton DJ (2012) Heavy metal toxicity and the environment. Experientia Suppl 101:133–164
20. He ZL, Yang XE, Stoffella PJ (2005) Trace elements in agroecosystems and impacts on the environment. J Trace Elem Med Biol Organ Soc Min Trace Elem 19(2–3):125–140
21. Tchounwou PB, Newsome C, Williams J, Glass K (2008) Copper-induced cytotoxicity and transcriptional activation of stress genes in human liver carcinoma (HepG(2)) cells. In: Metal ions in biology and medicine: proceedings of the international symposium on metal ions in biology and medicine held [Les ions metalliques en biologie et en medecine: symposium international sur les ions metalliques], vol 10, pp 285–290
22. Peng X, Dai C, Zhang M, Das GS (2020) Molecular mechanisms underlying protective role of quercetin on copper sulfate-induced nephrotoxicity in mice. Front Vet Sci 7:586033
23. Khairul I, Wang QQ, Jiang YH, Wang C, Naranmandura H (2017) Metabolism, toxicity and anticancer activities of arsenic compounds. Oncotarget 8(14):23905–23926
24. Hirano S, Cui X, Li S, Kanno S, Kobayashi Y, Hayakawa T et al (2003) Difference in uptake and toxicity of trivalent and pentavalent inorganic arsenic in rat heart microvessel endothelial cells. Arch Toxicol 77(6):305–312
25. Bencko V, Yan Li Foong F (2017) The history of arsenical pesticides and health risks related to the use of agent blue. Ann Agric Environ Med 24(2):312–316
26. Nurchi VM, Djordjevic AB, Crisponi G, Alexander J, Bjorklund G, Aaseth J (2020) Arsenic toxicity: molecular targets and therapeutic agents. Biomolecules 10(2)
27. Paul NP, Galvan AE, Yoshinaga-Sakurai K, Rosen BP, Yoshinaga M (2023) Arsenic in medicine: past, present and future. Biometals 36(2):283–301
28. Tchounwou PB, Wilson B, Ishaque A (1999) Important considerations in the development of public health advisories for arsenic and arsenic-containing compounds in drinking water. Rev Environ Health 14(4):211–229
29. Crinnion W (2017) Arsenic: the underrecognized common disease-inducing toxin. Integr Med (Encinitas) 16(2):8–13
30. Tchounwou PB, Centeno JA, Patlolla AK (2004) Arsenic toxicity, mutagenesis, and carcinogenesis—a health risk assessment and management approach. Mol Cell Biochem 255(1–2):47–55
31. Tsuji JS, Chang ET, Gentry PR, Clewell HJ, Boffetta P, Cohen SM (2019) Dose-response for assessing the cancer risk of inorganic arsenic in drinking water: the scientific basis for use of a threshold approach. Crit Rev Toxicol 49(1):36–84
32. Rehman K, Fatima F, Waheed I, Akash MSH (2018) Prevalence of exposure of heavy metals and their impact on health consequences. J Cell Biochem 119(1):157–184
33. Roy P, Mukherjee A, Giri S (2016) Evaluation of genetic damage in tobacco and arsenic exposed population of Southern Assam, India using buccal cytome assay and comet assay. Ecotoxicol Environ Saf 124:169–176
34. Anderson D, Yu TW, Phillips BJ, Schmezer P (1994) The effect of various antioxidants and other modifying agents on oxygen-radical-generated DNA damage in human lymphocytes in the COMET assay. Mutat Res 307(1):261–271
35. Liao YC, Chen YF, Lee TC (2015) Increased susceptibility of H-Ras(G12V)-transformed human urothelial cells to the genotoxic effects of sodium arsenite. Arch Toxicol 89(11):1971–1979
36. Tam LM, Price NE, Wang Y (2020) Molecular mechanisms of arsenic-induced disruption of DNA repair. Chem Res Toxicol 33(3):709–726
37. Zhao CQ, Young MR, Diwan BA, Coogan TP, Waalkes MP (1997) Association of arsenic-induced malignant transformation with DNA hypomethylation and aberrant gene expression. Proc Natl Acad Sci USA 94(20):10907–10912
38. Balali-Mood M, Naseri K, Tahergorabi Z, Khazdair MR, Sadeghi M (2021) Toxic mechanisms of five heavy metals: mercury, lead, chromium, cadmium, and arsenic. Front Pharmacol 12:643972

39. Sijko M, Kozlowska L (2021) Influence of dietary compounds on arsenic metabolism and toxicity. Part II-human studies. Toxics 9(10)
40. Bjorklund G, Rahaman MS, Shanaida M, Lysiuk R, Oliynyk P, Lenchyk L et al (2022) Natural dietary compounds in the treatment of arsenic toxicity. Molecules 27(15)
41. Richter P, Faroon O, Pappas RS (2017) Cadmium and cadmium/zinc ratios and tobacco-related morbidities. Int J Environ Res Public Health 14(10)
42. Cao ZR, Cui SM, Lu XX, Chen XM, Yang X, Cui JP et al (2018) Effects of occupational cadmium exposure on workers' cardiovascular system. Zhonghua lao dong wei sheng zhi ye bing za zhi = Zhonghua laodong weisheng zhiyebing zazhi = Chin J Ind Hyg Occup Dis 36(6):474–477
43. Rafati Rahimzadeh M, Rafati Rahimzadeh M, Kazemi S, Moghadamnia AA (2017) Cadmium toxicity and treatment: an update. Caspian J Intern Med 8(3):135–145
44. Sarwar N, Saifullah, Malhi SS, Zia MH, Naeem A, Bibi S et al (2010) Role of mineral nutrition in minimizing cadmium accumulation by plants. J Sci Food Agric 90(6):925–937
45. Kim K, Melough MM, Vance TM, Noh H, Koo SI, Chun OK (2018) Dietary cadmium intake and sources in the US. Nutrients 11(1)
46. Zhai Q, Narbad A, Chen W (2014) Dietary strategies for the treatment of cadmium and lead toxicity. Nutrients 7(1):552–571
47. Kim TH, Kim JH, Le Kim MD, Suh WD, Kim JE, Yeon HJ et al (2020) Exposure assessment and safe intake guidelines for heavy metals in consumed fishery products in the Republic of Korea. Environ Sci Pollut Res Int 27(26):33042–33051
48. Hartwig A (2013) Cadmium and cancer. Met Ions Life Sci 11:491–507
49. Stohs SJ, Bagchi D, Hassoun E, Bagchi M (2001) Oxidative mechanisms in the toxicity of chromium and cadmium ions. J Environ Pathol Toxicol Oncol Off Organ Int Soc Environ Toxicol Cancer 20(2):77–88
50. Skipper A, Sims JN, Yedjou CG, Tchounwou PB (2016) Cadmium chloride induces DNA damage and apoptosis of human liver carcinoma cells via oxidative stress. Int J Environ Res Public Health 13(1)
51. Vincent JB, Lukaski HC (2018) Chromium. Adv Nutr 9(4):505–506
52. Wong CC, Gamboni SE, Palmer AM, Nixon RL (2015) Occupational allergic contact dermatitis to chromium from cement: estimating the size of the problem in Australia. Australas J Dermatol 56(4):290–293
53. Thompson CM, Bichteler A, Rager JE, Suh M, Proctor DM, Haws LC et al (2016) Comparison of in vivo genotoxic and carcinogenic potency to augment mode of action analysis: case study with hexavalent chromium. Mutat Res Genet Toxicol Environ Mutagen 800–801:28–34
54. Junaid M, Hashmi MZ, Malik RN, Pei DS (2016) Toxicity and oxidative stress induced by chromium in workers exposed from different occupational settings around the globe: a review. Environ Sci Pollut Res Int 23(20):20151–20167
55. Nickens KP, Patierno SR, Ceryak S (2010) Chromium genotoxicity: a double-edged sword. Chem Biol Interact 188(2):276–288
56. Wu G. The molecular mechanism of Cr(VI)-induced carcinogenesis. Zhonghua lao dong wei sheng zhi ye bing za zhi = Zhonghua laodong weisheng zhiyebing zazhi = Chin J Ind Hyg Occup Dis 30(11):878–880
57. Proctor DM, Suh M, Campleman SL, Thompson CM (2014) Assessment of the mode of action for hexavalent chromium-induced lung cancer following inhalation exposures. Toxicology 325:160–179
58. Zhang XH, Zhang X, Wang XC, Jin LF, Yang ZP, Jiang CX et al (2011) Chronic occupational exposure to hexavalent chromium causes DNA damage in electroplating workers. BMC Public Health 11:224
59. Patlolla AK, Barnes C, Hackett D, Tchounwou PB (2009) Potassium dichromate induced cytotoxicity, genotoxicity and oxidative stress in human liver carcinoma (HepG2) cells. Int J Environ Res Public Health 6(2):643–653

60. Patlolla AK, Barnes C, Yedjou C, Velma V, Tchounwou PB (2009) Oxidative stress, DNA damage, and antioxidant enzyme activity induced by hexavalent chromium in Sprague-Dawley rats. Environ Toxicol 24(1):66–73
61. Nassar NT, Lederer GW, Brainard JL, Padilla AJ, Lessard JD (2022) Rock-to-metal ratio: a foundational metric for understanding mine wastes. Environ Sci Technol 56(10):6710–6721
62. Kim HC, Jang TW, Chae HJ, Choi WJ, Ha MN, Ye BJ et al (2015) Evaluation and management of lead exposure. Ann Occup Environ Med 27:30
63. Ara A, Usmani JA (2015) Lead toxicity: a review. Interdiscip Toxicol 8(2):55
64. Ettinger AS, Leonard ML, Mason J (2019) CDC's lead poisoning prevention program: a long-standing responsibility and commitment to protect children from lead exposure. J Public Health Manag Pract 25(Suppl 1):S5
65. Shaban NZ, Abdelrahman SA, El-Kersh MA, Mogahed FA, Talaat IM, Habashy NH et al (2020) The synergistic hepatoprotective potential of beta vulgaris juice and 2,3-dimercaptosuccinic acid in lead-intoxicated rats via improving the hepatic oxidative and inflammatory stress. BMC Complement Med Ther 20(1):1–15
66. Jirau-Colón H, González-Parrilla L, Martinez-Jiménez J, Adam W, Jiménez-Velez BJ (2019) Rethinking the dental amalgam dilemma: an integrated toxicological approach. Int J Environ Res Public Health 16(6):1036
67. Sigel A, Sigel H, Sigel RK (2015) Organometallics in environment and toxicology. Walter de Gruyter GmbH & Co KG
68. Novo JP, Martins B, Raposo RS, Pereira FC, Oriá RB, Malva JO et al (2021) Cellular and molecular mechanisms mediating methylmercury neurotoxicity and neuroinflammation. Int J Mol Sci 22(6):3101
69. Vassallo DV, Simões MR, Giuberti K, Azevedo BF, Ribeiro RF, Salaices M et al (2019) Effects of chronic exposure to mercury on angiotensin-converting enzyme activity and oxidative stress in normotensive and hypertensive rats. Arq Bras Cardiol 112:374–380
70. Zahra KF, Lefter R, Ali A, Abdellah E-C, Trus C, Ciobica A et al (2021) The involvement of the oxidative stress status in cancer pathology: a double view on the role of the antioxidants
71. Asbestos exposure and cancer risk (2021) National Cancer Institute. Available from: https://www.cancer.gov/about-cancer/causes-prevention/risk/substances/asbestos/asbestos-fact-sheet
72. Brandi G, Tavolari S (2020) Asbestos and intrahepatic cholangiocarcinoma. Cells 9(2):421
73. Yotsumoto T, Sano A, Fukuda T (2018) Clinical study of asbestos-related lung cancer diagnosed by asbestos medical examination. Cancer Rep (Hoboken) 1(3):e1124
74. Huh D-A, Kang M-S, Lee J, Choi JY, Moon KW, Lee Y-J (2021) Occupational and environmental asbestos exposure and the risk of lung cancer in Korea: a case-control study in South Chungcheong Province of Korea. PLoS ONE 16(4):e0249790
75. Kang D-M, Kim J-E, Kim Y-K, Lee H-H, Kim S-YJ (2018) Occupational burden of asbestos-related diseases in Korea, 1998–2013: asbestosis, mesothelioma, lung cancer, laryngeal cancer, and ovarian cancer. J Korean Med Sci 33(35):e226
76. Luberto F, Ferrante D, Silvestri S, Angelini A, Cuccaro F, Nannavecchia AM et al (2019) Cumulative asbestos exposure and mortality from asbestos related diseases in a pooled analysis of 21 asbestos cement cohorts in Italy. Environ Health 18(1):1–19
77. Vidican P, Perol O, Fevotte J, Fort E, Treilleux I, Belladame E et al (2022) Frequency of asbestos exposure and histological subtype of ovarian carcinoma. Int J Environ Res Public Health 19(9):5383
78. Dutheil F, Zaragoza-Civale L, Pereira B, Mermillod M, Baker JS, Schmidt J et al (2020) Prostate cancer and asbestos: a systematic review and meta-analysis. Perm J 24
79. Craighead JE (2008) Asbestos and its diseases. Oxford University Press
80. Matsuzaki H, Maeda M, Lee S, Nishimura Y, Kumagai-Takei N, Hayashi H et al (2012) Asbestos-induced cellular and molecular alteration of immunocompetent cells and their relationship with chronic inflammation and carcinogenesis

81. Kwon S-C, Lee S-S, Kang M-S, Huh D-A, Lee Y-J (2021) The epidemiologic characteristics of malignant mesothelioma cases in Korea: findings of the asbestos injury relief system from 2011–2015. Int J Environ Res Public Health 18(19):10007
82. Xue J, Patergnani S, Giorgi C, Suarez J, Goto K, Bononi A et al (2020) Asbestos induces mesothelial cell transformation via HMGB1-driven autophagy. Proc Natl Acad Sci USA 117(41):25543–25552
83. Li Y, Hecht SS (2022) Metabolism and DNA adduct formation of tobacco-specific *N*-nitrosamines. Int J Mol Sci 23(9):5109
84. Xia B, Blount BC, Guillot T, Brosius C, Li Y, Van Bemmel DM et al (2021) Tobacco-specific nitrosamines (NNAL, NNN, NAT, and NAB) exposures in the US population assessment of Tobacco and health (PATH) study wave 1 (2013–2014). Nicotine Tob Res 23(3):573–583
85. Hecht SS, Hatsukami DKJNRC (2022) Smokeless tobacco and cigarette smoking. Chem Mech Cancer Prev 22(3):143–155
86. Carreón T, Hein MJ, Hanley KW, Viet SM, Ruder AM (2014) Coronary artery disease and cancer mortality in a cohort of workers exposed to vinyl chloride, carbon disulfide, rotating shift work, and o-toluidine at a chemical manufacturing plant. Am J Ind Med 57(4):398-411
87. Mutlu E, Collins LB, Stout MD, Upton PB, Daye LR, Winsett D et al (2010) Development and application of an LC-MS/MS method for the detection of the vinyl chloride-induced DNA adduct N 2,3-ethenoguanine in tissues of adult and weanling rats following exposure to [13C2]-VC. 23(9):1485–1491
88. Choi YJ, Myung SK, Lee JH (2018) Light alcohol drinking and risk of cancer: a meta-analysis of cohort studies. Cancer Res Treat 50(2):474–487
89. Institute NC (2023) Diet and cancer risk
90. Donaldson MS (2004) Nutrition and cancer: a review of the evidence for an anti-cancer diet. Nutr J 3:19
91. Eslamian G, Jessri M, Hajizadeh B, Ibiebele TI, Rashidkhani B (2013) Higher glycemic index and glycemic load diet is associated with increased risk of esophageal squamous cell carcinoma: a case-control study. Nutr Res 33(9):719–725
92. Denley A, Carroll JM, Brierley GV, Cosgrove L, Wallace J, Forbes B et al (2007) Differential activation of insulin receptor substrates 1 and 2 by insulin-like growth factor-activated insulin receptors. Mol Cell Biol 27(10):3569–3577
93. Noto H, Tsujimoto T, Sasazuki T, Noda M (2011) Significantly increased risk of cancer in patients with diabetes mellitus: a systematic review and meta-analysis. Endocr Pract 17(4):616–628
94. Bouvard V, Loomis D, Guyton KZ, Grosse Y, Ghissassi FE, Benbrahim-Tallaa L et al (2015) Carcinogenicity of consumption of red and processed meat. Lancet Oncol 16(16):1599–1600
95. McGuire S (2016) World cancer report 2014. Geneva, Switzerland: World Health Organization, International Agency for Research on Cancer, WHO Press, 2015. Adv Nutr 7(2):418–419
96. Sugimura T, Wakabayashi K, Nakagama H, Nagao M (2004) Heterocyclic amines: mutagens/carcinogens produced during cooking of meat and fish. Cancer Sci 95(4):290–299
97. Pettersson A, Kasperzyk JL, Kenfield SA, Richman EL, Chan JM, Willett WC et al (2012) Milk and dairy consumption among men with prostate cancer and risk of metastases and prostate cancer death. Cancer Epidemiol Biomarkers Prev 21(3):428–436
98. Allen NE, Key TJ, Appleby PN, Travis RC, Roddam AW, Tjonneland A et al (2008) Animal foods, protein, calcium and prostate cancer risk: the European prospective investigation into cancer and nutrition. Br J Cancer 98(9):1574–1581
99. Sugimura T (2000) Nutrition and dietary carcinogens. Carcinogenesis 21(3):387–395
100. Schwab M (ed) (2011) Carcinogen metabolism. In: Encyclopedia of cancer. Springer, Berlin, pp 649–652

Understanding the Role of Polyunsaturated Fatty Acids in the Development and Prevention of Cancer

3

Samina Akbar, Abdur Rahman, Nazir Ahmad, Muhammad Imran, and Zeeshan Hafeez

Contents

S. Akbar (✉) · Z. Hafeez
CALBINOTOX, Université de Lorraine, 54000 Nancy, France
e-mail: samina.akbar@univ-lorraine.fr

A. Rahman
Atta ur Rahman School of Applied Biosciences, National University of Sciences and Technology, Islamabad, Pakistan

N. Ahmad
Faculty of Life Sciences, Institute of Home and Food Sciences, Government College University, Faisalabad, Pakistan

M. Imran
Department of Biosciences, Faculty of Sciences, COMSATS Institute of Information Technology, Park Road, Islamabad, Pakistan

R. F. Saeed and S. ul. Shaheed (eds.), *Nutrition and Dietary Interventions in Cancer*, Cancer Treatment and Research 191, https://doi.org/10.1007/978-3-031-55622-7_3

Abbreviations

ALA	α-Linolenic acid
CC	Cancer cachexia
COX	Cyclooxygenases
CRC	Colorectal cancer
CYP	Cytochrome P450
DHA	Docosahexaenoic acid
EPA	Eicosapentaenoic acid
LA	Linoleic acid
LDs	Lipid droplets
LOX	Lipoxygenases
PLA2	Phospholipase A2
PPARs	Peroxisome proliferator-activated receptors
PUFAs	Polyunsaturated fatty acids
ROS	Reactive oxygen species
SPM	Specialized presolving mediators
SREBPs	Sterol regulatory element binding proteins

3.1 Introduction

Lipids are the class of macromolecules, which are hydrophobic in nature and supply energy (9 kcal/mol) to living beings. They are the structural components of cell membranes and influence several biological functions including regulation of intracellular signaling pathways, membrane structure and function as well as production of bioactive lipid mediators [1].

3.1.1 Structure and Nomenclature of Fatty Acids

The simplest lipids are the fatty acids, which are long-chain molecules having a single carboxyl group attached to a hydrocarbon chain with a terminal methyl group. The carbon atom next to the carboxyl group is named α carbon while the subsequent one the β carbon.

Fatty acids are classified based on their chain length and saturation degree. They can be short chain (less than 6 carbons), medium chain (6–10 carbons) and long chain (12 or more carbons). The naturally occurring fatty acids mostly have straight carbon chains with even number of carbon atoms except for some bacterial ones [2]. Regarding saturation degree, saturated fatty acids have no double bond while monounsaturated fatty acids have a single double bond and polyunsaturated fatty acids (PUFAs) possess more than one double bond in their chain (Table 3.1). In margarines and oils, the concentration of certain fatty acids is higher than others, and the oils are primarily known as saturated, monounsaturated or polyunsaturated on the basis of predominant fatty acids present [3, 4].

Dr. Ralph Holman proposed another classification for unsaturated fatty acids, named omega (ω) system, since omega is the last letter of Greek alphabets; therefore, counting is started from methyl end rather than carboxyl end (Fig. 3.1). According to this system, unsaturated fatty acids are classified based on the first double bond position at the carbon atom from the methyl end of fatty acids. The first double bond is located between third and fourth carbon atoms of omega-3 (ω3 or n-3) fatty acids and between sixth and seventh of omega-6 (ω6 or n-6) fatty acids. The systematic nomenclature for fatty acids may also indicate the location of double bonds with reference to the carboxyl group (Table 3.1).

Furthermore, unsaturated fatty acids are also classified based on the stereochemistry of hydrogen atoms around double bonds, i.e., cis- or trans-configuration. In cis-configuration, hydrogen atoms on either side of the double bond are oriented in the same direction. In nature, most fatty acids have cis-configuration; however, the trans-configuration can also occur from industrial processing (hydrogenation) of unsaturated oils. For instance, trans-fatty acids are present in large amounts in margarine and have been shown to increase serum cholesterol levels [5]. Cis-double bonds are thermodynamically less stable due to a kink/bend generation in the molecules than trans-fatty acids which have the same straight chain three-dimensional structure as saturated fatty acids and may be partly involved in atherogenesis due to this similarity [3, 4].

Table 3.1 Nomenclature and structure of selected fatty acids

Common name	Systematic name	Carbon skeleton	Structural formula
Saturated fatty acids			
Butyric	n-Butanoic	4:0	$CH_3(–CH_2)_2–COOH$
Caproic	n-Hexanoic	6:0	$CH_3(–CH_2)_4–COOH$
Caprylic	n-Octanoic	8:0	$CH_3(–CH_2)_6–COOH$
Capric	n-Decanoic	10:0	$CH_3(–CH_2)_8–COOH$
Lauric	n-Dodecanoic	12:0	$CH_3(–CH_2)_{10}–COOH$
Myristic	n-Tetradecanoic	14:0	$CH_3(–CH_2)_{12}–COOH$
Palmitic	n-Hexadecanoic	16:0	$CH_3(–CH_2)_{14}–COOH$
Stearic	n-Octadecanoic	18:0	$CH_3(–CH_{22})_{16}–COOH$
Arachidic	n-Eicosanoic	20:0	$CH_3(–CH_2)_{18}–COOH$
Behenic	n-Docosanoic	22:0	$CH_3(–CH_2)_{20}–COOH$
Lignoceric	n-Tetracosanoic	24:0	$CH_3(–CH_2)_{22}–COOH$
Cerotic	n-Hexacosanoic	26:0	$CH_3(–CH_2)_{24}–COOH$
Montanic	n-Octacosanoic	28:0	$CH_3(–CH_2)_{26}–COOH$
Monounsaturated fatty acids			
Palmitoleic	9-hexadecenoic	16:1ω7	$CH_3(–CH_2)_4(–CH_2–CH=CH)(–CH_2)_7–COOH$
Cis-vaccenic	11-octadecenoic	18:1ω7	$CH_3(–CH_2)_4(–CH_2–CH=CH)(–CH_2)_9–COOH$
Oleic	9-octadecenoic	18:1ω9	$CH_3(–CH_2)_6(–CH_2–CH=CH)(–CH_2)_7–COOH$

(continued)

Table 3.1 (continued)

Common name	Systematic name	Carbon skeleton	Structural formula
Eicosenoic	11-eicosenoic	20:1ω9	$CH_3(-CH_2)_6(-CH_2-CH=CH)(-CH_2)_9-COOH$
Nervonic	15-tetracosenoic	24:1ω9	$CH_3(-CH_2)_6(-CH_2-CH=CH)(-CH_2)_{13}-COOH$
Polyunsaturated fatty acids			
α-Linolenic, ALA	9,12,15-octadecatrienoic	18:3ω3	$CH_3(-CH_2-CH=CH)_3(-CH_2)_7-COOH$
Stearidonic	6,9,12,15-octadecatetraenoic	18:4ω3	$CH_3(-CH_2-CH=CH)_4(-CH_2)_4-COOH$
Mead's	5,8,11-eicosatrienoic	20:3ω9	$CH_3(-CH_2)_6(-CH_2-CH=CH)_3(-CH_2)_3-COOH$
Timnodonic, EPA	5,8,11,14,17-eicosapentaenoic	20:5ω3	$CH_3(-CH_2-CH=CH)_5(-CH_2)_3-COOH$
Clupanodonic, DPA	7,10,13,16,19-docosapentaenoic	22:5ω3	$CH_3(-CH_2-CH=CH)_5(-CH_2)_5-COOH$
Cervonic, DHA	4,7,10,13,16,19-docosahexaenoic	22:6ω3	$CH_3(-CH_2-CH=CH)_6(-CH_2)_2-COOH$
Linoleic, LA	9,12-octadecadienoic	18:2ω6	$CH_3(-CH_2)_3(-CH_2-CH=CH)_2(-CH_2)_7-COOH$
γ-Linolenic, GLA	6,9,12-octadecatrienoic	18:3ω6	$CH_3(-CH_2)_3(-CH_2-CH=CH)_3(-CH_2)_4-COOH$
Dihomolinoleic	11,14-eicosadienoic	20:2ω6	$CH_3(-CH_2)_3(-CH_2-CH=CH)_2(-CH_2)_9-COOH$
Dihomo-γ-linolenic, DGLA	8,11,14-eicosatrienoic	20:3ω6	$CH_3(-CH_2)_3(-CH_2-CH=CH)_3(-CH_2)_6-COOH$
Arachidonic, AA	5,8,11,14-eicosatetraenoic	20:4ω6	$CH_3(-CH_2)_3(-CH_2-CH=CH)_4(-CH_2)_3-COOH$
Adrenic	7,10,13,16-docosatetraenoic	22:4ω6	$CH_3(-CH_2)_3(-CH_2-CH=CH)_4(-CH_2)_5-COOH$
DPA	4,7,10,13,16-docosapentaenoic	22:5ω6	$CH_3(-CH_2)_3(-CH_2-CH=CH)_5(-CH_2)_2-COOH$

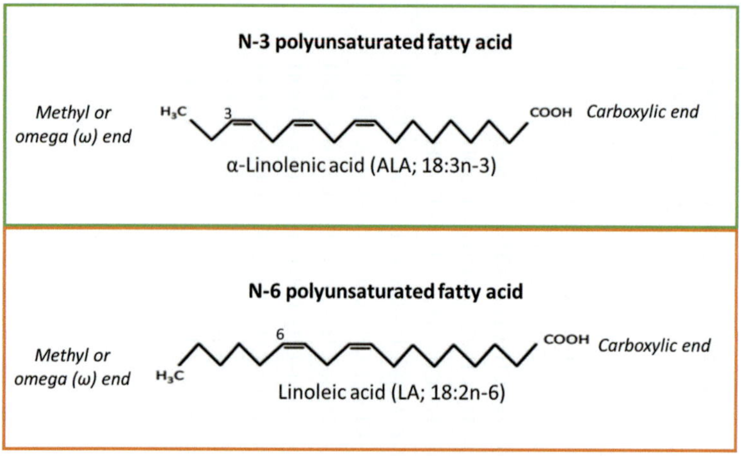

Fig. 3.1 Schematic representation of n-3 and n-6 polyunsaturated fatty acids

3.1.2 N-3 and n-6 Fatty Acids

PUFAs are classified mainly into four families designated as n-3, n-6, n-7 and n-9. Among them, n-3 and n-6 families predominate in plants and animals. Both n-3 and n-6 fatty acids are the essential fatty acids because they cannot be synthesized by human beings and therefore must be obtained through dietary intake. The main distinction between n-3 and n-6 fatty acids is based on the location of the first double bond while counting from the methyl end of the fatty acid molecule. The first double bond of n-3 and n-6 fatty acids is located at three and six carbon atoms, respectively, from the methyl end and represents the cis-configuration. Linoleic acid (LA; 18:2n-6) is the principal precursor of n-6 family in which a single methylene group CH2 separates two double bonds, whereas alpha-linolenic acid (ALA; 18:3n-3) is the precursor of n-3 family and has two CH2 groups between the three double bonds [6, 7]. Both families are not interconvertible and are metabolically and functionally distinct, often having the opposite physiological functions [8].

3.1.3 Sources of Polyunsaturated Fatty Acids

The n-6 and n-3 fatty acids are essentially obtained from plants and animals, however, their relative proportion in the food is source-dependent. The vegetable oils such as sunflower, safflower and corn oils are the significant source of LA, the parent n-6 PUFA. LA is found in medium quantities in soybean, almonds and sesame, in small amounts in canola, peanut and olive oils and in very low quantity in palm kernel and coconut oils. Among the other n-6 PUFAs, gamma-linolenic acid (GLA) is found in human breast milk and some botanical seed oils as blackcurrant, borage oil and evening primrose oil and is typically consumed as dietary supplement, while arachidonic acid (ARA) is obtained from diet rich in organ meats, poultry, and eggs.

The n-3 fatty acids are abundantly present in the chloroplast of green leafy vegetables such as purslane and spinach in the form of ALA, and the latter is mainly obtained from flax seed but also present in small quantities in walnut, soybean, hemp and canola oil [6, 9]. The long-chain n-3 PUFAs, i.e., eicosapentaenoic acid (EPA) and docosahexaenoic acid (DHA), are found in breastmilk, fish oils such as mackerel, sardines, salmon, black cod, bluefish, anchovies and rainbow trout and algae [6, 10]. The marine fish are rich in n-3 PUFAs as they feed mostly on zooplankton and phytoplankton, whereas the farmed fish contain more n-6 fatty acids as they are fed on the meal made of cereal and vegetable oils [6, 10]. In addition to the natural dietary sources, the supplements enriched with n-3 PUFAs, such as krill oils obtained from Antarctic krill, have also gained significance due to the presence of more bioavailable form of DHA (phospholipids) compared to fish oil (triglycerides) [10, 11]. Furthermore, algal and fish oils enriched in n-3 PUFAs have also been used in infant formulas, health supplements and conventional food products in order to attain a wide range of health benefits [12].

3.1.4 Synthesis and Metabolism of PUFAs in Mammals

Diet is the principal precursor of LA and ALA as the enzymes required to synthesize these PUFAs from oleic acid lack in human beings and animals contrary to plants. Nearly, all the higher plants, algae and lower animals such as *Caenorhabditis elegans* and some fungi possess Δ12-desaturases to convert oleic acid (C18:1n-9) into LA and Δ15-desaturases to convert LA to ALA [13]. However, as mammalian cells lack the desaturase enzymes required to produce n-6 or n-3 fatty acids de novo, these fatty acids are considered essential and must be obtained through diet [14].

The n-6 and n-3 fatty acids are present in different foods in the form of triglycerides. When such foods are consumed, triglycerides undergo digestion in the small intestine, and the released PUFAs are absorbed and transported in the blood. Subsequently, they are assimilated in different body tissues (brain, heart and retina ...,) and can undergo diverse metabolic pathways. They are either β-oxidized to provide energy in the form of ATP or esterified into cellular lipids including triglycerides, phospholipids and cholesterol esters and are converted into their important longer chain and more unsaturated products. The latter are principally obtained from the LA and ALA by a series of desaturation and elongation reactions, which take place, particularly in the liver of animals (Fig. 3.2) [6, 9]. In endoplasmic reticulum of liver, LA and ALA are first converted to GLA (18:3n-6) and stearidonic acid (18:4n-3), respectively, by Δ6-desaturase which are then elongated by Δ6 specific elongase (ELOVL 5) to generate dihomo-gamma-linolenic acid (DGLA; 20:3n-6) and eicosatetraenoic acid (20:4n-3), respectively. These long-chain PUFAs are again desaturated via Δ5-desaturase to produce ARA

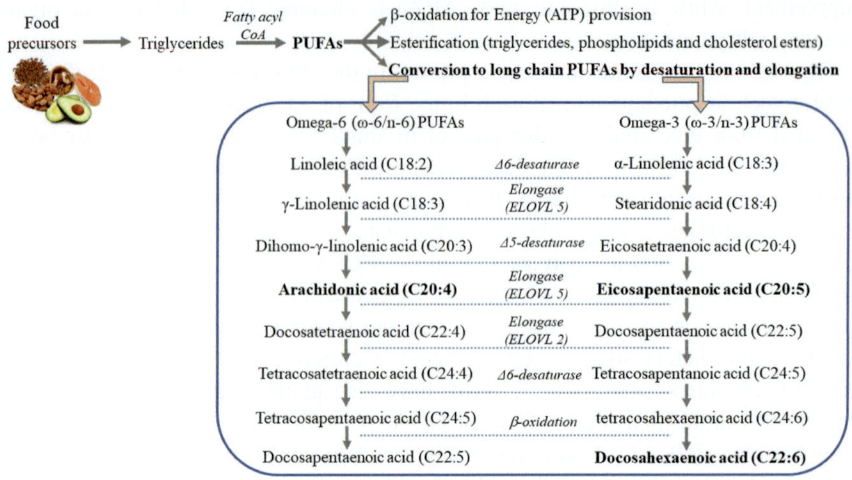

Fig. 3.2 Metabolic pathways of long-chain omega-3 and omega-6 fatty acids through a cascade of desaturation-elongation reactions to produce arachidonic acid (ARA; C20:4n-6) from linoleic acid (LA; C18:2n-6) and eicosapentaenoic acid (EPA; C20:5n-3) and docosahexaenoic acid (DHA; C22:6n-3) from α-linolenic acid (ALA; C18:3n-3)

(20:4n-6) and EPA (20:5n-3). Both ARA and EPA undergo two successive elongations via ELOVL 5 and 2 and a subsequent desaturation (Δ6-desaturase) to yield tetracosatetraenoic acid (24:4n-6) and tetracosapentanoic acid (C24:5n-3), respectively. Both these PUFAs are then subjected to peroxisomal β-oxidation resulting in short-chain final products, i.e., docosapentaenoic acid (C22:5n-6) and docosahexaenoic acid (DHA; 22:6n-3) (Fig. 3.2) [15].

DHA production in mammals takes place via another pathway named ‘Sprecher’s shunt.’ During this, DHA precursor tetracosahexaenoic acid (C24:6n-3) is β-oxidized in peroxisome through the successive actions of acyl-coenzyme A oxidases, D-bifunctional protein and peroxisomal thiolases [16, 17]. DHA produced is then transported back to endoplasmic reticulum to be incorporated into membrane phospholipids by esterification or diacylation reacylation reaction. These translocations between endoplasmic reticulum and peroxisomes are supposed to be responsible in part for the low efficiency of DHA biosynthesis in mammals [18, 19].

The significant long-chain PUFAs (DGLA, ARA, EPA, DHA) obtained from LA and ALA metabolism are stored in esterified form in membrane phospholipids or as neutral glycerides after esterification with hydroxyl groups of the glycerol backbone of phospholipids or glycerides. When needed, they can be mobilized by phospholipase A2 as free (unesterified) PUFAs to form eicosanoids (pro- or anti-inflammatory signaling molecules) or other autacoids by various oxygenase enzymes [10], which will be discussed in detail in Sect. 1.5.2.

3.1.5 Biological Significance of PUFAs

3.1.5.1 Regulation of Membrane Structural and Functional Dynamics

PUFAs are essential structural components of the cell as well as organelle membranes, primarily incorporated at sn-2 position into membrane phospholipids. They are crucial in regulating the membrane structure, fluidity, phase transitions and permeability as well as in controlling the membrane-associated signaling cascades [20, 21].

Different types of membranes present in eukaryotic cells (plasma, mitochondrial, nuclear and endosomal) perform diverse biological functions that may largely be influenced by their specific lipid composition. Unlike membrane proteins that are encoded by the genome, the membrane lipid composition depends upon the activities of the enzymes involved and the availability of the substrate [22]. Therefore, the modifications in the membrane composition of long-chain n-PUFAs, such as EPA and DHA, significantly affect the membrane biophysical properties such as the membrane permeability, fluidity and rigidity. The number of cis-double bonds in fatty acids is of great significance in determining the membrane fluidity. The increasing cis-double bonds produce a higher kink or curve in carbon skeleton of the fatty acid that consequently occupies more space in the membrane, thereby increasing its fluidity [23]. N-3 PUFAs further increase the membrane fluidity by eliminating cholesterol from the highly ordered and tightly packed membrane microdomains called 'lipid rafts' that have been recognized as important platforms to control the downstream signal transduction, apoptosis and immune response. This in turn alters the membrane architecture and the organization of various membrane-associated proteins (transporters, receptors and enzymes), thereby playing a vital role in the pathogenesis and the prevention of various diseases including cancer [24, 25]. For instance, DHA exerts its anti-cancer effects via reduced membrane rigidity and epidermal growth factor receptor (EGFR) signaling [26], suggesting the membrane lipid therapy as a valuable therapeutic target against cancer risk.

3.1.5.2 Eicosanoid Synthesis

Eicosanoids are the signaling mediators derived through the enzymatic oxidation of PUFAs by cyclooxygenases (COX), lipoxygenases (LOX) and cytochrome P450 (CYP). Since PUFAs are mainly present in esterified form at the *sn*-2 position in phospholipids, they are released and utilized as substrates by the enzymes to produce eicosanoids. The Ca^{2+}-dependent cytosolic phospholipase enzyme ($cPLA_2$) and secreted phospholipase A2 ($sPLA_2$) function to release the PUFAs mainly from the *sn*-2 position of phosphatidylinositol and phosphatidylcholine, which is the major phospholipid in most mammalian cell membranes. After being released, these PUFAs can be metabolized by COX, LOX or CYP to produce various lipid mediators of biological significance. Three main classes of eicosanoids are generated: prostaglandins (PGs) and thromboxanes (TXs) are produced through COX pathways, leukotrienes (LTs) and lipoxins (LXs) via LOX pathways, whereas several epoxy, hydroxy and dihydroxy derivatives are derived from CYP pathways [27] (Fig. 3.3). For instance, ARA is transformed into 2-series prostaglandins (PGD2, PGE2, PGF2 and PGI2), thromboxanes (TxA2), 4-series of leukotrienes (LtC4) and hydroxyeicosatetraenoic acid (HETEs) (5-, 12-, 15-HETE). It is important to note that the ARA-derived eicosanoids lead toward enhanced inflammation and oxidative stress, thereby exerting pro-carcinogenic properties (Fig. 3.3). However, ARA can also be converted to anti-inflammatory and pro-resolving lipoxins, (LXA4, LXB4) [28].

The metabolites derived from EPA consist of 3-series prostaglandins (PGE3, PGD3, PGF3 and PGI3) and thromboxane A3 (TxA3), 5-series leukotrienes (LtA5, LtB5, LtC5, LtD5, LtE5) and E-series resolvins (RvE1, RvE2 and RvE3). Furthermore, DHA-derived oxylipins include the resolvins of the D series (RvD1, RvD2, RvD3, RvD4, RvD5 and RvD6), protectins, (PD1/NPD1 and PDX) and maresins (MaR1 and MaR2). In addition, these bioactive mediators derived from n-3 PUFAs display anti-inflammatory and pro-resolving properties [10], leading to a reduced oxidative stress (Fig. 3.3). These metabolites interact with different receptors including peroxisome proliferator-activated receptors (PPARs) and G

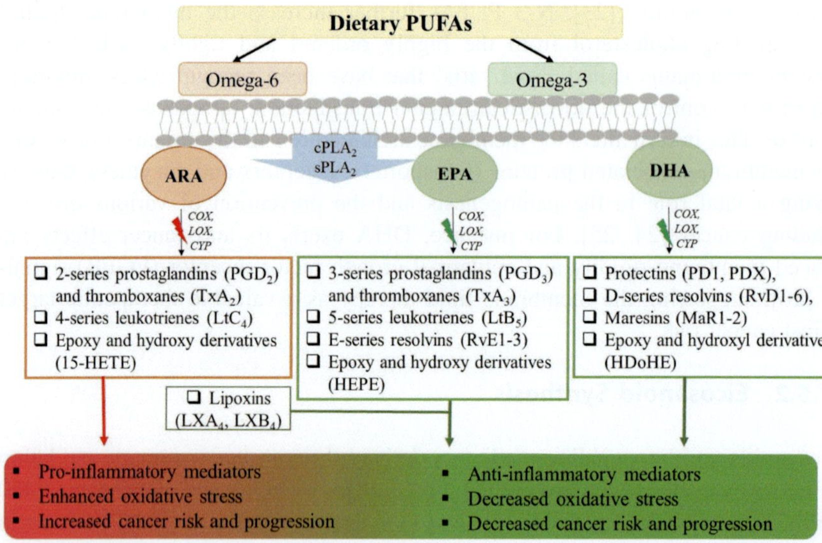

Fig. 3.3 Pathways of synthesis of oxylipins from arachidonic acid (ARA), eicosapentaenoic acid (EPA) and docosahexaenoic acid (DHA). N-6 and n-3 PUFAs are first released from the cell membrane phospholipids by cytosolic ($cPLA_2$) and secretory phospholipases A2 ($sPLA_2$). These PUFAs are then metabolized via a panel of enzymes (COX, LOX and CYP) into various signaling mediators (few examples are mentioned in parenthesis) which exert anti- or pro-inflammatory activities and also function to regulate the cellular oxidative stress. Cyclooxygenases (COX), lipoxygenases (LOX), cytochrome P450 (CYP), hydroxyeicosatetraenoic acids (HETE), hydroxyeicosapentaenoic acid (HEPE), HDoHE (hydroxydocosahexanoic acid)

protein-coupled receptors (GPCRs) to modulate various physiological responses including tumorigenesis. It is important to mention that n-3 and n-6 PUFAs compete for their binding with different enzymes involved in eicosanoid production and may, therefore, modulate various biological processes involved either in the maintenance of healthy state or in the pathogenesis [28, 29].

3.1.5.3 Modulation of Gene Expression

PUFAs regulate gene expression in various tissues including liver, adipose tissue, heart and brain where they are implicated in the prevention/development of various pathologies including cancer, diabetes, cardiovascular and neurodegenerative disorders. Numerous studies have highlighted the role of PUFAs in the modification of a wide array of genes, which may account for their influence on lipid metabolism [30]. PUFAs control gene expression either by regulating the signaling pathways or directly as ligands by binding to the transcription factors.

Numerous signaling networks and cellular mediators related to carcinogenesis are differentially regulated by n-3 and n-6 PUFAs. For instance, the protein kinase C, ras, ERK 1/2 and NF-κB [31–34] were upregulated by n-6 PUFAs, whereas n-3 PUFAs have shown the opposite effects. Furthermore, these PUFAs also inversely affect the expression of a wide array of genes associated with various biological processes, highlighting the complexity of PUFAs-mediated transcriptional regulation [35].

Moreover, considerable evidence suggests that PUFAs directly regulate the transcription of genes related to lipid metabolism through their interaction with nuclear receptors including PPARs, nuclear factor-kappa B (NF-κB) and sterol regulatory element binding proteins (SREBPs) [36]. Interestingly, PUFAs bind differently to these transcription factors to control their nuclear abundance, ultimately regulating a variety of cellular functions including lipid metabolism, cell differentiation and proliferation, apoptosis and inflammation [37].

3.1.6 The Importance of the Omega-6/Omega-3 Fatty Acid Ratio in Health Maintenance

Although both n-6 and n-3 fatty acids are essentials, there is a need to find the right balance between n-6 and n-3 fatty acids intake, as n-6 and n-3 ratio in the diet can play a pivotal role in the overall health of an individual. For adolescents, children and infants older than six months, the daily recommended combined dose of EPA and DHA in the diet ranges from 40 to 250 mg. For adults, it ranges from 250 to 1000 mg per day [38, 39]. However, n-6 and n-3 fatty acids ratio varies depending upon the diet source. For instance, one consuming n-6-rich plant oils has higher n-6 and n-3 ratio than those living near coastal areas where fish is mainly consumed in the diet and serves as the primary source of n-3 fatty acids. In Japan, people take an ideal ratio (1:2–4) of n-6 and n-3 fatty acids, and this is due to higher consumption of seafood [40]. According to nutrition experts, a diet containing n-6 and n-3 fatty acids in a ratio of less than 5:1 is highly recommended [41]. During the last three decades, the intake of total fat and saturated fat as a percentage of total calories in the diet has continuously decreased while that of n-6 consumption has increased largely. Consequently, an increase in n-6 and n-3 ratio from 1–2:1 during evolution to 20–50:1 today has been observed [42, 43]. Accumulating evidence suggests that an increased n-6 consumption and a lower n-3 intake contribute to the development chronic inflammation and related disorders such as cancer, cardiovascular and neurodegenerative diseases [42–48].

3.2 PUFAs and Cancer

3.2.1 Cancer and Its Hallmarks

Cancer is a multifactorial disease in which growth and development of some body cells go beyond control, and this may affect any tissue or organ of the body. In normal conditions, human cells grow and multiply through an organized process of cell division where old and damaged cells are cleared by the process called apoptosis. An imbalance or dysfunction of this system leads to uncontrolled multiplication of abnormal/damaged cells. As a result, the cells may form tumors, lumps of tissue, that can be malignant (cancerous) or benign (not cancerous). Unlike benign tumors, cancerous tumors may metastasize, i.e., they can invade adjacent tissues and can travel to remote areas in the body to form new tumors [49].

There are over 100 different types of cancers that are categorized on the basis of the affected tissue or organ of the human body. Many biological and biochemical features are displayed by cancer cells in vitro or in vivo, and among them, some are common to most cancers while others are tumor-dependent. These common features include origin from normal cells, aberrant proliferation, loss of differentiation and invasion of adjacent tissues in situ that leads to extravasation and metastasis to other sites in the body. Cancer involves a diverse series of genetic changes due to interactions with an individual's environment [50].

The hallmarks of cancer are defined as a set of functional capabilities acquired by human cells that are crucial for their ability to form malignant tumors. Initially, six cancer hallmarks were proposed which were then expanded to eight (Table 3.2), as the knowledge about multi-step processes involved in carcinogenesis has progressed [51, 52]. These eight core attributes comprise the acquired functional capabilities for sustaining proliferative signaling, resisting apoptosis, reprogramming of energy metabolism, activating invasion and metastasis, enabling replicative immortality, inducing angiogenesis and evading growth suppressors [53].

It is evident that these hallmarks are not able to explain the underlying complicated cellular and molecular mechanisms involved in the tumor development and its progression. Therefore, the concept of 'enabling characteristics' has been introduced in recent years to highlight the neoplastic mechanisms essential to acquire

Table 3.2 Summary of core and emerging cancer hallmark capabilities and enabling characteristics of cancer cells

Core cancer hallmarks	Proposed emerging hallmarks
1. Sustaining proliferative signaling	• Unlocking phenotypic plasticity
2. Resisting apoptosis	• Senescent cells
3. Reprogramming of energy metabolism	• The ability of cells to regress from a specific specialized functional state
4. Activating invasion and metastasis	• Epigenetic changes that can affect gene expression
5. Enabling replicative immortality	• The role of microorganisms
6. Inducing angiogenesis	• Neuronal signaling
7. Evading growth suppressors	
8. Avoiding immune destruction	
Enabling characteristics	***Proposed emerging enabling characteristics***
• Genome instability and mutation	• Non-mutational epigenetic reprogramming
• Tumor-promoting inflammation	• Polymorphic microbiomes

the hallmark traits. In this regard, two enabling characteristics, i.e., 'genome stability and mutation' and 'tumor-promoting inflammation,' have been incorporated for their role in activating the eight hallmark capabilities essential for carcinogenesis [50]. Recently, Senga et al. [54] have suggested four novel cancer hallmarks including, 'the ability of cells to regress from a specific specialized functional state,' 'epigenetic changes that can affect gene expression,' 'the role of microorganisms' and 'neuronal signaling.' Additionally, some other emerging hallmarks 'unlocking phenotypic plasticity' and 'senescent cells' and enabling characteristics 'non-mutational epigenetic reprogramming' and 'polymorphic microbiomes' have also been proposed to be added [53] (Table 3.2). This conceptualization of the complex tumorigenic pathways is widely accepted and has played a crucial role in developing cancer therapeutics through hallmark targeting.

3.2.2 Rewiring of Fatty Acid Metabolism in Cancer Cells

Aberrant metabolism in cancer biology has emerged as a major hallmark, which results in the deregulation or abnormal metabolic activation of various signaling pathways involved in cancer development, progression as well as in drug resistance. Furthermore, due to the heterogeneous nature of the disease, the cellular metabolic requirements can change from tumor to tumor and even in different cells from the same tumor, i.e., intra-tumor heterogeneity [55].

Cancer cells are known to reprogram their metabolic activities related to lipid metabolism by modulating the synthesis of lipids and cholesterol [56]. These metabolic activities favor an enhanced production of cellular building blocks such as lipids, proteins and nucleic acids, which is a prerequisite for the rapid cancer cell growth and proliferation [57]. The term lipid encompasses a variety of lipid classes including fatty acids, glycerolipids, glycerophospholipids, sphingolipids and sterols. Here, we focus on fatty acid metabolism in cancer cells.

3.2.2.1 Fatty Acid Synthesis

It is widely accepted that rewiring of lipid metabolism in cancer cells broadly includes the alterations in fatty acid synthesis, storage and degradation [58]. The rapidly proliferating cancer cells require fatty acids in order to sustain their high energy demands and to generate metabolic intermediates for membrane biosynthesis and signaling mediators [59]. Normal mammalian cells obtain fatty acids either endogenously from the surrounding microenvironment or through de novo synthesis by using nutrients, such as glucose or glutamine. Unlike normal human cells, tumor cells obtain majority of fatty acids required for their rapid proliferation through de novo synthesis [60]. In cancer cells, fatty acid synthesis is fueled by the upregulation of key enzymes such as fatty acid synthase, acetyl-CoA carboxylase and ATP citrate lyase [61–63]. For instance, an increased expression of fatty acid synthase was reported to enhance cancer growth in lung cancer cells [64] and to stimulate angiogenic pathways in colorectal cancer [65]. Cancer cells produce acetyl-CoA from the cytosolic citrate, which is produced from the mitochondrial tricarboxylic acid cycle (TCA). One molecule of palmitic acid (C16:0) is generated via the condensation of acetyl groups through fatty acid synthase. Palmitic acid is further transformed to the long-chain fatty acids through the action of elongases and desaturases in the endoplasmic reticulum [66]. It is important to mention that fatty acid synthesis is a highly coordinated and controlled process regulated by the SREBPs. SREBPs constitute a family of transcription factors that are vital for maintaining cellular lipid homeostasis and whose expression has been shown to increase in many cancers [67, 68].

3.2.2.2 Fatty Acid Uptake

Cancer cells meet their overwhelming needs for fatty acids by increasing their uptake from the extracellular medium. The enhanced lipid uptake is made possible through the upregulation of different proteins that function as transporters and display increased expression in tumors [67, 69]. These specialized transporters include the cluster of differentiation 36 (CD36), fatty acid transport protein family (FATPs), plasma membrane-associated fatty acid-binding proteins (FABP) and lipoprotein binding receptors [70, 71]. It has also been shown that triglycerides and cholesteryl esters could represent key sources of lipids for cancer cells that express receptors for lipoproteins [72].

3.2.2.3 Fatty Acid Storage and Degradation

Due to their continuous exposure to fluctuations in nutrient and oxygen supply, cancer cells display an adaptation mechanism to strive stressful conditions, whereby they can switch between alternative nutrient sources and metabolic pathways [73]. The excessive uptake and/or biosynthesis of fatty acids often leads to the production of lipid droplets (LDs). In the absence of exogenous nutrient supply, these LDs undergo degradation mediated by the process of lipolysis to release fatty acids that fulfill the exaggerating needs of cancer cells. During this process, the triglycerides in the LDs are hydrolyzed by the sequential action of different lipases, driving the production of free fatty acids. The free fatty acids, thus produced, undergo mitochondrial or peroxisomal β-oxidation to produce energy and could serve as substrates for membrane synthesis and signaling lipid mediators. In comparison with healthy tissues, high content of LDs has been reported in various cancer types including breast, prostate, liver, colorectal, hepatocellular carcinoma and glioblastoma [67, 74]. Interestingly, LDs formation is frequently linked with tumor invasiveness and metastatic spreading, which could be suppressed by inhibiting the mobilization of fatty acids from LDs [75, 76]. This indicates that the reprogramming of lipid metabolic pathways in cancer cells could provide valuable targets in cancer pathogenesis.

3.3 Role of PUFAs in Various Cancer Types

There is an increasing evidence that PUFAs play a significant role in the pathogenesis, progression and management of various types of cancers through their control over multiple biological pathways. Here, we have focused on the cancer types that are more prevalent and cause high mortality among male and female individuals [77].

3.3.1 Gastrointestinal Cancer

Gastrointestinal cancers include esophageal, gastric, colon and rectal tumors. In 2018, World Health Organization (WHO) has recorded approximately 3.5 million new gastrointestinal cancer cases worldwide. Whereas the esophageal cancer is less frequent, the gastric cancer (GC) is the fifth most common cancer and the third leading cause of cancer death worldwide. Colorectal cancer (CRC) is the third most commonly diagnosed cancer worldwide after lung and breast cancer with 1.8 million new cases reported in 2018 [78].

A large body of evidence has suggested dietary fats to influence significantly the risk of developing the gastrointestinal cancers. Higher n-3 PUFAs intake in subjects with Barrett's esophagus was negatively associated with esophageal adenocarcinoma [79, 80] as well as other digestive system cancers including oral cavity/pharyngeal cancers, gastric cancer, large bowel cancer and CRC [81, 82]. Several prospective studies including Cancer Prevention Study II (CPS II) and Nutrition Cohort and the European Prospective Investigation into Cancer and Nutrition (EPIC) have reported the significance of fish intake in reducing CRC risk [83, 84]. Moreover, the total long-chain n-3 PUFAs plasma levels were associated with the reduced CRC risk [85, 86], whereas high ARA plasma levels were found to be positively correlated with the colon cancer pathogenesis [87, 88]. However, the findings remain insufficient and inconsistent with additional complications and differences due to the gender, subjects' origin, follow-up duration, cancer location, stage and characteristics and need further investigation in large clinical trials [89–91].

3.3.2 Prostate Cancer

Prostate cancer is known as the most frequently diagnosed cancer in men, accounting for almost 375,000 deaths worldwide [92]. Most prostate cancers are less aggressive and curable when the malignancy is limited to prostate; however, the outcomes can vary in view of the metastasis. Epidemiological data have supported the association between the incidence as well the progression of the disease with the intake and metabolism of PUFAs [93–95]. Particularly, the Mediterranean diet that comprises of plant-based foods and high content of fish-derived n-3 PUFAs has gained significant attention in lowering prostate cancer aggressiveness [96] as well as its progression [97]. In addition, the blood n-3 PUFA levels were reported to be inversely correlated with the prostate cancer risk in a randomized, double-blind, placebo-controlled trial on 476 patients diagnosed with prostate cancer [98]. Interestingly, a high n-6 to n-3 ratio in 79 prostate cancer patients was associated with an increase in prostate cancer risk [48].

In contrast, a randomized, placebo-controlled trial (SELECT) consisting of 834 subjects, diagnosed with low- or high-grade prostate cancer indicated that high plasma n-3 PUFA concentrations in these patients are linked to an increased prostate cancer risk [99]. Similar results were obtained from another trial, the Prostate Cancer Prevention Trial, comprising of 1658 participants with low- and high-grade prostate cancer [100]. This indicates the existence of complex interactions between these PUFAs and a particular cancer type and requires further investigation using larger clinical trials and cohort studies [101].

3.3.3 Lung Cancer

Lung cancer is the leading cause of cancer-related deaths globally, with an estimated 1.8 million deaths [77]. The pathophysiology of this cancer is not well known; however, it is hypothesized that it may be caused by an increased as well as repeated exposure to carcinogens, most importantly the cigarette smoke. This leads to the lung epithelium dysplasia and, in severe cases, results in genetic mutations, which possibly interfere with the cell cycle and promote carcinogenesis [102]. The non-small cell lung carcinomas (NSCLC) account for the majority (85%) of all lung malignant neoplasms [78].

Several studies have highlighted the roles of PUFAs as potential biomarkers in the diagnosis, progression or prevention of lung cancer. Increased levels of free fatty acids ARA and LA and their metabolites (HETE) have been observed in lung adenocarcinoma and squamous cell carcinoma patients (n = 37) compared with control subjects (n = 111) without cancer [103]. Furthermore, the diet rich in n-6 PUFAs in murine model of lung cancer has been shown to be associated with an increased cancer risk by increasing the markers related to cell proliferation, angiogenesis and inflammation such as NF-κB, p65, YY1, COX-2 and TGF-β [104]. Moreover, n-3 PUFAs have also been shown to improve the nutritional and inflammatory status in lung cancer patients undergoing chemotherapy and radiotherapy [105].

However, a study on two population-based cohorts, the Shanghai Women's Health Study (SWHS) and Shanghai Men's Health Study (SMHS) with 121,970 study participants, has shown that the DHA and EPA intake was associated with an increased lung cancer risk in Chinese women who were all never-smokers. Interestingly, the total PUFAs intake and the ratio of n-6 to n-3 PUFAs (7:1) were inversely associated with the risk of lung cancer, particularly in adenocarcinoma patients and in never-smokers [106]. This could explain the genetic variability among the individuals from different ethnic differences in metabolizing PUFAs and hence modulating the disease risk [107].

3.3.4 Breast Cancer

Breast cancer is the most frequently diagnosed cancer in women and is considered as the second most common cause of death from cancer worldwide among women [77]. Several factors have been recognized as important in the development and progression of breast cancer including hormonal, physiological and genetic. In the past few decades, numerous epidemiological studies have emphasized upon the use of healthy diet, and the n-3 PUFAs have been the most intensively studied factors to reduce carcinogenesis. The dietary n-3 PUFAs intake was found to be inversely associated with breast cancer risk in different large prospective cohort studies, such as the Japan Collaborative Cohort Study [108] and the Singapore Chinese Health Study [109]. Furthermore, in addition to the dietary PUFA intake, the tissue or erythrocyte n-3 PUFA composition has also been inversely associated to the breast cancer risk, as suggested by various case–control studies [110–112]. In contrast, the results from the multicenter EPIC cohort [113], the VITamin D and OmegA-3Trial (VITAL) study [114] and the meta-analyses reported no association between the fish or marine n-3 PUFA intake and the breast cancer incidence [115, 116]. This necessitates further investigation to confirm the findings.

3.3.5 Brain Tumors

Brain cancer is an aggressive form of cancer, causing high mortality rates in children and adults. It includes malignant and non-malignant tumors that arise from the brain parenchyma and associated structures. Benign brain cancer comprises of cells that grow relatively slowly, rarely invade the surrounding cells and, therefore, can be surgically removed, as in the case of meningiomas, pituitary tumors and low-grade astrocytoma. However, the malignant brain tumors such as high-grade astrocytoma and oligodendroglia have faster growth rates and spread quickly to other brain parts and spinal cord. The unique and complex brain microenvironment renders cancer treatment highly challenging. Furthermore, most of the anti-tumor drugs are unable to cross the blood–brain barrier (BBB), a semipermeable barrier that protects brain from exposure to the molecules in the bloodstream [82, 117]. This emphasizes upon the need to develop novel treatment strategies as well as the preventive measures. Several studies support the use of PUFAs to limit the progression of brain cancer. PUFAs are found in the brain where they function to regulate the neuronal membrane fluidity and integrity, thus playing crucial role in neurotransmission and signal transduction, mainly due to their ability to cross the BBB, unlike most of the chemotherapeutic drugs. In vivo studies have shown that dietary PUFAs supplementation alters their composition in brain tissues. Among PUFAs, n-3 PUFAs have been reported to exert anti-tumor properties, whereas n-6 could increase the risk of brain tumor development [117]. Several epidemiological studies have suggested the association of dietary fish intake with a reduced brain tumor risk [118]. An increased level of pro-inflammatory cytokines was reported during cancer, ultimately leading toward neuroinflammation and promoting brain cancer growth [119]. Grade IV glioblastoma patients show high levels of ARA and pro-inflammatory prostanoids including PGD2, PGE2, TXB2 and PGF2α along with decreased survival rates, compared to patients with grade II/III tumors [120]. In contrast, n-3 PUFAs-derived molecules such as oxylipins (LXA4), resolvins (D1) and docosanoids (17RS-HpDHA) inhibit pro-inflammatory cytokine production in astrocytes and glial cells, thereby reducing brain tumor development [121–123].

3.4 Potential Mechanisms Defining the Role of PUFAs (Omega-3 vs. Omega 6) in Carcinogenesis

This section aims to explore the mechanism or actions through which PUFAs control the growth of tumor cells, angiogenesis, metastasis, apoptosis, signal transduction as well as cancer-related inflammation and oxidative stress.

3.4.1 Alteration of the Biological Membrane Physicochemical Properties and Functions

Proper functioning of the cellular membranes requires the organization of lipid and protein assemblies into micro- and nano-domains that facilitate the signal transduction and transport mechanisms. Indeed, the role of membrane lipid composition in maintaining the cellular functions and, therefore, human health has become more apparent in the past few decades. Alterations in lipid metabolism and an increased cholesterol synthesis have been considered as one of the hallmarks in cancer biology (see Sect. 2.1). Interestingly, the membrane lipid composition and the structural and functional dynamics are largely influenced by the dietary factors. The incorporation of PUFAs results in an increased membrane unsaturation in breast cancer cells [124]. Furthermore, a high membrane ARA content increased, whereas the EPA and DHA levels decreased the risk of developing different cancer types including colorectal cancer [125], breast cancer [112], hepatocellular carcinoma [126], prostate cancer [127] and brain tumors [128]. However, the results remain inconclusive since the lipid rich-microenvironment could also facilitate the cancerous cell proliferation by providing energy to these rapidly dividing cells [129], thereby rendering lipid metabolism as a promising therapeutic target in oncology.

3.4.2 Regulation of the Inflammatory Pathways

While acute inflammation refers to the normal physiological response of the body against microbial infections and other harmful events, chronic inflammation leads toward the tumor development due to the genome instability, DNA damage, epigenetic alterations and modifications in signal transduction. This inflammatory microenvironment needs to be disrupted with anti-inflammatory mediators in order to restore the tissue homeostasis. N-3 PUFAs exert beneficial effects in cancer in part through their anti-inflammatory properties, in contrast to the n-6 PUFAs that exhibit pro-inflammatory effects [130]. This is mainly ascribed to the ability of n-3 PUFAs to compete with n-6 PUFAs for their metabolic conversion into n-3 eicosanoids, resulting in reduced levels of pro-inflammatory and pro-carcinogenic n-6 eicosanoids. Supplementation with fish oil rich in n-3 PUFAs has been reported to cure a number of illnesses including different cancer types, possibly through increased n-3 eicosanoids and reduced n-6 eicosanoids concentrations [28, 131].

Substantial effort has been made in the recent years to develop the pharmacological strategies that target cancer-related inflammation. Recently, the PUFAs derivatives referred as the specialized pro-resolving mediators (SPMs) have emerged as novel potential therapeutic agents against the development of chronic inflammation. SPMs are a group of endogenously synthesized lipid mediators from n-3 and n-6 PUFAs, including lipoxins, resolvins, protectins and maresins (see Sect. 1.5.2) [132]. These bioactive molecules have gained great significance due to their ability to reduce chronic inflammation without exerting side effects and immunosuppression [133], in contrast to the anti-inflammatory drugs, such as NSAID [134]. In colon cancer patients, high levels of serum inflammatory cytokines (IL-1β, IL-6, IL-10 and TNF-α) were observed along with the low levels of RvD1 in association with pathological staging of colon cancer [135]. However, opposite or no association was observed in some studies [136, 137]. The effects of SPMs have been shown to be mediated via specific G-protein-coupled receptors, though the clinical studies are still lacking to establish SPMs as an effective line of intervention for cancer-derived inflammation [138].

3.4.3 Effects on Cellular Oxidative Stress and Related Molecular Pathways

Oxidative stress results from an imbalance between the production of reactive oxygen species (ROS) in cells and tissues and the capacity of the biological system to eliminate these reactive products. This imbalance is mainly caused by various physiological and environmental factors (pollutants, UV, ionizing radiations, heavy metals) that increase the ROS production, resulting in cellular damage and playing a significant role in the pathogenesis of various inflammation-related disorders including neurodegenerative diseases and cancer [139]. In addition, chronic oxidative stress can also lead to a continuous local inflammation, inducing tissue destruction and regeneration, and consequently the development of chronic inflammation that fuels tumor development and its progression. Elevated levels of biomarkers related to DNA oxidative damage (8-oxo-dG) and lipid peroxidation (4-HNE) and the reduced activities of antioxidant enzymes (SOD, CAT, GST and GPx) were observed in different cancer types including head and neck, ovarian, gastric CRC and breast cancers [139].

The antioxidant properties of PUFAs have largely been exploited in the development and progression of different cancer types [140]. Epidemiological studies have found that the n-3 PUFAs supplementation was associated with lower levels of lipid peroxidation in patients with advanced lung cancer [141] and an increased antioxidant levels in cancer patients with acute lymphoblastic leukemia [142]. In addition, a significant increase in the activities of antioxidant enzymes including catalase, superoxide dismutase and glutathione reductase in red blood cell has been reported in breast cancer patients undergoing chemotherapy [143].

3.4.4 Effects on Apoptosis and Cell Cycle

Apoptosis or programmed cell death functions to eliminate the unwanted, damaged or infected cells. The pro-apoptotic effects of n-3 PUFAs, particularly EPA and DHA, have been reported in different breast cancer cell lines, mostly through an increased apoptosis via the activation of caspase 8 [117, 144], and an increased production of ROS in cancerous cells [145].

Moreover, the treatment with DHA and EPA causes an increased ROS formation, accompanying with the caspase-3 and caspase-9 activation in different colorectal cancer cell lines [146]. Furthermore, DHA also inhibited the growth of gastric cancer both in in vivo and in vitro models through an increased pro-apoptotic miRNA expression along with caspase-9 activation [147]. In human brain tumor cells, EPA and DHA significantly induce apoptosis and G0/G1 cell cycle arrest via an increased Bax and decreased Bcl-Xl protein expression, together with an activation of caspase-3 and caspase-9 [148]. Studies using cell lines and mouse models have shown that these n-3 PUFAs suppressed cell growth and enhanced cell death in pancreatic cancer through WNT/β-catenin pathway [149] and in hepatocellular carcinoma through the simultaneous suppression of COX-2 and β-catenin, along with caspase-3 and caspase-9 activation [150]. Moreover, DHA also exhibits the anti-proliferative effects by downregulating the anti-apoptotic (Mcl-1) and cell cycle proteins (CDK6, CDK4, cyclin D1) in ovarian cancer cells [151].

3.4.5 Effects on Metastasis and Angiogenesis

Cancerous cells have the ability to penetrate the blood or lymphatic vessels and therefore spread to the other parts of the body (metastatic tumors) caused by the loss of cell polarity as well as the cell–cell adhesion resulting in invasiveness. The metastatic spreading is promoted by the neoangiogenesis, which requires the synthesis of vascular endothelial growth factor (VEGF) and metalloproteinase (MMP) activity [152]. The antiangiogenic properties of n-3 PUFAs have been supported by several studies demonstrating that n-3 PUFAs supplementation suppressed angiogenesis via reduced MMP expression thereby inhibiting the metastasis in patients with colon cancer [153, 154] and in gastric cancer patients treated with cisplatin [155]. In addition, DHA-derived lipid mediators, produced by cytochrome P450 epoxygenases, such as epoxydocosapentaenoic acids (EDPs) prevent angiogenesis by suppressing VEGF and fibroblast growth factor 2 along with endothelial cell migration in in vivo and in vitro models. On the contrary, the ARA metabolites epoxyeicosatrienoic acids (EETs) promote angiogenesis and tumorigenesis [156]. Furthermore, in breast cancer cell lines (MDA-MB-231 MCF-7), DHA reduced the expression of colony stimulating factor-1, a potent activator of metastasis, through PI 3 kinase/Akt signaling [157]. Moreover, high EPA cellular levels and its metabolites (F4-neuroprostanes and resolvins) along with reduced levels of ARA-derived pro-angiogenic prostaglandins (PGE2) were associated with reduced tumor growth in the mice model of prostate cancer [158].

3.4.6 Regulation of the Transcription Factor Activity and Signal Transduction

Several studies have shown that n-3 and n-6 PUFAs and their derivatives regulate the expression and activity of a wide array of transcription factors and their target genes involved in carcinogenesis [159]. Indeed, different PUFAs such as ARA, EPA and DHA interact directly with certain transcription factors including the PPARs. PPARs are the nuclear receptor proteins consisting of three subtypes (α, β/δ and γ) with organ-specific expression. PPARs are the ligand-activated transcription factors that are involved in the regulation of lipid metabolism and homeostasis as well as in cell proliferation, cell differentiation and inflammatory pathways [160]. PUFAs are known as the natural ligands and activators of PPARs since these PUFAs may control carcinogenesis through the activation of different signaling pathways associated with various cellular responses including cell growth and differentiation, apoptosis, hormonal regulation and membrane function [161]. Sustained PPAR-α activation through ligands leads to liver carcinogenesis, possibly due to the accumulation of lipid peroxidation products [162]. Several studies using different cancer cell lines and animal models have supported the anti-neoplastic properties of PPARs, mainly due to their control of the cell cycle progression and apoptosis [163]. The anti-inflammatory and anti-proliferative properties of PPARα and PPARγ may contribute to their role in the suppression of carcinogenesis [164]. However, PPARδ has been found to induce the cell proliferation and the development of certain cancer types, though further investigation is required to address the controversies [161].

Apart from direct binding, PUFAs can also indirectly interact with the transcription factors by modulating different regulatory pathways and signaling molecules, which participate in a variety of cellular processes including cell cycle regulation, cell differentiation, apoptosis and gene expression [159]. For instance, the n-3 and n-6 PUFAs compete to regulate the activity of protein kinase C (PKC), which is a calcium-activated serine/threonine kinase. PKC consists of 11 isoforms including α, βI, βII and γ with unique structure and biological functions. Interestingly, the dietary n-3 PUFAs prevent colon cancer by inhibiting the PKCβII-mediated cell proliferation and colon carcinogenesis [165].

Another family of transcription factors, the nuclear transcription factor κB (NF-κB), controls the cytokine gene expression, proliferation, apoptosis, the adaptive immune response, the stress response and tissue remodeling. Studies have shown a constitutive NF-κB activation in most cancer cells (prostate, hematopoietic, breast cancers). However, the n-3 PUFAs-mediated suppression of NF-κB signaling appears to play an anti-proliferative and anti-apoptotic role in different cancer types including prostate and breast cancer [166, 167]. Moreover, PUFAs appear to have a more complex effect on the Toll-like receptor (TLR) family, which provides an important interface to modulate the downstream NF-κB activity [159]. In addition, PUFAs may also control carcinogenesis-related signal transduction through another checkpoint that involves the SREBPs, consisting of three members, SREBP-1a, SREBP-1c and SREBP-2. This class of transcription factors mediate the expression of target genes involved in the metabolism of cholesterol, fatty acids, triglycerides and phospholipids, thereby playing an important role in tumorigenesis [168]. The increased SREBP1 expression promotes the cancer cell proliferation and metastasis through metabolic reprogramming of tumor cells [169]. N-3 PUFAs inhibit cell proliferation in breast cancer cells by suppressing protein kinase B (pAKT) signaling network along with reduced SREBP-1 and fatty acid synthase expression [170]. This indicates that a comprehensive understanding is necessary in order to explore the mechanisms of transcription factor regulation through PUFAs in cancer.

3.5 Anti-neoplastic Effects of Omega-3 PUFA

3.5.1 Chemopreventive and Chemotherapeutic Agents

In recent years, several improvements have been made in cancer treatment using chemotherapy, nevertheless, little or no satisfactory response to treatment has been obtained in long-term clinical trials. Studies have shown that the chemotherapy promotes chemoresistance due to prolonged exposure that favors a pro-metastatic tumor microenvironment, consequently leading toward the tumor relapse [171]. Furthermore, the chemotherapeutic agents target rapidly dividing cells and therefore are not capable of distinguishing normal cells from the tumor cells. Consequently, these agents may damage or destroy normal cells such as the bone marrow cells, hair follicles, the red blood cells and gut epithelia leading to systemic toxicity, hair loss and impaired organ functioning [172]. Therefore, the tumor-targeting drugs should be carefully designed to improve their specificity and minimize the life-threatening secondary effects.

Increasing evidence based on clinical data suggests the use of a combination of natural bioactive molecules and chemotherapeutic agents to cure tumorigenesis with reduced adverse effects of chemotherapy. In recent years, n-3 PUFAs have emerged as the appropriate candidates for chemoprevention or combinational chemotherapy due to their anti-neoplastic properties [141, 173].

The cancer cells are characterized by their rapid proliferation, which is largely dependent on the availability of nutrients. After being taken up by the tumor cells, PUFAs are readily integrated into the membrane lipid rafts that causes significant modulation in their biophysical characteristics. This influences the functions of various transmembrane proteins, including receptors, transporters and growth factors that are essential for the growth of tumor cells [174–177]. Various studies have shown that EPA and DHA function as adjuvants to enhance the chemosensitivity and improve multidrug resistance in various cancer cells through their anti-proliferative, anti-inflammatory and anti-neoplastic properties [175, 178]. Furthermore, n-3 PUFAs overcome chemoresistance via reduced tumor vascularization in cancer cells treated with chemotherapeutic drugs such as anthracyclines and taxanes [179–181]. Importantly, the enhanced cholesterol synthesis in tumor cells is one the important mechanisms leading toward the multidrug resistance via upregulation of the ATP-binding cassette (ABC) transporters, which resist to the toxic effects of several anti-cancer agents [182]. Importantly, n-3 PUFAs treatment produces changes in lipid composition, reduces the transporters activity and restores the effectiveness of anti-cancer drugs with no adverse effects [176, 183].

3.5.2 Secondary Cancer Complications

Cancer-related complications can be highly variable depending upon the type and stage of cancer, the patient's response to treatment, and generally include pain, infection, nausea, fatigue, anxiety and cachexia [184]. In addition, the malnutrition in cancer causes increased complications and worse clinical outcomes [105]. Chemotherapeutic drugs alter the nutritional and inflammatory status in cancer patients, which greatly affects their quality of life. Studies have shown that n-3 PUFAs may also ameliorate the oxidative status in patients undergoing chemotherapy, leading to better clinical outcome and management of side effects, thereby reducing cancer incidence and mortality [143, 185].

Moreover, the depression in cancer patients cannot be overlooked, as it is highly prevalent (10–30%) and greatly influences the effectiveness of chemotherapeutic drugs [186]. The enhanced inflammation in cancer patients is a major factor that induces depression-like behavior [187]. Cumulative evidence suggests n-3 PUFA as a promising dietary approach to manage depression in cancer. An inverse association was observed between the erythrocyte n-3 PUFA levels and depression, which may be associated with the anti-inflammatory properties of these PUFAs [188, 189].

Cancer cachexia (CC) is a complicated condition that occurs in about 70% of cancer patients with an advanced stage of cancer and is responsible for 20% of deaths [190]. CC is a multifactorial 'wasting' complication characterized by an involuntary weight loss of skeletal muscle and/or fat mass, systemic inflammation and metabolic changes that may lead to impaired functions of different organs including liver, brain, gut, heart and adipose tissue [191]. It causes severe fatigue and weakness, critically affects the quality of life and has profound effects on disease prognosis [192]. Several studies have reported n-3 PUFAs supplementation as a promising dietary approach in cancer patients with cachexia. It has been shown that the use of fish oil improves body fat, lean body mass, pain, appetite and quality of life in pancreatic and lung cancer patients with cachexia [189, 193–195]. Furthermore, n-3 PUFAs used either alone or as an adjuvant to chemotherapy provide better response to treatment with decreased secondary complications associated with chemotherapy. However, the anti-cachectic effects of EPA supplementation were more pronounced in the case of early intervention rather than later, when muscle loss is accelerated [184, 196, 197].

3.6 Safety Concerns of PUFAs

According to the European Society for Clinical Nutrition and Metabolism (ESPEN) guidelines on nutrition in cancer patients (2021) [198], the fish oil or n-3 PUFAs supplementation is beneficial in cancer patients undergoing chemotherapy and therefore presentings great risk towards malnutrition and cachexia. The adverse effects that have been associated with high EPA and DHA intakes in humans include bleeding complications, enhanced lipid peroxidation, immunosuppression and impaired glucose and lipid homeostasis [199]. To date, no acceptable upper intake level has yet been set for EPA and DHA by any authoritative body due to insufficient data for any population group. However, the US Food and Drug Administration (FDA) has recommended not exceeding a daily intake of 3 g of

EPA and DHA combined in order to avoid any possible side effects [200]. Likewise, the European Food Safety Authority (EFSA) recognizes the daily doses of EPA and DHA combined up to 5 g as safe, the supplemental intake of EPA alone up to 1.8 g/day and that of DHA alone up to 1 g/day as safe. It is important to note that no side effects were reported with n-3 PUFAs supplementation in healthy volunteers using doses as high as 17.6 g/day for about 24 days [201]. At the usual PUFAs intake levels, consumption of n-3 long-chain PUFA was tolerable in healthy children or adults [199]. However, mild gastrointestinal disturbances along with the unpleasant taste, fishy smell and regurgitations were also associated with fish oil supplementation [202]. Furthermore, the increased bleeding risk was reported in patients on simultaneous treatment with anti-cancer drugs (ibrutinib) and fish oil supplements [203], suggesting the need to carefully consider the use of n-3 PUFAs supplements in cancer patients.

3.7 Future Perspectives and Challenges

A large body of evidence from pre-clinical, clinical and epidemiological studies demonstrates the efficacy of n-3 PUFA dietary supplements in combatting against various cancer types. N-3 PUFAs also present an effective and non-toxic mode of chemoprevention and treatment, either alone or in combination with anticancer drugs. However, the inconsistent and contradictory findings from clinical data have raised questions about the efficacy of these fatty acids that need to be addressed. Various factors such as the small population number, PUFAs dose and n-6 to n-3 ratio selection and the disease complexity and heterogeneity may lead toward inconsistent results. Moreover, the optimum dose and treatment duration for each stage of cancer prevention need yet to be determined, emphasizing upon the necessity to conduct larger and quality clinical trials. It is also evident that under certain pathological conditions, the absorption and the metabolism of n-3 PUFAs are highly impaired, resulting in an increased risk of developing cancer. On the other hand, the maximum protective effects of n-3 PUFAs supplementation were observed in patients who showed greater incorporation of these PUFAs in circulation and at tissue levels. In addition, the inter-individual genetic, metabolic and gut microbiota variabilities are among the crucial factors that determine an individual's response to PUFAs treatment. This may also provide important biomarkers for the personalized PUFAs supplementation in further human intervention trials, potentially clarifying the inconsistencies regarding the anti-cancer role of PUFAs.

3.8 Conclusion

Considerable debate exists regarding the opposing effects of n-3 and n-6 PUFAs in modulating cancer pathogenesis. N-3 PUFAs exhibit anti-tumor effects through their anti-proliferative, pro-apoptotic and anti-inflammatory properties, without raising serious safety concerns. In cancer patients, n-3 PUFAs exert multifaceted roles by ameliorating the chemotherapy response with reduced side effects, increasing overall survival rates and reducing postoperative infections, improving the quality of life and organ functioning (liver, pancreas) and treating cancer-related cachexia. Moreover, numerous epidemiological studies and clinical trials have also highlighted the cancer-promoting role of n-6 PUFAs and their bioactive lipid mediators. This emphasizes upon maintaining the optimal balance of n-6 to n-3 ratio in the diet, since human population is exposed to a diet with a higher proportion of n-6 PUFAs. Furthermore, larger clinical trials should be conducted with careful dose selection, keeping into consideration the genetic variability among the individuals, in order to develop the valuable therapeutic strategies for the management of this devastating disease.

References

1. Calder PC (2015) Functional roles of fatty acids and their effects on human health. JPEN J Parenter Enteral Nutr 39(1 Suppl):18S–32S. https://doi.org/10.1177/0148607115595980
2. Zarate R, El Jaber-Vazdekis N, Tejera N, Perez JA, Rodriguez C (2017) Significance of long chain polyunsaturated fatty acids in human health. Clin Transl Med 6(1):25. https://doi.org/10.1186/s40169-017-0153-6
3. Rustan AC, Drevon CA (2005) Fatty acids: structures and properties. In: Encyclopedia of life sciences (ELS). Wiley
4. Laposata M (1995) Fatty acids. Biochemistry to clinical significance. Am J Clin Pathol 104(2):172–179. https://doi.org/10.1093/ajcp/104.2.172
5. Mensink RP, Katan MB (1990) Effect of dietary trans fatty acids on high-density and low-density lipoprotein cholesterol levels in healthy subjects. N Engl J Med 323(7):439–445. https://doi.org/10.1056/NEJM199008163230703
6. Balic A, Vlasic D, Zuzul K, Marinovic B, Bukvic Mokos Z (2020) Omega-3 versus omega-6 polyunsaturated fatty acids in the prevention and treatment of inflammatory skin diseases. Int J Mol Sci 21(3). https://doi.org/10.3390/ijms21030741
7. Ferreri C, Chatgilialoglu C (2015) Membrane lipidomics for personalized health. Wiley, Chichester
8. Akbar S, Bhatti MZ, Saeed RF, Qazi AS (2021) Polyunsaturated fatty acids: impact on health and disease status. Life Sci 2(2):71–82. https://doi.org/10.37185/LnS.1.1.85
9. Kaur N, Chugh V, Gupta AK (2014) Essential fatty acids as functional components of foods—a review. J Food Sci Technol 51(10):2289–2303. https://doi.org/10.1007/s13197-012-0677-0
10. Saini RK, Keum YS (2018) Omega-3 and omega-6 polyunsaturated fatty acids: dietary sources, metabolism, and significance—a review. Life Sci 203:255–267. https://doi.org/10.1016/j.lfs.2018.04.049
11. Mariamenatu AH, Abdu EM (2021) Overconsumption of omega-6 polyunsaturated fatty acids (PUFAs) versus deficiency of omega-3 PUFAs in modern-day diets: the disturbing factor for their "balanced antagonistic metabolic functions" in the human body. J Lipids 2021:8848161. https://doi.org/10.1155/2021/8848161
12. Winwood RJ (2013) Recent developments in the commercial production of DHA and EPA rich oils from micro-algae. OCL 20(6). https://doi.org/10.1051/ocl/2013030
13. Ruiz-Lopez N, Usher S, Sayanova OV, Napier JA, Haslam RP (2015) Modifying the lipid content and composition of plant seeds: engineering the production of LC-PUFA. Appl Microbiol Biotechnol 99(1):143–154. https://doi.org/10.1007/s00253-014-6217-2

14. Lee JM, Lee H, Kang S, Park WJ (2016) Fatty acid desaturases, polyunsaturated fatty acid regulation, and biotechnological advances. Nutrients 8(1). https://doi.org/10.3390/nu8010023
15. Abedi E, Sahari MA (2014) Long-chain polyunsaturated fatty acid sources and evaluation of their nutritional and functional properties. Food Sci Nutr 2(5):443–463. https://doi.org/10.1002/fsn3.121
16. Moore SA, Hurt E, Yoder E, Sprecher H, Spector AA (1995) Docosahexaenoic acid synthesis in human skin fibroblasts involves peroxisomal retroconversion of tetracosahexaenoic acid. J Lipid Res 36(11):2433–2443. https://doi.org/10.1016/s0022-2275(20)39724-8
17. Su HM, Moser AB, Moser HW, Watkins PA (2001) Peroxisomal straight-chain Acyl-CoA oxidase and D-bifunctional protein are essential for the retroconversion step in docosahexaenoic acid synthesis. J Biol Chem 276(41):38115–38120. https://doi.org/10.1074/jbc.M106326200
18. Sprecher H, Chen Q, Yin FQ (1999) Regulation of the biosynthesis of 22:5n-6 and 22:6n-3: a complex intracellular process. Lipids 34:S153–S156. https://doi.org/10.1007/BF02562271
19. Sprecher H (2000) Metabolism of highly unsaturated n-3 and n-6 fatty acids. Biochim Biophys Acta 1486(2–3):219–231. https://doi.org/10.1016/s1388-1981(00)00077-9
20. Gill I, Valivety R (1997) Polyunsaturated fatty acids, part 1: occurrence, biological activities and applications. Trends Biotechnol 15(10):401–409. https://doi.org/10.1016/S0167-7799(97)01076-7
21. Berdanier CD (2000) In: Chow CK (ed) Fatty acids in foods and their health implications, 2nd edn. Marcel Dekker Inc, New York, pp 569–584
22. Fuentes NR, Kim E, Fan YY, Chapkin RS (2018) Omega-3 fatty acids, membrane remodeling and cancer prevention. Mol Aspects Med 64:79–91. https://doi.org/10.1016/j.mam.2018.04.001
23. Naudi A, Jove M, Ayala V, Portero-Otin M, Barja G, Pamplona R (2013) Membrane lipid unsaturation as physiological adaptation to animal longevity. Front Physiol 4:372. https://doi.org/10.3389/fphys.2013.00372
24. Corsetto PA, Cremona A, Montorfano G, Jovenitti IE, Orsini F, Arosio P et al (2012) Chemical-physical changes in cell membrane microdomains of breast cancer cells after omega-3 PUFA incorporation. Cell Biochem Biophys 64(1):45–59. https://doi.org/10.1007/s12013-012-9365-y
25. Sorensen LS, Rasmussen HH, Aardestrup IV, Thorlacius-Ussing O, Lindorff-Larsen K, Schmidt EB et al (2014) Rapid incorporation of omega-3 fatty acids into colonic tissue after oral supplementation in patients with colorectal cancer: a randomized, placebo-controlled intervention trial. JPEN J Parenter Enteral Nutr 38(5):617–624. https://doi.org/10.1177/0148607113491782
26. Fuentes NR, Mlih M, Wang X, Webster G, Cortes-Acosta S, Salinas ML et al (2021) Membrane therapy using DHA suppresses epidermal growth factor receptor signaling by disrupting nanocluster formation. J Lipid Res 62:100026. https://doi.org/10.1016/j.jlr.2021.100026
27. Liput KP, Lepczynski A, Ogluszka M, Nawrocka A, Polawska E, Grzesiak A et al (2021) Effects of dietary n-3 and n-6 polyunsaturated fatty acids in inflammation and cancerogenesis. Int J Mol Sci 22(13). https://doi.org/10.3390/ijms22136965
28. Serhan CN, Petasis NA (2011) Resolvins and protectins in inflammation resolution. Chem Rev 111(10):5922–5943. https://doi.org/10.1021/cr100396c
29. Calder PC (2020) Eicosanoids. Essays Biochem 64(3):423–441. https://doi.org/10.1042/EBC20190083
30. Desvergne B, Michalik L, Wahli W (2006) Transcriptional regulation of metabolism. Physiol Rev 86(2):465–514. https://doi.org/10.1152/physrev.00025.2005
31. Reddy BS, Simi B, Patel N, Aliaga C, Rao CV (1996) Effect of amount and types of dietary fat on intestinal bacterial 7 alpha-dehydroxylase and phosphatidylinositol-specific phospholipase C and colonic mucosal diacylglycerol kinase and PKC activities during stages of colon tumor promotion. Cancer Res 56(10)

32. Singh J, Hamid R, Reddy BS (1997) Dietary fat and colon cancer: modulating effect of types and amount of dietary fat on ras-p21 function during promotion and progression stages of colon cancer. Cancer Res 57(2):253–258
33. Sauer LA, Blask DE, Dauchy RT (2007) Dietary factors and growth and metabolism in experimental tumors. J Nutr Biochem 18(10):637–649. https://doi.org/10.1016/j.jnutbio.2006.12.009
34. Novak TE, Babcock TA, Jho DH, Helton WS, Espat NJ (2003) NF-kappa B inhibition by omega-3 fatty acids modulates LPS-stimulated macrophage TNF-alpha transcription. Am J Physiol Lung Cell Mol Physiol 284(1):184–189. https://doi.org/10.1152/ajplung.00077.2002
35. Berger A, Roberts MA, Hoff B (2006) How dietary arachidonic- and docosahexaenoic-acid rich oils differentially affect the murine hepatic transcriptome. Lipids Health Dis 5:10. https://doi.org/10.1186/1476-511X-5-10
36. Georgiadi A, Kersten S (2012) Mechanisms of gene regulation by fatty acids. Adv Nutr 3(2):127–134. https://doi.org/10.3945/an.111.001602
37. Berquin IM, Edwards IJ, Chen YQ (2008) Multi-targeted therapy of cancer by omega-3 fatty acids. Cancer Lett 269(2):363–377. https://doi.org/10.1016/j.canlet.2008.03.044
38. Weylandt KH, Serini S, Chen YQ, Su HM, Lim K, Cittadini A et al (2015) Omega-3 polyunsaturated fatty acids: the way forward in times of mixed evidence. Biomed Res Int 2015:143109. https://doi.org/10.1155/2015/143109
39. Amjad Khan W, Chun-Mei H, Khan N, Iqbal A, Lyu SW, Shah F (2017) Bioengineered plants can be a useful source of omega-3 fatty acids. Biomed Res Int 2017:7348919. https://doi.org/10.1155/2017/7348919
40. Aleksandra A, Niveska P, Vesna V, Jasna T, Tamara P, Vrvic M et al (2009) Milk in human nutrition: comparison of fatty acid profiles. Acta Vet 59(5–6):569–578. https://doi.org/10.2298/avb0906569a
41. Moynihan P (2000) Nutrition: the British nutrition foundation oral task force report—issues relevant to dental health professionals. Br Dent J 188(6):308–312. https://doi.org/10.1038/sj.bdj.4800464
42. Chaves H, Singh RB, Khan S, Wilczynska A, Takahashi T (2019) High omega-6/omega-3 fatty acid ratio diets and risk of noncommunicable diseases. In: The role of functional food security in global health, pp 217–259
43. Simopoulos AP (2016) An increase in the omega-6/omega-3 fatty acid ratio increases the risk for obesity. Nutrients 8(3):128. https://doi.org/10.3390/nu8030128
44. Sokola-Wysoczanska E, Wysoczanski T, Wagner J, Czyz K, Bodkowski R, Lochynski S et al (2018) Polyunsaturated fatty acids and their potential therapeutic role in cardiovascular system disorders—a review. Nutrients 10(10). https://doi.org/10.3390/nu10101561
45. Simopoulos AP, DiNicolantonio JJ (2016) The importance of a balanced omega-6 to omega-3 ratio in the prevention and management of obesity. Open Heart. 3(2):e000385. https://doi.org/10.1136/openhrt-2015-000385
46. Molfino A, Amabile MI, Monti M, Muscaritoli M (2017) Omega-3 polyunsaturated fatty acids in critical illness: anti-inflammatory, proresolving, or both? Oxid Med Cell Longev 2017:5987082. https://doi.org/10.1155/2017/5987082
47. Nindrea RD, Aryandono T, Lazuardi L, Dwiprahasto I (2019) Association of dietary intake ratio of n-3/n-6 polyunsaturated fatty acids with breast cancer risk in Western and Asian countries: a meta-analysis. Asian Pac J Cancer Prev 20(5):1321–1327. https://doi.org/10.31557/APJCP.2019.20.5.1321
48. Williams CD, Whitley BM, Hoyo C, Grant DJ, Iraggi JD, Newman KA et al (2011) A high ratio of dietary n-6/n-3 polyunsaturated fatty acids is associated with increased risk of prostate cancer. Nutr Res 31(1):1–8. https://doi.org/10.1016/j.nutres.2011.01.002
49. Diori Karidio I, Sanlier SH (2021) Reviewing cancer's biology: an eclectic approach. J Egypt Natl Canc Inst 33(32). https://doi.org/10.1186/s43046-021-00088-y
50. Floor SL, Dumont JE, Maenhaut C, Raspe E (2012) Hallmarks of cancer: of all cancer cells, all the time? Trends Mol Med 18(9):509–515. https://doi.org/10.1016/j.molmed.2012.06.005

51. Hanahan D, Weinberg RA (2011) Hallmarks of cancer: the next generation. Cell 144(5):646–674. https://doi.org/10.1016/j.cell.2011.02.013
52. Hanahan D, Weinberg RA (2000) The hallmarks of cancer. Cell 100(1):57–70. https://doi.org/10.1016/s0092-8674(00)81683-9
53. Hanahan D (2022) Hallmarks of cancer: new dimensions. Cancer Discov 12(1):31–46. https://doi.org/10.1158/2159-8290.CD-21-1059
54. Senga SS, Grose RP (2021) Hallmarks of cancer—the new testament. Open Biol 11:200358200358. https://doi.org/10.1098/rsob.200358
55. Caiado F, Silva-Santos B, Norell H (2016) Intra-tumour heterogeneity—going beyond genetics. FEBS J 283(12):2245–2258. https://doi.org/10.1111/febs.13705
56. Swinnen JV, Brusselmans K, Verhoeven G (2006) Increased lipogenesis in cancer cells: new players, novel targets. Curr Opin Clin Nutr Metab Care 9(4):358–365. https://doi.org/10.1097/01.mco.0000232894.28674.30
57. Beloribi-Djefaflia S, Vasseur S, Guillaumond F (2016) Lipid metabolic reprogramming in cancer cells. Oncogenesis 5:e189. https://doi.org/10.1038/oncsis.2015.49
58. Koundouros N, Poulogiannis G (2020) Reprogramming of fatty acid metabolism in cancer. Br J Cancer 122(1):4–22. https://doi.org/10.1038/s41416-019-0650-z
59. Rohrig F, Schulze A (2016) The multifaceted roles of fatty acid synthesis in cancer. Nat Rev Cancer 16(11):732–749. https://doi.org/10.1038/nrc.2016.89
60. Medes G, Thomas A, Weinhouse S (1953) Metabolism of neoplastic tissue. IV. A study of lipid synthesis in neoplastic tissue slices in vitro. Cancer Res 13(1):27–29, 61
61. Luo X, Cheng C, Tan Z Li N, Tang M, Yang L et al (2017) Emerging roles of lipid metabolism in cancer metastasis. Mol Cancer 16:76. https://doi.org/10.1186/s12943-017-0646-3
62. Liu Q, Luo Q, Halim A, Song G (2017) Targeting lipid metabolism of cancer cells: a promising therapeutic strategy for cancer. Cancer Lett 401:39–45. https://doi.org/10.1016/j.canlet.2017.05.002
63. Currie E, Schulze A, Zechner R, Walther TC, Farese RV Jr (2013) Cellular fatty acid metabolism and cancer. Cell Metab 18(2):153–161. https://doi.org/10.1016/j.cmet.2013.05.017
64. Chen WL, Jin X, Wang M, Liu D, Luo Q, Tian H et al (2020) GLUT5-mediated fructose utilization drives lung cancer growth by stimulating fatty acid synthesis and AMPK/mTORC1 signaling. JCI Insight 5(3). https://doi.org/10.1172/jci.insight.131596
65. Zaytseva YY, Elliott VA, Rychahou P, Mustain WC, Kim JT, Valentino J et al (2014) Cancer cell-associated fatty acid synthase activates endothelial cells and promotes angiogenesis in colorectal cancer. Carcinogenesis 35(6):1341–1351. https://doi.org/10.1093/carcin/bgu042
66. Baenke F, Peck B, Miess H, Schulze A (2013) Hooked on fat: the role of lipid synthesis in cancer metabolism and tumour development. Dis Model Mech 6(6):1353–1363. https://doi.org/10.1242/dmm.011338
67. Dierge E, Larondelle Y, Feron O (2020) Cancer diets for cancer patients: lessons from mouse studies and new insights from the study of fatty acid metabolism in tumors. Biochimie 178:56–68. https://doi.org/10.1016/j.biochi.2020.08.020
68. Griffiths B, Lewis CA, Bensaad K, Ros S, Zhang Q, Ferber EC et al (2013) Sterol regulatory element binding protein-dependent regulation of lipid synthesis supports cell survival and tumor growth. Cancer Metab. 1(1):3. https://doi.org/10.1186/2049-3002-1-3
69. Amiri M, Yousefnia S, Seyed Forootan F, Peymani M, Ghaedi K, Nasr Esfahani MH (2018) Diverse roles of fatty acid binding proteins (FABPs) in development and pathogenesis of cancers. Gene 676:171–183. https://doi.org/10.1016/j.gene.2018.07.035
70. Fu Y, Zou T, Shen X, Nelson PJ, Li J, Wu C et al (2020) Lipid metabolism in cancer progression and therapeutic strategies. MedComm 2(1):27–59. https://doi.org/10.1002/mco2.27
71. Su X, Abumrad NA (2009) Cellular fatty acid uptake: a pathway under construction. Trends Endocrinol Metab 20(2):72–77. https://doi.org/10.1016/j.tem.2008.11.001
72. Long J, Zhang CJ, Zhu N, Du K, Yin YF, Tan X et al (2018) Lipid metabolism and carcinogenesis, cancer development. Am J Cancer Res 8(5):778–791

73. Petan T (2020) Lipid droplets in cancer. Rev Physiol Biochem Pharmacol. https://doi.org/10.1007/112_2020_51
74. Li Z, Liu H, Luo X (2020) Lipid droplet and its implication in cancer progression. Am J Cancer Res 10(12):4112–4122
75. Corbet C, Bastien E, Santiago de Jesus JP, Dierge E, Martherus R, Vander Linden C et al (2020) TGFbeta2-induced formation of lipid droplets supports acidosis-driven EMT and the metastatic spreading of cancer cells. Nat Commun 11(1):454. https://doi.org/10.1038/s41467-019-14262-3
76. Menard JA, Christianson HC, Kucharzewska P, Bourseau-Guilmain E, Svensson KJ, Lindqvist E et al (2016) Metastasis stimulation by hypoxia and acidosis-induced extracellular lipid uptake is mediated by proteoglycan-dependent endocytosis. Cancer Res 76(16):4828–4840. https://doi.org/10.1158/0008-5472.CAN-15-2831
77. Sung H, Ferlay J, Siegel RL, Laversanne M, Soerjomataram I, Jemal A et al (2021) Global cancer statistics 2020: GLOBOCAN sstimates of incidence and mortality worldwide for 36 cancers in 185 countries. CA Cancer J Clin 71(3):209–249. https://doi.org/10.3322/caac.21660
78. Bray F, Ferlay J, Soerjomataram I, Siegel RL, Torre LA, Jemal A (2018) Global cancer statistics 2018: GLOBOCAN estimates of incidence and mortality worldwide for 36 cancers in 185 countries. CA Cancer J Clin 68(6):394–424. https://doi.org/10.3322/caac.21492
79. Kubo A, Block G, Quesenberry CP Jr, Buffler P, Corley DA (2009) Effects of dietary fiber, fats, and meat intakes on the risk of Barrett's esophagus. Nutr Cancer 61(5):607–616. https://doi.org/10.1080/01635580902846585
80. Zamani SA, McClain KM, Graubard BI, Liao LM, Abnet CC, Cook MB et al (2020) Dietary polyunsaturated fat intake in relation to head and neck, esophageal, and gastric cancer incidence in the national institutes of health-AARP diet and health study. Am J Epidemiol 189(10):1096–1113. https://doi.org/10.1093/aje/kwaa024
81. Wang J, Zhang Y, Zhao L (2020) Omega-3 PUFA intake and the risk of digestive system cancers: a meta-analysis of observational studies. Medicine (Baltimore) 99(19):e20119. https://doi.org/10.1097/MD.0000000000020119
82. Lee S, Lee J, Choi IJ, Kim YW, Ryu KW, Kim YI et al (2018) Dietary n-3 and n-6 polyunsaturated fatty acids, the FADS gene, and the risk of gastric cancer in a Korean population. Sci Rep 8(1):3823. https://doi.org/10.1038/s41598-018-21960-3
83. Norat T, Bingham S, Ferrari P, Slimani N, Jenab M, Mazuir M et al (2005) Meat, fish, and colorectal cancer risk: the European prospective investigation into cancer and nutrition. J Natl Cancer Inst 97(12):906–916. https://doi.org/10.1093/jnci/dji164
84. Chao A, Thun MJ, Connell CJ, McCullough ML, Jacobs EJ, Flanders WD et al (2005) Meat consumption and risk of colorectal cancer. JAMA 293(2):172–182. https://doi.org/10.1001/jama.293.2.172
85. Aglago EK, Huybrechts I, Murphy N, Casagrande C, Nicolas G, Pischon T et al (2020) Consumption of fish and long-chain n-3 polyunsaturated fatty acids is associated with reduced risk of colorectal cancer in a large European cohort. Clin Gastroenterol Hepatol 18(3):654–666, e6. https://doi.org/10.1016/j.cgh.2019.06.031
86. Kim Y, Kim J (2020) Intake or blood levels of n-3 polyunsaturated fatty acids and risk of colorectal cancer: a systematic review and meta-analysis of prospective studies. Cancer Epidemiol Biomarkers Prev 29(2):288–299. https://doi.org/10.1158/1055-9965.EPI-19-0931
87. Butler LM, Yuan JM, Huang JY, Su J, Wang R, Koh WP et al (2017) Plasma fatty acids and risk of colon and rectal cancers in the Singapore Chinese health study. NPJ Precis Oncol 1(1):38. https://doi.org/10.1038/s41698-017-0040-z
88. May-Wilson S, Sud A, Law PJ, Palin K, Tuupanen S, Gylfe A et al (2017) Pro-inflammatory fatty acid profile and colorectal cancer risk: a Mendelian randomisation analysis. Eur J Cancer 84:228–238. https://doi.org/10.1016/j.ejca.2017.07.034
89. Kojima M, Wakai K, Tokudome S, Suzuki K, Tamakoshi K, Watanabe Y et al (2005) Serum levels of polyunsaturated fatty acids and risk of colorectal cancer: a prospective study. Am J Epidemiol 161(5):462–471. https://doi.org/10.1093/aje/kwi066

90. Shen XJ, Zhou JD, Dong JY, Ding WQ, Wu JC (2012) Dietary intake of n-3 fatty acids and colorectal cancer risk: a meta-analysis of data from 489 000 individuals. Br J Nutr 108(9):1550–1556. https://doi.org/10.1017/S0007114512003546
91. Chen GC, Qin LQ, Lu DB, Han TM, Zheng Y, Xu GZ et al (2015) N-3 polyunsaturated fatty acids intake and risk of colorectal cancer: meta-analysis of prospective studies Cancer Causes Control 26(1):133–141. https://doi.org/10.1007/s10552-014-0492-1
92. Mattiuzzi C, Lippi G (2019) Current cancer epidemiology. J Epidemiol Glob Health 9(4):217–222. https://doi.org/10.2991/jegh.k.191008.001
93. Berquin IM, Edwards IJ, Kridel SJ, Chen YQ (2011) Polyunsaturated fatty acid metabolism in prostate cancer. Cancer Metastasis Rev 30(3–4):295–309. https://doi.org/10.1007/s10555-011-9299-7
94. Di Sebastiano KM, Mourtzakis M (2014) The role of dietary fat throughout the prostate cancer trajectory. Nutrients 6(12):6095–6109. https://doi.org/10.3390/nu6126095
95. Lin PH, Aronson W, Freedland SJ (2015) Nutrition, dietary interventions and prostate cancer: the latest evidence. BMC Med 13:3. https://doi.org/10.1186/s12916-014-0234-y
96. Castello A, Boldo E, Amiano P, Castano-Vinyals G, Aragones N, Gomez-Acebo I et al (2018) Mediterranean dietary pattern is associated with low risk of aggressive prostate cancer: MCC-Spain study. J Urol 199(2):430–437. https://doi.org/10.1016/j.juro.2017.08.087
97. Gregg JR, Zhang X, Chapin BF, Ward JF, Kim J, Davis JW et al (2021) Adherence to the Mediterranean diet and grade group progression in localized prostate cancer: an active surveillance cohort. Cancer 127(5):720–728. https://doi.org/10.1002/cncr.33182
98. Chavarro JE, Stampfer MJ, Li H, Campos H, Kurth T, Ma J (2007) A prospective study of polyunsaturated fatty acid levels in blood and prostate cancer risk. Cancer Epidemiol Biomarkers Prev 16(7):1364–1370. https://doi.org/10.1158/1055-9965.EPI-06-1033
99. Brasky TM, Darke AK, Song X, Tangen CM, Goodman PJ, Thompson IM et al (2013) Plasma phospholipid fatty acids and prostate cancer risk in the SELECT trial. J Natl Cancer Inst 105(15):1132–1141. https://doi.org/10.1093/jnci/djt174
100. Brasky TM, Till C, White E, Neuhouser ML, Song X, Goodman P et al (2011) Serum phospholipid fatty acids and prostate cancer risk: results from the prostate cancer prevention trial. Am J Epidemiol 173(12):1429–1439. https://doi.org/10.1093/aje/kwr027
101. Aucoin M, Cooley K, Knee C, Fritz H, Balneaves LG, Breau R et al (2017) Fish-derived omega-3 fatty acids and prostate cancer: a systematic review. Integr Cancer Ther 16(1):32–62. https://doi.org/10.1177/1534735416656052
102. Siddiqui F, Vaqar S, Siddiqui AH (2022) Lung cancer. In: StatPearls [Internet]. StatPearls Publishing, Treasure Island
103. Liu J, Mazzone PJ, Cata JP, Kurz A, Bauer M, Mascha EJ et al (2014) Serum free fatty acid biomarkers of lung cancer. Chest 146(3):670–679. https://doi.org/10.1378/chest.13-2568
104. Montecillo-Aguado M, Tirado-Rodriguez B, Antonio-Andres G, Morales-Martinez M, Tong Z, Yang J et al (2022) Omega-6 polyunsaturated fatty acids enhance tumor aggressiveness in experimental lung cancer model: important role of oxylipins. Int J Mol Sci 23(11). https://doi.org/10.3390/ijms23116179
105. Tao X, Zhou Q, Rao Z (2022) Efficacy of ω-3 polyunsaturated fatty acids in patients with lung cancer undergoing radiotherapy and chemotherapy: a meta-analysis. Int J Clin Pract 2022:6564466. https://doi.org/10.1155/2022/6564466
106. Luu HN, Cai H, Murff HJ, Xiang YB, Cai Q, Li H et al (2018) A prospective study of dietary polyunsaturated fatty acids intake and lung cancer risk. Int J Cancer 143(9):2225–2237. https://doi.org/10.1002/ijc.31608
107. Azrad M, Turgeon C, Demark-Wahnefried W (2013) Current evidence linking polyunsaturated fatty acids with cancer risk and progression. Front Oncol 3:224. https://doi.org/10.3389/fonc.2013.00224
108. Wakai K, Tamakoshi K, Date C, Fukui M, Suzuki S, Lin Y et al (2005) Dietary intakes of fat and fatty acids and risk of breast cancer: a prospective study in Japan. Cancer Sci 96(9):590–599. https://doi.org/10.1111/j.1349-7006.2005.00084.x

109. Gago-Dominguez M, Yuan JM, Sun CL, Lee HP, Yu MC (2003) Opposing effects of dietary n-3 and n-6 fatty acids on mammary carcinogenesis: the Singapore Chinese health study. Br J Cancer 89(9):1686–1692. https://doi.org/10.1038/sj.bjc.6601340
110. Kim J, Lim SY, Shin A, Sung MK, Ro J, Kang HS et al (2009) Fatty fish and fish omega-3 fatty acid intakes decrease the breast cancer risk: a case-control study. BMC Cancer 9:216. https://doi.org/10.1186/1471-2407-9-216
111. Maillard V, Bougnoux P, Ferrari P, Jourdan ML, Pinault M, Lavillonniere F et al (2002) N-3 and N-6 fatty acids in breast adipose tissue and relative risk of breast cancer in a case-control study in Tours, France. Int J Cancer 98(1):78–83. https://doi.org/10.1002/ijc.10130
112. Kuriki K, Hirose K, Wakai K, Matsuo K, Ito H, Suzuki T et al (2007) Breast cancer risk and erythrocyte compositions of n-3 highly unsaturated fatty acids in Japanese. Int J Cancer 121(2):377–385. https://doi.org/10.1002/ijc.22682
113. Engeset D, Alsaker E, Lund E, Welch A, Khaw KT, Clavel-Chapelon F et al (2006) Fish consumption and breast cancer risk. The European prospective investigation into cancer and nutrition (EPIC). Int J Cancer 119(1):175–182. https://doi.org/10.1002/ijc.21819
114. Manson JE, Cook NR, Lee IM, Christen W, Bassuk SS, Mora S et al (2019) Marine n-3 fatty acids and prevention of cardiovascular disease and cancer. N Engl J Med 380(1):23–32. https://doi.org/10.1056/NEJMoa1811403
115. Cao Y, Hou L, Wang W (2016) Dietary total fat and fatty acids intake, serum fatty acids and risk of breast cancer: a meta-analysis of prospective cohort studies. Int J Cancer 138(8):1894–1904. https://doi.org/10.1002/ijc.29938
116. Liu J, Li X, Hou J, Sun J, Guo N, Wang Z (2021) Dietary intake of N-3 and N-6 polyunsaturated fatty acids and risk of cancer: meta-analysis of data from 32 studies. Nutr Cancer 73(6):901–913. https://doi.org/10.1080/01635581.2020.1779321
117. Montecillo-Aguado M, Tirado-Rodriguez B, Tong Z, Vega OM, Morales-Martinez M, Abkenari S et al (2020) Importance of the role of omega-3 and omega-6 polyunsaturated fatty acids in the progression of brain cancer. Brain Sci 10(6):381. https://doi.org/10.3390/brainsci10060381
118. Lian W, Wang R, Xing B, Yao Y (2017) Fish intake and the risk of brain tumor: a meta-analysis with systematic review. Nutr J 16(1):1. https://doi.org/10.1186/s12937-016-0223-4
119. Joffre C, Rey C, Laye S (2019) N-3 polyunsaturated fatty acids and the resolution of neuroinflammation. Front Pharmacol 10:1022. https://doi.org/10.3389/fphar.2019.01022
120. Ferreira MT, Gomes RN, Panagopoulos AT, de Almeida FG, Veiga JCE, Colquhoun A (2018) Opposing roles of PGD2 in GBM. Prostaglandins Other Lipid Mediat 134:66–76. https://doi.org/10.1016/j.prostaglandins.2017.10.002
121. Serhan CN, Hong S, Gronert K, Colgan SP, Devchand PR, Mirick G et al (2002) Resolvins: a family of bioactive products of omega-3 fatty acid transformation circuits initiated by aspirin treatment that counter proinflammation signals. J Exp Med 196(8):1025–1037. https://doi.org/10.1084/jem.20020760
122. Hong S, Gronert K, Devchand PR, Moussignac RL, Serhan CN (2003) Novel docosatrienes and 17S-resolvins generated from docosahexaenoic acid in murine brain, human blood, and glial cells. Autacoids in anti-inflammation. J Biol Chem 278(17):14677–14687. https://doi.org/10.1074/jbc.M300218200
123. Svensson CI, Zattoni M, Serhan CN (2007) Lipoxins and aspirin-triggered lipoxin inhibit inflammatory pain processing. J Exp Med 204(2):245–252. https://doi.org/10.1084/jem.20061826
124. Corsetto PA, Montorfano G, Zava S, Jovenitti IE, Cremona A, Berra B et al (2011) Effects of n-3 PUFAs on breast cancer cells through their incorporation in plasma membrane. Lipids Health Dis 10:73. https://doi.org/10.1186/1476-511X-10-73
125. Rifkin SB, Shrubsole MJ, Cai Q, Smalley WE, Ness RM, Swift LL et al (2017) PUFA levels in erythrocyte membrane phospholipids are differentially associated with colorectal adenoma risk. Br J Nutr 117(11):1615–1622. https://doi.org/10.1017/S0007114517001490

126. Sawada N, Inoue M, Iwasaki M, Sasazuki S, Shimazu T, Yamaji T et al (2012) Consumption of n-3 fatty acids and fish reduces risk of hepatocellular carcinoma. Gastroenterology 142(7):1468–1475. https://doi.org/10.1053/j.gastro.2012.02.018
127. Shannon J, O'Malley J, Mori M, Garzotto M, Palma AJ, King IB (2010) Erythrocyte fatty acids and prostate cancer risk: a comparison of methods. Prostaglandins Leukot Essent Fatty Acids 83(3):161–169. https://doi.org/10.1016/j.plefa.2010.06.003
128. Kökoğlu E, Tüter Y, Yazici Z, Sandikci KS, Sönmez H, Ulakoğlu EZ et al (1998) Profiles of the fatty acids in the plasma membrane of human brain tumors. Cancer Biochem Biophys 16(4):301–312
129. Mika A, Kobiela J, Pakiet A, Czumaj A, Sokolowska E, Makarewicz W et al (2020) Preferential uptake of polyunsaturated fatty acids by colorectal cancer cells. Sci Rep 10(1):1954. https://doi.org/10.1038/s41598-020-58895-7
130. Tu M, Wang W, Zhang G, Hammock BD (2020) Omega-3 polyunsaturated fatty acids on colonic inflammation and colon cancer: roles of lipid-metabolizing enzymes involved. Nutrients 12(11). https://doi.org/10.3390/nu12113301
131. Bagga D, Wang L, Farias-Eisner R, Glaspy JA, Reddy ST (2003) Differential effects of prostaglandin derived from omega-6 and omega-3 polyunsaturated fatty acids on COX-2 expression and IL-6 secretion. Proc Natl Acad Sci U S A 100(4):1751–1756. https://doi.org/10.1073/pnas.0334211100
132. Basil MC, Levy BD (2016) Specialized pro-resolving mediators: endogenous regulators of infection and inflammation. Nat Rev Immunol 16(1):51–67. https://doi.org/10.1038/nri.2015.4
133. Lavy M, Gauttier V, Poirier N, Barille-Nion S, Blanquart C (2021) Specialized pro-resolving mediators mitigate cancer-related inflammation: role of tumor-associated macrophages and therapeutic opportunities. Front Immunol 12:702785. https://doi.org/10.3389/fimmu.2021.702785
134. Ungprasert P, Cheungpasitporn W, Crowson CS, Matteson EL (2015) Individual non-steroidal anti-inflammatory drugs and risk of acute kidney injury: a systematic review and meta-analysis of observational studies. Eur J Intern Med 26(4):285–291. https://doi.org/10.1016/j.ejim.2015.03.008
135. Zhuang Q, Meng Q, Xi Q, Wu G (2018) Association of serum inflammatory cytokines and Resolvin D1 concentration with pathological stage of colon cancer. Zhonghua Wei Chang Wai Ke Za Zhi 21(11):1285–1290
136. Fedirko V, McKeown-Eyssen G, Serhan CN, Barry EL, Sandler RS, Figueiredo JC et al (2017) Plasma lipoxin A4 and resolvin D1 are not associated with reduced adenoma risk in a randomized trial of aspirin to prevent colon adenomas. Mol Carcinog 56(8):1977–1983. https://doi.org/10.1002/mc.22629
137. Blogowski W, Dolegowska K, Deskur A, Dolegowska B, Starzynska T (2022) Lipoxins and resolvins in patients with pancreatic cancer: a preliminary report. Front Oncol 11:757073. https://doi.org/10.3389/fonc.2021.757073
138. Ungaro F, D'Alessio S, Danese S (2020) The role of pro-resolving lipid mediators in colorectal cancer-associated inflammation: implications for therapeutic strategies. Cancers (Basel) 12(8). https://doi.org/10.3390/cancers12082060
139. Jelic MD, Mandic AD, Maricic SM, Srdjenovic BU (2021) Oxidative stress and its role in cancer. J Cancer Res Ther 17(1):22–28. https://doi.org/10.4103/jcrt.JCRT_862_16
140. Kawanishi S, Hiraku Y, Pinlaor S, Ma N (2006) Oxidative and nitrative DNA damage in animals and patients with inflammatory diseases in relation to inflammation-related carcinogenesis. Biol Chem 387(4):365–372. https://doi.org/10.1515/BC.2006.049
141. Finocchiaro C, Segre O, Fadda M, Monge T, Scigliano M, Schena M et al (2012) Effect of n-3 fatty acids on patients with advanced lung cancer: a double-blind, placebo-controlled study. Br J Nutr 108(2):327–333. https://doi.org/10.1017/S0007114511005551

142. Elbarbary NS, Ismail EA, Farahat RK, El-Hamamsy M (2016) Omega-3 fatty acids as an adjuvant therapy ameliorates methotrexate-induced hepatotoxicity in children and adolescents with acute lymphoblastic leukemia: a randomized placebo-controlled study. Nutrition 32(1):41–47. https://doi.org/10.1016/j.nut.2015.06.010
143. Mansara P, Ketkar M, Deshpande R, Chaudhary A, Shinde K, Kaul-Ghanekar R (2015) Improved antioxidant status by omega-3 fatty acid supplementation in breast cancer patients undergoing chemotherapy: a case series. J Med Case Rep 9:148. https://doi.org/10.1186/s13256-015-0619-3
144. Kang KS, Wang P, Yamabe N, Fukui M, Jay T, Zhu BT (2010) Docosahexaenoic acid induces apoptosis in MCF-7 cells in vitro and in vivo via reactive oxygen species formation and caspase 8 activation. PLoS ONE 5(4):e10296. https://doi.org/10.1371/journal.pone.0010296
145. Leaver HA, Bell HS, Rizzo MT, Ironside JW, Gregor A, Wharton SB et al (2002) Antitumour and pro-apoptotic actions of highly unsaturated fatty acids in glioma. Prostaglandins Leukot Essent Fatty Acids 66(1):19–29. https://doi.org/10.1054/plef.2001.0336
146. Jayathilake AG, Kadife E, Luwor RB, Nurgali K, Su XQ (2019) Krill oil extract suppresses the proliferation of colorectal cancer cells through activation of caspase 3/9. Nutr Metab (Lond) 16:53. https://doi.org/10.1186/s12986-019-0382-3
147. Sun HMX, Han J, Zhang Z, Wang B, Bai X, Zhang X (2013) Anti-cancer activity of DHA on gastric cancer—an in vitro and in vivo study. Tumour Biol 34(6):3791–3800. https://doi.org/10.1007/s13277-013-0963-0
148. So WW, Liu WN, Leung KN (2015) Omega-3 polyunsaturated fatty acids trigger cell cycle arrest and induce apoptosis in human neuroblastoma LA-N-1 cells. Nutrients 7(8):6956–6973. https://doi.org/10.3390/nu7085319
149. Song KS, Jing K, Kim JS, Yun EJ, Shin S, Seo KS et al (2011) Omega-3-polyunsaturated fatty acids suppress pancreatic cancer cell growth in vitro and in vivo via downregulation of Wnt/Beta-catenin signaling. Pancreatology 11(6):574–584. https://doi.org/10.1159/000334468
150. Lim K, Han C, Dai Y, Shen M, Wu T (2009) Omega-3 polyunsaturated fatty acids inhibit hepatocellular carcinoma cell growth through blocking beta-catenin and cyclooxygenase-2. Mol Cancer Ther 8(11):3046–3055. https://doi.org/10.1158/1535-7163.MCT-09-0551
151. West L, Yin Y, Pierce SR, Fang Z, Fan Y, Sun W et al (2020) Docosahexaenoic acid (DHA), an omega-3 fatty acid, inhibits tumor growth and metastatic potential of ovarian cancer. Am J Cancer Res 10(12):4450–4463
152. Nishida N, Yano H, Nishida T, Kamura T, Kojiro M (2006) Angiogenesis in cancer. Vasc Health Risk Manag 2(3):213–219. https://doi.org/10.2147/vhrm.2006.2.3.213
153. Iigo M, Nakagawa T, Ishikawa C, Iwahori Y, Asamoto M, Yazawa K et al (1997) Inhibitory effects of docosahexaenoic acid on colon carcinoma 26 metastasis to the lung. Br J Cancer 75(5):650–655. https://doi.org/10.1038/bjc.1997.116
154. Suzuki I, Iigo M, Ishikawa C, Kuhara T, Asamoto M, Kunimoto T et al (1997) Inhibitory effects of oleic and docosahexaenoic acids on lung metastasis by colon-carcinoma-26 cells are associated with reduced matrix metalloproteinase-2 and -9 activities. Int J Cancer. 73: 607–12. https://doi.org/10.1002/(SICI)1097-0215(19971114)73:4<607::AID-IJC24>3.0.CO;2-4
155. Khojastehfard M, Dolatkhah H, Somi MH, Nazari Soltan Ahmad S, Estakhri R, Sharifi R et al (2019) The effect of oral administration of PUFAs on the matrix metalloproteinase expression in gastric adenocarcinoma patients undergoing chemotherapy. Nutr Cancer 71(3):444–451. https://doi.org/10.1080/01635581.2018.1506494
156. Zhang G, Panigrahy D, Mahakian LM, Yang J, Liu JY, Stephen Lee KS et al (2013) Epoxy metabolites of docosahexaenoic acid (DHA) inhibit angiogenesis, tumor growth, and metastasis. Proc Natl Acad Sci U S A 110(16):6530–6535. https://doi.org/10.1073/pnas.1304321110
157. Mandal CC, Ghosh-Choudhury T, Dey N, Choudhury GG, Ghosh-Choudhury N (2012) MiR-21 is targeted by omega-3 polyunsaturated fatty acid to regulate breast tumor CSF-1 expression. Carcinogenesis 33(10):1897–1908. https://doi.org/10.1093/carcin/bgs198

158. Bilodeau JF, Gevariya N, Larose J, Robitaille K, Roy J, Oger C et al (2021) Long chain omega-3 fatty acids and their oxidized metabolites are associated with reduced prostate tumor growth. Prostaglandins Leukot Essent Fatty Acids 164:102215. https://doi.org/10.1016/j.plefa.2020.102215
159. Comba A, Lin YH, Eynard AR, Valentich MA, Fernandez-Zapico ME, Pasqualini ME (2011) Basic aspects of tumor cell fatty acid-regulated signaling and transcription factors. Cancer Metastasis Rev 30:325–342. https://doi.org/10.1007/s10555-011-9308-x
160. Wagner N, Wagner KD (2020) The role of PPARs in disease. Cells 9(11). https://doi.org/10.3390/cells9112367
161. Cheng HS, Yip YS, Lim EKY, Wahli W, Tan NS (2021) PPARs and tumor microenvironment: the emerging roles of the metabolic master regulators in tumor stromal-epithelial crosstalk and carcinogenesis. Cancers (Basel) 13(9). https://doi.org/10.3390/cancers13092153
162. Peters JM, Cheung C, Gonzalez FJ (2005) Peroxisome proliferator-activated receptor-alpha and liver cancer: where do we stand? J Mol Med (Berl) 83(10):774–785. https://doi.org/10.1007/s00109-005-0678-9
163. Grommes C, Landreth GE, Heneka MT (2004) Antineoplastic effects of peroxisome proliferatoractivated receptor γ agonists. Lancet Oncol 5(7):419–429. https://doi.org/10.1016/s1470-2045(04)01509-8
164. Maggiora M, Oraldi M, Muzio G, Canuto RA (2010) Involvement of PPARα and PPARγ in apoptosis and proliferation of human hepatocarcinoma HepG2 cells. Cell Biochem Funct 28(7):571–577. https://doi.org/10.1002/cbf.1691
165. Murray NR, Weems C, Chen L, Leon J, Yu W, Davidson LA et al (2002) Protein kinase C betaII and TGFbetaRII in omega-3 fatty acid-mediated inhibition of colon carcinogenesis. J Cell Biol 157(6):915–920. https://doi.org/10.1083/jcb.200201127
166. Schley PD, Jijon HB, Robinson LE, Field CJ (2005) Mechanisms of omega-3 fatty acid-induced growth inhibition in MDA-MB-231 human breast cancer cells. Breast Cancer Res Treat 92(2):187–195. https://doi.org/10.1007/s10549-005-2415-z
167. Cavazos DA, Price RS, Apte SS, deGraffenried LA (2011) Docosahexaenoic acid selectively induces human prostate cancer cell sensitivity to oxidative stress through modulation of NF-κB. Prostate 71(13):1420–1428. https://doi.org/10.1002/pros.21359
168. Jiang T, Zhang G, Lou Z (2020) Role of the sterol regulatory element binding protein pathway in tumorigenesis. Front Oncol 10:1788. https://doi.org/10.3389/fonc.2020.01788
169. Cheng C, Geng F, Cheng X, Guo D (2018) Lipid metabolism reprogramming and its potential targets in cancer. Cancer Commun (Lond) 38(1):27. https://doi.org/10.1186/s40880-018-0301-4
170. Huang LH, Chung HY, Su HM (2017) Docosahexaenoic acid reduces sterol regulatory element binding protein-1 and fatty acid synthase expression and inhibits cell proliferation by inhibiting pAkt signaling in a human breast cancer MCF-7 cell line. BMC Cancer 17(1):890. https://doi.org/10.1186/s12885-017-3936-7
171. D'Alterio C, Scala S, Sozzi G, Roz L, Bertolini G (2020) Paradoxical effects of chemotherapy on tumor relapse and metastasis promotion. Semin Cancer Biol 60:351–361. https://doi.org/10.1016/j.semcancer.2019.08.019
172. Wang J, Luo T, Li S, Zhao J (2012) The powerful applications of polyunsaturated fatty acids in improving the therapeutic efficacy of anticancer drugs. Expert Opin Drug Deliv 9(1):1–7. https://doi.org/10.1517/17425247.2011.618183
173. Gu Z, Shan K, Chen H, Chen YQ (2015) N-3 polyunsaturated fatty acids and their role in cancer chemoprevention. Curr Pharmacol Rep 1(5):283–294. https://doi.org/10.1007/s40495-015-0043-9
174. Miccadei S, Masella R, Mileo AM, Gessani S (2016) Omega3 polyunsaturated fatty acids as immunomodulators in colorectal cancer: new potential role in adjuvant therapies. Front Immunol 7:486. https://doi.org/10.3389/fimmu.2016.00486
175. Corsetto PA, Colombo I, Kopecka J, Rizzo AM, Riganti C (2017) Omega-3 long chain polyunsaturated fatty acids as sensitizing agents and multidrug resistance revertants in cancer therapy. Int J Mol Sci 18(12). https://doi.org/10.3390/ijms18122770

176. Gelsomino G, Corsetto PA, Campia I, Montorfano G, Kopecka J, Castella B et al (2013) Omega 3 fatty acids chemosensitize multidrug resistant colon cancer cells by down-regulating cholesterol synthesis and altering detergent resistant membranes composition. Mol Cancer 12:137. https://doi.org/10.1186/1476-4598-12-137
177. Slagsvold JE, Pettersen CH, Storvold GL, Follestad T, Krokan HE, Schonberg SA (2010) DHA alters expression of target proteins of cancer therapy in chemotherapy resistant SW620 colon cancer cells. Nutr Cancer 62(5):611–621. https://doi.org/10.1080/01635580903532366
178. Wei L, Wu Z, Chen YQ (2022) Multi-targeted therapy of cancer by omega-3 fatty acids-an update. Cancer Lett 526:193–204. https://doi.org/10.1016/j.canlet.2021.11.023
179. Colas S, Maheo K, Denis F, Goupille C, Hoinard C, Champeroux P et al (2006) Sensitization by dietary docosahexaenoic acid of rat mammary carcinoma to anthracycline: a role for tumor vascularization. Clin Cancer Res 12(19):5879–5886. https://doi.org/10.1158/1078-0432.CCR-06-0386
180. Hardman WE, Avula CP, Fernandes G, Cameron IL (2001) Three percent dietary fish oil concentrate increased efficacy of doxorubicin against MDA-MB 231 breast cancer xenografts. Clin Cancer Res 7(7):2041–2049
181. Kornfeld S, Goupille C, Vibet S, Chevalier S, Pinet A, Lebeau J et al (2012) Reducing endothelial NOS activation and interstitial fluid pressure with n-3 PUFA offset tumor chemoresistance. Carcinogenesis 33(2):260–267. https://doi.org/10.1093/carcin/bgr274
182. Gottesman MM, Fojo T, Bates SE (2002) Multidrug resistance in cancer: role of ATP-dependent transporters. Nat Rev Cancer 2(1):48–58. https://doi.org/10.1038/nrc706
183. Siddiqui RA, Harvey KA, Xu Z, Bammerlin EM, Walker C, Altenburg JD (2011) Docosahexaenoic acid: a natural powerful adjuvant that improves efficacy for anticancer treatment with no adverse effects. BioFactors 37(6):399–412. https://doi.org/10.1002/biof.181
184. Vaughan VC, Hassing MR, Lewandowski PA (2013) Marine polyunsaturated fatty acids and cancer therapy. Br J Cancer 108(3):486–492. https://doi.org/10.1038/bjc.2012.586
185. Arshad A, Chung WY, Steward W, Metcalfe MS, Dennison AR (2013) Reduction in circulating pro-angiogenic and pro-inflammatory factors is related to improved outcomes in patients with advanced pancreatic cancer treated with gemcitabine and intravenous omega-3 fish oil. HPB (Oxford) 15(6):428–432. https://doi.org/10.1111/hpb.12002
186. Caruso R, Nanni MG, Riba M, Sabato S, Mitchell AJ, Croce E et al (2017) Depressive spectrum disorders in cancer: prevalence, risk factors and screening for depression: a critical review. Acta Oncol 56(2):146–155. https://doi.org/10.1080/0284186X.2016.1266090
187. Young K, Singh G (2018) Biological mechanisms of cancer-induced depression. Front Psychiatry 9:299. https://doi.org/10.3389/fpsyt.2018.00299
188. Bigornia SJ, Harris WS, Falcon LM, Ordovas JM, Lai CQ, Tucker KL (2016) The omega-3 index is inversely associated with depressive symptoms among individuals with elevated oxidative stress biomarkers. J Nutr 146(4):758–766. https://doi.org/10.3945/jn.115.222562
189. Freitas RDS, Campos MM (2019) Protective effects of omega-3 fatty acids in cancer-related complications. Nutrients 11(5). https://doi.org/10.3390/nu11050945
190. Ryan AM, Power DG, Daly L, Cushen SJ, Ni Bhuachalla E, Prado CM (2016) Cancer-associated malnutrition, cachexia and sarcopenia: the skeleton in the hospital closet 40 years later. Proc Nutr Soc 75(2):199–211. https://doi.org/10.1017/S002966511500419X
191. Argilés JM, Busquets S, Stemmler B, López-Soriano FJ (2014) Cancer cachexia: understanding the molecular basis. Nat Rev Cancer 14(11):754–762. https://doi.org/10.1038/nrc3829
192. Bachmann J, Heiligensetzer M, Krakowski-Roosen H, Buchler MW, Friess H, Martignoni ME (2008) Cachexia worsens prognosis in patients with resectable pancreatic cancer. J Gastrointest Surg 12(7):1193–1201. https://doi.org/10.1007/s11605-008-0505-z
193. Fearon KC, Von Meyenfeldt MF, Moses AG, Van Geenen R, Roy A, Gouma DJ et al (2003) Effect of a protein and energy dense n-3 fatty acid enriched oral supplement on loss of weight and lean tissue in cancer cachexia: a randomised double blind trial. Gut 52(10):1479–1486. https://doi.org/10.1136/gut.52.10.1479

194. Sanchez-Lara K, Turcott JG, Juarez-Hernandez E, Nunez-Valencia C, Villanueva G, Guevara P et al (2014) Effects of an oral nutritional supplement containing eicosapentaenoic acid on nutritional and clinical outcomes in patients with advanced non-small cell lung cancer: randomised trial. Clin Nutr 33(6):1017–1023. https://doi.org/10.1016/j.clnu.2014.03.006
195. Taylor LA, Pletschen L, Arends J, Unger C, Massing U (2010) Marine phospholipids—a promising new dietary approach to tumor-associated weight loss. Support Care Cancer 18(2):159–170. https://doi.org/10.1007/s00520-009-0640-4
196. Murphy RA, Yeung E, Mazurak VC, Mourtzakis M (2011) Influence of eicosapentaenoic acid supplementation on lean body mass in cancer cachexia. Br J Cancer 105(10):1469–1473. https://doi.org/10.1038/bjc.2011.391
197. Murphy RA, Mourtzakis M, Mazurak VC (2012) N-3 polyunsaturated fatty acids: the potential role for supplementation in cancer. Curr Opin Clin Nutr Metab Care 15(3):246–251. https://doi.org/10.1097/MCO.0b013e328351c32f
198. Muscaritoli M, Arends J, Bachmann P, Baracos V, Barthelemy N, Bertz H et al (2021) ESPEN practical guideline: clinical nutrition in cancer. Clin Nutr 40(5):2898–2913. https://doi.org/10.1016/j.clnu.2021.02.005
199. EFSA (2012) EFSA panel on dietetic products. Nutrition and allergy (NDA). Scientific opinion on the tolerable upper intake level of eicosapentaenoic acid (EPA), docosahexaenoic acid (DH) and docosapentaenoic acid (DPA). EFSA J 10(7):2815
200. Food and Drug Administration (FDA) (1997) 62(108):62 FR 30751, 6 pp
201. Skarke C, Alamuddin N, Lawson JA, Li X, Ferguson JF, Reilly MP et al (2015) Bioactive products formed in humans from fish oils. J Lipid Res 56(9):1808–1820. https://doi.org/10.1194/jlr.M060392
202. Malinowski SS, Barber KE, Kishk OA, Mays AA, Jones SR, Turner AL et al (2019) Effect of fish oil supplement administration method on tolerability and adherence: a randomized pilot clinical trial. Pilot Feasibility Stud 5:3. https://doi.org/10.1186/s40814-018-0387-0
203. Treon SP, Tripsas CK, Meid K, Warren D, Varma G, Green R et al (2015) Ibrutinib in previously treated Waldenstrom's macroglobulinemia. N Engl J Med 372(15):1430–1440. https://doi.org/10.1056/NEJMoa1501548

Role of Natural Antioxidants in Cancer

4

Faizah Jabr Alsulami and Sadr ul Shaheed

Contents

4.1 Introduction

4.1.1 Oxidation Process

Neutrons, protons, and electrons are subatomic particles. Protons are positively charged particles near the nucleus and electrons are negatively charged particles around an atom. Chemical reactions usually involve the activation of electrons,

F. J. Alsulami (✉)
Department of Academic Affairs and Training Centre, King Fahad Armed Forces Hospital, Jeddah, Saudi Arabia
e-mail: FAlSulami@kfafh.med.sa

Susan Wakil School of Nursing and Midwifery, University of Sydney, Sydney, Australia

S. ul Shaheed
Nuffield Department of Surgical Sciences, University of Oxford, Oxford, UK

R. F. Saeed and S. ul. Shaheed (eds.), *Nutrition and Dietary Interventions in Cancer*, Cancer Treatment and Research 191, https://doi.org/10.1007/978-3-031-55622-7_4

leading to the formation or breaking of chemical bonds. Oxidation is a term that refers to the loss of one or more electrons. These electron-losing molecules are said to be oxidized. Oxidation and reduction occur simultaneously and cannot be done separately. The gain or loss of electrons are explicitly used to balance the charges. The combination of half-reactions to make the net chemical equation often cancel out electrons [1]. The processes of oxidation and reduction occur together and cannot be carried out independently. Redox reactions are the collective term for oxidation and reduction processes. The oxidising agent is the reactant that causes the oxidation, while the reducing agent itself reduces this reagent. In the above-mentioned cases, the oxidising agents are mercury (II) oxide, oxygen, and copper (II) ion, while reducing agents are carbon, hydrazine, and zinc. In biological process, the initial step for every heterotrophic organism is glycolysis and then fermentation occur in anaerobes. Next steps are oxidation of pyruvate, Krebs cycle and oxidative phosphorylation. The oxidation process of a substance can be summarised as, the substrate releases hydrogen which is called dehydration process, oxygen attaches to the substrate and electrons are released from substrate.

All of the forms of oxidation reactions are found in the cells of living organisms, and they are catalysed by corresponding enzymes called oxidoreductases. The oxidation reaction is linked to the reduction reaction: hydrogen or electron combination reactions occur simultaneously, resulting in oxidation–reduction reactions. Oxidation is the name given to any chemical reaction that results in the loss of electrons and an increase in oxidation states (the oxidised atom has a higher oxidation state). Reduction can occur when a substance undergoes oxidation, in which electrons attach to the atoms of another substance [1]. Fatty acid oxidation, citric acid cycle, and amino acid oxidation all result in NADH and $FADH_2$ production which are reducing equivalents which act as electron donors for the ETC. Many important processes require a redox response. Oxygen and carbon dioxide molecules are produced in response to glycolysis during cellular respiration. Cellular respiration also relies heavily on reducing NAD^+ to NADH and retardation (NADH oxidation to NAD^+) reactions. Both photosynthesis and cellular respiration are related; however, in cellular photosynthesis, it is not the opposite of a redox reaction [2]. In response to redox, biological energy is often collected and released.

4.1.2 The Formulation of Free Radicals

4.1.2.1 Reactive Oxygen Species

Reactive oxygen species (ROS) are small molecules present in oxygen atoms along with loose radicals in oxygen, which include ozone (O_3), superoxide ($O_2\cdot-$), hydroxyl ($\cdot OH$), alkoxyl (RO–) and hypochlorous acid (HOCl), peroxyl ($RO_2\cdot$), hydrogen peroxide (H_2O_2), and singlet oxygen ($^1O_2$) which are radicals. And the non-radicals can be oxidising or converted to radicals [3]. ROS was first identified as the product of cellular activity, particularly mitochondrial respiration, and its high regeneration is linked to the disruption of macromolecules such as proteins, lipids, and DNA. ROS are also produced through metabolism of xenobiotic compounds, microsomal cytochrome P450, promotion of bacterial phagocytosis or lipopolysaccharides, peroxisomal β-oxidation of fatty acids, arginine metabolism, and cellular enzymes tissue-specific [4]. Large amounts of oxygen, not only has the ability to produce more ATP through aerobic respiration, but also increase the risk of ROS formation. Major aerobic organisms for survival through the action of antioxidant defence mechanisms, exhibiting a protective role against high ROS level [5]. Most of the immune systems are involved in the fight against these highly reactive molecules, the most important of which are the antioxidative system [6].

Antioxidants are used to protect cells against ROS and the oxidative stress. Studies recently introduced the idea that ROS are a trigger for carcinogenesis in the 1990s. High level of ROS is a crucial difference between cancer cells and normal cells, which are followed by high level of antioxidant levels that detoxify the accumulated ROS and restore a redox equilibrium. As signalling molecules that promote abnormal cell growth and metastasis, proto-oncogene activation, tumour suppressor gene inactivation, and proto-oncogene activation are all considered to be ways whereby ROS play oncogenic functions [7–9]. For a better knowledge of cell pathophysiology, intracellular ROS production and their localised redox status are important. Endoplasmic reticulum, lysosomes, and peroxisomes are examples of subcellular compartments that are more oxidising than others (mitochondria, nuclei). As a result, ROS levels may vary between subcellular compartments and result in either disease or positive effects [10]. ROS control strategies are used to treat diseases mainly antioxidant therapy initiated by ROS scavengers.

4.1.2.2 Reactive Nitrogen Species

Various endogenous systems, exposure to different physiochemical conditions, or pathological conditions are the major source of production of Reactive nitrogen species (RNS). In most of the diseases, Reactive oxygen/nitrogen species (RONS) are also produced as metabolic products. The production of RONS within living cells is due to the electron mitochondrial transport system, NADH oxidase, and cytochrome P450, all of which play a key contribution in numerous important developmental processes, such as cell signalling pathways and cell division. Recently, RONS has received much focus because of its use on a broader range in many biological and pharmaceutical fields, including wound healing, an upper limb closure, cancer treatment, dental treatment, and dermatology. Peroxiredoxins (Prxs) and glutathione peroxidases (GPx) catalyse the conversion of H_2O_2 to H_2O. Metabolic activity or other stressors, including as chemokines, growth hormones, and physical stressors, encourage the formation of H_2O_2, while an efficient reduction system drives its elimination [11, 12]. Reactive oxygen species (ROS) and reactive nitrogen species (RNS) are produced by all eukaryotic cells These atoms regulate several physiological functions, such as differentiation, migration, hypertrophy, cytoskeletal dynamics, proliferation, and metabolism, but when overused, they interact with lipids, proteins, and nucleic acids, respectively. How to change the structure and behaviour of certain molecules in a way that damages and dysfunctions tissues.

ROS and RNS have been associated to a number of heart conditions, including hypertension, coronary heart disease, heart failure, and diabetes-related cardiovascular and kidney problems. Cardiovascular damage from an excessive build-up of ROS and RNS is accompanied by ischaemia–reperfusion injury or exposure to toxins, cigarette smoke, and ionising radiation. Many physiological processes are performed by mitochondrial RONS [13–16], and also associated with the tissue homeostasis and disease progression [17, 18]. Based on different studies on oxidative stress in animal models of cardiovascular disease and dysfunction, there is no conclusive evidence that ROS/RNS is primarily associated with the pathogenesis of heart disease in humans, and there is no such evidence that antioxidants are drugs effective for the treatment of cardiovascular diseases. But still it is believed that oxidative stress is a factor in many cardiovascular pathologies. The underlying cause of this disorder is incomplete understanding of complex cellular processes in which ROS causes pathological changes, additional complications found from experimental models to clinical situations, and related functional challenges in the cardiovascular system.

Numerous cells continuously produce chemical molecules including ROS or RNS throughout healthy metabolism, when a disease develops, and in reaction to tissue damage. Additionally, these species (ROS and RNS) are produced when subjected to external dangers including ionising radiation, cigarette smoke, and environmental pollutants. However, these species also include stable species like peroxides and S-Nitrosothiols (SNO).

4.1.2.3 Reactive Sulfur Species

Reactive sulfur species (RSS) are a group of chemical substances with a sulfur base that have the ability to oxidise and inhibit thiol-proteins and enzymes. They are often created when strong oxidation conditions are applied to the oxidation of thiols and disulfides. Persulfides, polysulfides, and thiosulfate are a few examples of RSS. When hydrogen sulphide (H_2S) undergoes an electron-one oxidation sequence, three molecules are created: the pure radical (HS·), hydrogen persulfide (H_2S_2), and the persulfide "supersulfide" radical. RSS's significance beyond the cellular antioxidant systems has gotten a lot of attention recently, but it's still unclear. RSS is made up of sulfide metabolites that come in a variety of chemical types [19].

Reactive sulfur species (RSS) act as strong antioxidants and produce various biological responses to animals and bacteria. RSS is considered to be those molecules produced from the oxidation of one consecutive H_2S electron. This production of thiyl radical (HS·), hydrogen persulfide (H_2S_2) and persulfide "supersulfide" radical (S^{2-}) oxidation of H_2S to persulfide in combination produces a powerful antioxidant. RSS is very efficient and versatile and can be stored and reused. Both ROS and RSS signals respond to oxidation with protein cysteine sulfur and produce similar effect responses, but RSS appears to work better. RSS in the form of persulfidated cysteines (Cys-S–S) is produced endogenously and by translation into proteins, and there is growing evidence that most cell proteins are persulfidated. Oxidation levels of sulfur range from − 2 to + 6, and sulfur contains more than 30 allotropes.

4.1.3 Effect of Free Radicals on the Body

Important macromolecules including lipids, carbohydrates, nucleic acids, and proteins can be destroyed by ROS, which are naturally created in living organisms as part of regular cellular metabolism [20]. In fact, the majority of ROS are produced at low levels during normal aerobic metabolism and play a vital role in the redox-dependent regulation of several signalling events in living organisms [21]. Low and moderately produced molecular signals that regulate a variety of physiological processes, including infection defence, vascular tone maintenance, ventilation regulation, and erythropoietin production, as well as signal transduction from membrane receptors in numerous physiological processes. Oxidative stress can lead to a variety of abnormalities, such as mitochondrial DNA mutation, mitochondrial respiratory chain dysfunction, and alteration in membrane permeability that alters $Ca2^+$ homeostasis [22].

Reactive oxidants, which can react with other biological molecules in your body including DNA, proteins, and lipids, are formed both inside our body tissues and in the environment. When it does, the molecules are damaged, which leads to sickness and inflammation. The oxidation of lipids, proteins, and DNA by ROS and other oxidants can result in tissue damage. The toxic by-products of oxidation continue to have cytostatic effects, damage membranes, and cause mobile death through necrosis or apoptosis. Free radical damage plays a role in the genesis of many chronic health issues, such as cancer, cataracts, and inflammatory and cardiovascular diseases. Inflammatory conditions such as coronary heart disease, malignancies, strokes, respiratory illnesses, immune system deficiencies, Parkinson's disorders, and other inflammatory conditions have all been linked to oxidative pressure, which refers to cell and tissue damage. Excessive amounts of these free radicals can lead to cell damage and apoptosis, contributing to many diseases such as cancer, stroke [23], myocardial infarction, diabetes, and other significant conditions [24].

The theory of free radicals of oxygen has been known for over 50 years, however, it is only in the last two decades that their role in the development of diseases were discovered and, thus, the beneficial effects of antioxidants have been widely observed [25].

4.1.4 Antioxidants

Antioxidants are compounds that can help in preventing cell damage caused by free radicals, unstable molecules produced by the body in response to environmental and other stress conditions.

Antioxidants are abundant in vegetables, nuts, seeds, and fruits, which are beneficial to our health Vitamins E and C are two examples of vitamins that include antioxidants. Since they increase food's shelf life, antioxidant preservatives are also significant in the processing of food. Antioxidants are also known as "free-radical scavengers," and their sources might be natural or synthetic. Some plant-based foods are known to have high levels of antioxidants. Phytonutrients, or nutrients derived from plants, include plant-based antioxidants. Endogenous antioxidants are those that the body produces on its own. Antioxidants that come from outside the body are known as exogenous antioxidants [26].

4.1.4.1 Antioxidant Defence System

At low concentrations, antioxidants prevent or delay lipid oxidation. Natural antioxidants found in diet include tocopherols, ascorbic acid, carotenoids, flavonoids, amino acids, phospholipids, and sterols. By scavenging free radicals, chelating prooxidative metals, quenching singlet oxygen and photosensitizers, and inactivating lipoxygenase, antioxidants prevent food from oxidising. The NADPH and NADP+ ratio are important for antioxidant defence; NADPH acts as a donor of reductive potential to glutathione and thioredoxin reductases. The main source of NADPH is the oxidative branch of the pentose phosphate pathway (ox-PPP) [27]. The transcription factor p53 is a well-known tumour suppressor gene that regulates the expression of genes that code for both ROS-producing and antioxidant components. The intracellular antioxidant defence system includes superoxide dismutase (SOD), catalase (CAT), and glutathione peroxidase [28]. When the production of reactive oxygen species (ROS) and reactive nitrogen species (RNS) exceeds the antioxidant defence system's ability to neutralise them, oxidative stress occurs and can damage DNA and proteins.

4.1.4.2 Antioxidants Mechanism

There are numerous antioxidant strategies to choose from. To begin, there is an effort to reduce free radical production by lowering oxygen availability, decreasing the activities of enzymes that produce ROS and RNS (e.g. NADPH oxidase, xanthine oxidase), and keeping iron and copper bound to proteins and preventing their participation in new radical formation. Second, maintaining mitochondrial integrity, which is the principal source of free radicals in biological systems, is critical. Third, critical elements of an antioxidant defence strategy include scavenging free radicals (e.g. vitamin E, vitamin C, GSH, and coenzyme Q) and detoxification and decomposition of free radicals and non-radical harmful chemicals (SOD, GPx, catalase, etc.). Fourth, the biological antioxidant activity of vitamin E can be increased by the vitamin E recycling system, which includes ascorbic acid, thioredoxin reductase (TrxR), vitamins B1, and B2. Fifth, the primary components of the anti-stress strategy are redox signalling, transcription factor (Nrf2), and vitagene activation, as well as the additional manufacture of protective molecules with antioxidant and detoxifying properties. The enzymatic systems involved in damaged molecules repair (heat shock proteins and methionine sulfoxide reductase) and removal (phospholipases, phospholipid hydroperoxide

GPX, proteasomes, etc.) are critical in preventing the accumulation of damaged molecules and maintaining proteostasis. Finally, apoptosis, autophagy, and other processes that deal with terminally damaged cells in order to eliminate them and prevent damage from spreading to other cells and tissues are important elements of the antioxidant defence network [29].

Antioxidants produced by the body are important for supporting healthy cellular processes. The natural antioxidants, however, are insufficient under some circumstances that encourage oxidative stress. In order to sustain optimal cellular activities, exogenous antioxidants must be provided. The biomedical research community paid a great deal of attention to antioxidants as a class of substances that can combat oxidative stress and lessen its effects on individual's health. This is because antioxidants not only demonstrated a high level of efficacy in terms of disease prevention and treatment, but also because there is a widespread belief that they have no significant side effects. Antioxidants are capable of being highly helpful in preventing, controlling, or curing human diseases, but they are also capable of having negative consequences. However, some prooxidant substances or agents may also be beneficial to human health, notably in the treatment of cancer.

4.1.4.3 Types of Antioxidants

Natural antioxidants are of two types: enzymatic and non-enzymatic antioxidants. Enzymatic antioxidants include catalase, glutathione peroxidase (GSHPx), superoxide dismutase (SOD), and Glutaredoxins (Grxs); while non-enzymatic antioxidants include β-carotene, ubiquinone, lipoic acid, reduced glutathione, and vitamins C and E [30]. Fruits are a valuable source of vitamins, minerals, and other nutrients, and they frequently have high antioxidant activity. Consuming fruit helps maintain good health by preventing the body from being damaged by oxidative stress. The identification, quantitative determination, and measurement of the antioxidant activity of diverse compounds in fruits are therefore of widespread interest.

Enzymatic Antioxidants

Superoxide Dismutase

The first enzyme involved in detoxification and most potent antioxidant in a cell is superoxide dismutase (SOD). The only enzyme known to directly scavenge a free radical is superoxide dismutase. With great specificity and efficiency, SOD converts superoxide to oxygen and hydrogen peroxide. Over the past 50 years, it has been increasingly clear that SOD is crucial for cellular health maintenance and that when SOD is dysregulated, a number of illnesses can develop [31].

Catalase

Almost all biological tissues that utilise oxygen, contain the antioxidant enzyme catalase. Using either iron or manganese as a cofactor, the enzyme catalyses the conversion of hydrogen peroxide (H_2O_2) to water and molecular oxygen. Millions of hydrogen peroxide molecules can be oxidised by catalase in a single second, making it a potent antioxidant. Catalase, for example, has been found in mouse oocytes, where it is thought to protect the genome from oxidative damage during meiotic maturation [31].

Glutathione Peroxidase

An essential intracellular enzyme called glutathione peroxidase (GPx) breaks down lipid peroxides to their corresponding alcohols and hydrogen peroxides (H_2O_2) to water, primarily in the mitochondria and occasionally in the cytoplasm. Cells are protected from oxidative stress by this enzyme's more important function of suppressing the lipid peroxidation process [31].

Non-enzymatic Antioxidants

Vitamin C

Vitamin C (also known as ascorbic acid) is essential antioxidant for maintaining bodily health. A vital complement for rapid intestine absorption is ascorbic acid, a water-soluble vitamin. During oxidative stress, ascorbic acid is quickly used up and oxidised [32]. Vitamin C and its derivatives perform very well in chemical and medical applications because of their antioxidant activity [33]. Vitamin C is a water-soluble vitamin, antioxidant, and crucial cofactor for the metabolism of carnitine and catecholamines, the production of collagen, and the absorption of dietary iron. Vitamin C cannot be synthesised by humans, so they must consume fruits and vegetables to consume it. Citrus fruits, potatoes, pepper, strawberries, gooseberries, broccoli, kiwi fruit, and paprika are a few examples of foods that naturally have a lot of vitamin C [34].

Vitamin D

The fat-soluble vitamin D is known to play a significant role in calcium and bone homeostasis and operate as an anti-inflammatory agent by suppressing the expression of cell cytokines and inducing monocyte and macrophages to release molecules with a strong antibacterial effect. Oily fish has the highest concentration of vitamin D in food; other sources include milk and oranges [35]. By preserving calcium absorption from the intestine, vitamin D primarily serves to ensure a constant amount of calcium. Additionally, this equilibrium maintains a constant quantity of phosphorus. These functions elucidate vitamin D's significance for bone density and for the growth of the musculoskeletal system [36].

Vitamin E

A fat-soluble vitamin, vitamin E is also known by the name tocopherol. When it comes to protecting biological membranes and nucleic acids in the body from the effects of free radicals, vitamin E has an incredibly broad range of applications. In humans, vitamin E has antioxidant, anti-inflammatory, anticancer, and anti-atherogenic properties, as well as direct impacts on enzyme activity and gene transcription modulation. Vitamin E is the most important lipid-soluble antioxidant for preventing oxidation of cell membrane lipids by free oxygen radicals. It can scavenge ROS such as lipid peroxyl radicals and break the antioxidant chain [37]. The optimal levels of vitamin E have been found to improve growth performance, antioxidant properties, and tolerance against oxidative stress. Vegetables, vegetable oil, almonds, walnuts, and other foods are high in vitamin E. Tumour-suppressing properties of vitamin E have been found [38].

Carotenoids

The carotenoids antioxidants from food have been shown to have photoprotective effects. Among the carotenoids, tomato, carrots, and other plants are good providers of β-Carotene, lycopene, and lutein [39]. B-Carotene (β-C) is an unsaturated compound that is susceptible to isomerization, oxidation, and degradation. β-C is a famous oil-soluble natural pigment, which has anticancer and antioxidant properties, as well as the ability to reduce the incidence of colorectal adenomas, heart disease, and cataracts [40].

Polyphenols

Polyphenols are micronutrients that are widespread in plant-based food and are also powerful antioxidants. Polyphenols can be found in a variety of fruits and beverages, including coffee, chocolate, and tea, among others. Polyphenols have been found to have neuroprotective properties. Recent evidence suggests that they have a positive impact on oxidative stress, defensive signalling, and the production of genes that code for antioxidant enzymes, neurotrophic factors, and protective proteins [38]. The bioavailability of plant-derived phenolic chemicals, such as flavonoids, determines their antioxidant potential and effectiveness. Numerous flavonoids found in plants are important for reducing the spread of infections. Anthocyanins, isoflavones, and flavones, are examples of basic flavonoid compounds. After giving lipid compound radicals hydrogen, flavonoids eliminate free radicals by converting them into phenolic radicals, which are inactive. Herbs, onions, blueberries, bananas, all citrus fruits, and others are foods that contain a lot of flavonoids [36].

Selenium

Selenium (Se) is an important micronutrient involved in a variety of biological activities. Many organs, including the thyroid, brain, muscle, prostate, and testis, require Se to function properly. Se acts as an antioxidant, protecting cells and tissues from oxidative stress and thereby preserving cellular redox balance [41].

4.1.5 Oxidative Stress in Human Health

Cardiovascular Diseases

ROS are essential for maintaining cell homeostasis and regulate a number of physiological signalling pathways and biological processes in the heart. The most significant ROS generators in the heart are mitochondria, cytochrome P450, uncoupled nitric oxide synthases, xanthine oxidoreductase, NADPH oxidase, and monoamine oxidases. Multiple antioxidant defence systems scavenge and convert ROS to harmless chemicals to prevent ROS build-up. ROS are important second messengers in the heart because they are involved in a variety of physiological processes such differentiation, proliferation, and excitation–contraction coupling. ROS has been linked to some problems associated with particular clinical situations, including chemotherapy-induced cardiotoxicity, postoperative atrial fibrillation, and diabetic cardiomyopathy. When ROS levels are too high, they can cause DNA, protein, and lipid damage, as well as NO inactivation and organelle dysfunction, which can result in cardiomyocyte apoptosis and dysfunction, ventricular hypertrophy, myocardial ischaemia–reperfusion, and heart failure. In addition to their glucose-lowering actions, sodium-glucose cotransporter 2 (SGLT2) inhibitors, a new family of antidiabetic medications, have recently been found to reduce myocardial oxidative stress in animal models [42].

Neurological Diseases

Oxidative stress-induced homeostatic dysregulation is a characteristic of a number of neurodegenerative diseases, including Alzheimer's disease, Parkinson's disease, and Amyotrophic lateral sclerosis, Stroke, Spinal cord injury, Peripheral nerve injury, and other injury-related neurodegenerative disorders [43]. Through mitochondrial malfunction, neuroinflammation, apoptosis, and tissue necrosis, cell damage sets off a chain of degenerative processes [44].

Respiratory Diseases

Pulmonary disorders, which account for huge rates of morbidity and mortality in western countries, are one pathological consequence of high levels of ROS generation. Mitochondrial dysfunction is one of the most important pathways involved in the pathophysiology of pulmonary illness. Because of the significance of oxidative stress produced by ROS in lung disorders, antioxidants may be useful as a supplemental therapy strategy for COPD and other respiratory diseases [45].

Rheumatoid Arthritis

Oxidative stress (OS) and inflammation are hypothesised to have an impact on the pathogenesis of rheumatoid arthritis (RA). OS-mediated damage to lipids, proteins, and DNA, as well as alterations in enzymatic and non-enzymatic antioxidant defence, are being investigated in human rheumatoid arthritis. Because free radicals play a function as secondary messengers in the inflammatory and immunological cellular responses in RA, they are indirectly implicated in joint damage. In RA patients, there is a significant increase in ROS production, DNA damage, protein oxidation, and a decrease in antioxidant defence system activity, which clearly results in tissue damage and chronic disease condition [46].

Kidney Diseases

In numerous types of studies, it has been studied that reducing oxidative stress and inflammation in dialysis patients improves long-term survival. There is some evidence that these medicines may play a protective function in the treatment of chronic kidney disease (CKD) and dialysis-induced oxidative stress and inflammation. In particular for dialysis patients, oxidative stress is critical in the development of CKD into ESRD [47]. These natural antioxidants, notably polyphenols and carotenoids, have been shown to have a number of essential biological activities, including antibacterial, antiviral, anti-ageing, anticancer, and anti-inflammatory activities [48].

Sexual Maturation

Oxidative stress, which is a major factor in the aetiology of many human diseases, is produced by an imbalance between ROS and antioxidants. There is a lot of evidence that oxidative stress has a role in male infertility because of sperm DNA breakage and aberrant semen parameters [49]. Antioxidants could be used as a treatment to lower ROS and increase sperm quality and sexual development. Antioxidants are appealing since they are easily bought over the counter and are deemed all-natural and thus healthful. Glutathione peroxidase, catalase, and glutathione-S-transferase activities were all significantly reduced in men with OS, resulting in a reduction in overall antioxidant capacity (TAC). The rapid replication of spermatogonia and high rate of mitochondrial oxygen consumption in the testis, which is connected to a high level of unsaturated fatty acids, make it particularly susceptible to oxidative damage. Free radical-induced oxidative stress has a significant impact on male reproductive function [50].

4.1.6 Oxidative Stress in Cancer

ROS play a dual role in cancer because of their cellular signalling capabilities. On the one side, ROS can promote pro-tumorigenic signalling, facilitating cancer cell proliferation, survival, and adaptation to hypoxia. On the other side, ROS can promote antitumorigenic signalling and trigger oxidative stress-induced cancer cell death. To accelerate the cell signalling pathways necessary for cellular transformation and tumorigenesis, cancer cells increase their rate of ROS production compared to normal cells. Concurrently, in order to maintain ROS homeostasis and evade cell death, cancer cells increase their antioxidant capacity compared with normal cells. The deregulation of specific mitochondrial metabolic pathways and mitochondrial function in cancer cells are hypothesised to play a key role in determining which adaptive mechanisms are "accessible" in the later stages of carcinogenesis. This altered redox microenvironment of cancer cells may decrease their susceptibility to ROS-based therapies. By increasing their antioxidant status to optimise ROS-driven proliferation and avoiding ROS thresholds that would trigger senescence, apoptosis, or ferroptosis, tumour cells achieve this. Specifically, hyperproliferation of tumour cells is accompanied by high ROS production, but they are adapted to thrive under conditions where this oxidative burden pushes redox balance away from a reduced state [51]. Changes in redox homeostasis have been linked to the genesis and progression of cancer. As a result, inhibiting tumour antioxidant defences reduces tumours' ability to manage oxidative stress, leading to cell death [52]. Indeed, decreased levels of antioxidant enzymes activity such as SOD, GSH, and CAT have been documented in groups of patients with breast cancer prostate cancer and malignant lymphoma in children [53, 54].

4.1.6.1 Antioxidants and Cancer Prevention

ROS deposition in normal cells is one of the initial factors in the early stages of the neoplastic process and excess of ROS levels promote cancer cells proliferation, angiogenesis, metastasis, and survival. By using antioxidants, the effects of oxidative stress can be avoided, and a malignant transformation of normal cells can be prevented. Humans have evolved complex antioxidant systems that work in tandem to scavenge ROS, protect cells from free radical damage, and maintain normal mitochondrial activity. These systems also work to block the oxidation process by neutralising free radicals. Antioxidants have been shown to lower the occurrence of several processes such as cancer, inflammation, ageing, and liver disease since the middle of the twentieth century. Cancer is a broad term that refers to a variety of diseases that can start in practically any organ or tissue of the body. Hereditary factors, mode of life, nutrition, exposure to a variety of synthetic substances, and radiation are all potential causes of cancer. Antioxidants can be used as dietary supplements, preventative treatments for a variety of illnesses, or even to alleviate the side effects of chemotherapy and radiotherapy by lowering oxidative stress in cancer patients [55, 56]. Antioxidants are naturally abundant in food sources, and their consumption has several positive health effects. Dietary antioxidants reduce oxidative stress, which is a major contributor to a variety of diseases. Plant-derived nutrients, such as organic foods, red wine, nuts, vegetables, tea, cereals, and spices can provide a large quantity and variety of antioxidants. In recent years, there has been an increase in the use of natural products, and reports have suggested that eating antioxidant-rich fruits and vegetables may be linked to a reduction in the frequency of diseases like cancer and cardiovascular disease that are brought on by reactive oxygen species. The natural antioxidants like polyphenols and carotenoids, have anti-atherosclerosis, anti-ageing, anti-inflammatory, and anticancer properties [57]. The Supplementation in Vitamines et Mineraux Antioxydants study (SU.VI.MAX), one of a few registered phase III studies, examined the impact of antioxidant intake on the prevalence of cancer in 12,741 adults between the ages of 35 and 60 using a randomised, double-blind, and placebo-controlled model [58]. A total of 6364 participants got the daily dose of 120 mg of vitamin C, 30 mg of vitamin E, 100 UI (unit international) of beta carotene, 6 mg of selenium, and 100 mg of zinc, while 6377 subjects comprised of the control group. No differences in the cancer incidence was seen during the course of the 7.5 years of data collecting between the placebo and control groups; however, when the data were grouped by sex, there was a reduction in cancer incidence and death incidence in men (risk 0.69 vs. 1.06) (relative risk 0.63 vs. 1.03). However, in another randomised interventional phase III study, 14,641 over-50-year-old males who took a mixture of vitamins were examined for the onset of cancer and other disorders. The 8-year analysis found no evidence of a preventive effect of 500 mg of vitamin C and 400 IU of vitamin E administered daily, either alone or in combination with beta carotene (50 mg of lurotin daily), on the prevention of prostate cancer or in the incidence of all cancers over the subsequent 14 years [59].

Vitamin C causes upregulation of the tumour necrosis factor-related apoptosis-inducing ligand, and low levels of vitamin C are linked to a decrease in this route and an increased risk of cancer, indicating that normal serum vitamin C may play a role in breast cancer prevention [60]. A total of 57 meta-analyses examining the association between vitamin C consumption and malignancies and reported a lower risk of many malignancies affecting various systems; bladder cancer, breast cancer, cervical neoplasms, endometrial carcinoma, oesophageal cancer, gastric cancer, glioma, lung cancer, pancreatic cancer, prostate cancer, and renal cell cancer [61].

Consuming polyphenols for the prevention of breast cancer (BC) is truly debatable because only high quantities can stop ER and ER+ BC cells from proliferating, while lesser concentrations can even encourage ER+cell growth. Carnosol is one of the polyphenols whose inhibitory effects on breast cancer cell lines are being investigated. An in vivo experiment showed that this substance can lessen BC cell line proliferation. Particularly, it has been demonstrated that carnosol inhibits invasion and metastasis of MDA-MB-231 breast cancer cell lines by downregulating Matrix Metalloproteinase-9 (MMP 9) activity, as well as by inhibiting the signal transducer and activator of transcription-3 (STAT3) signalling pathway by ROS-dependent proteasome degradation of the STAT3 protein [62]. A recent large-scale prospective study even found a positive correlation between vegetable intake and pancreatic cancer incidence in smokers [63], while a meta-analysis published in 2018 of 12 prospective studies revealed no association between the consumption of fruits and vegetables and the incidence of pancreatic cancer [64]. Four prospective studies have examined the relationship between total antioxidant capacity (TAC) and overall cancer mortality in the general population to date; one of these studies found negative relationship [65], while the other three found no relationship [66–68]. A meta-analysis of fourteen randomised controlled trials, found vitamin and antioxidant supplements have no preventive effect against bladder cancer [69]. These findings suggest that further controlled trails are required to establish a clear link between diet rich in antioxidants and incidence of pancreatic cancer, which has significant implications for the general public's health. According to the World Cancer Research Fund/American Institute for Cancer Research (WCRF/

AICR) Diet and Cancer Report, it is strongly advised to increase your intake of the vital nutrients through your regular diet, foods and beverages, dietary supplements are not the best source of antioxidants.

4.1.6.2 Cancer Chemotherapy and Antioxidants

Chemotherapy is the process of using medications, commonly referred to as anti-cancer drugs, to kill or destroy cancer cells. These medications stop tumours from growing and even cause cancer cells to die. Chemotherapy is often regarded as a potent cancer treatment, but it can have major side effects because it can damage healthy cells or tissues. Chemotherapy side effects vary depending on the type of cancer, its location, and how the patient reacts to different types of chemotherapy. Cancer patients' side effects are not indicative of the treatment's feasibility, and these side effects disappear once the treatment is ended. Chemotherapy medications are typically prescribed to a patient in little doses over a period. Combination chemotherapy refers to the administration of at least two distinct medications at the same time during chemotherapy [70].

Exogenous or endogenous ROS created by chemotherapeutics or cancer cells, respectively, have the ability to inhibit cell division and maintain the G_0 phase of the cell cycle. High amounts of ROS interact with chemotherapy medicines in this way because chemotherapy agents can only kill cells that are reproducing. Antioxidants may be able to minimise the high amount of ROS in cancer cells, which is necessary for tumour function, metastasis, and angiogenesis. Antioxidant chemicals are commonly ingested as dietary supplements, and their efficiency in the prevention of several diseases, including malignant tumours, has been researched. According to recent research, antioxidant chemicals may be ineffective or even hazardous in the prevention and treatment of cancer [71].

Antioxidant supplements are used during chemotherapy to compensate for antioxidant depletion caused by the treatment or disease. There isn't much evidence for such depletion. Some research has looked at how conventional therapy affects antioxidant status (as defined by serum micronutrients and/or total antioxidant capacity) in cancer patients. The findings could indicate that antioxidant enzymes, especially Manganese superoxide dismutase (MnSOD), play a significant role in the early stages of colorectal melanoma in both types of colorectal tissues, and that they could be used as new individual biomarkers to advance Colorectal cancer (CRC) detection [72]. Another study found that women who used antioxidant supplements both before and during chemotherapy had an increased risk of recurrence. This study compared the chemotherapy schedules for breast cancer patients [73]. Additionally, it appears that all cell types of antioxidant-modified cell signalling should be compared, and a threshold should be established in this regard. The nutrigenomics of each antioxidant should also be thoroughly investigated in order to draw firm conclusions about whether patients should use antioxidants or not. Antioxidants can reduce ROS levels, induce cancer cells to emerge from dormancy, and make them more susceptible to chemotherapeutic treatments.

In addition to lowering the incidence of cancer, antioxidants inhibit its growth and combat drug resistance. The location, composition, and amount of antioxidants that cells absorb, or the role that antioxidants play in cell signalling may all lead to contradictions between antioxidants and chemotherapy. It is advised that the screening of orally administered antioxidants, the comparative study of various types of cancer cells, and the comparison of cancer, chemotherapeutic agents be accepted in order to determine which type of chemotherapy agent and which type of antioxidant should be specified for each type of cancer.

In later stages, when cancer develops a malignant and invasive character, the activity of antioxidant enzymes and the intracellular pool of NADPH and GSH rise to limit oxidative damage produced by excessive ROS synthesis; hence, antioxidants at late stages of cancer are expected to aid excrescence cells in avoiding ROS-induced oxidative cuts and apoptosis. A study also claimed that antioxidants should be avoided in cases of advanced cancer and/or those receiving radiotherapy [74]. Patients with systemic deficits may benefit from nutritional supplementation once anticancer therapies are finished. When antioxidants are given in combination with chemotherapeutic drugs, the results were attempted to be replicated in humans, however, the efficacy was a major question. Natural antioxidants, in addition to medicinal compounds, surely help in preventing and treating a variety of diseases due to their chemical diversity, multi-targeting activities, and good safety profiles. Some natural antioxidants are currently being studied in clinical trials, while others have been approved for use in humans. Although natural antioxidants are normally made up of a variety of biological compounds in varying amounts and proportions, calculating their safe concentrations is a major concern because no such safety analysis have been performed. With synthetic antioxidants, it is easily understood which antioxidants are safer, owing to the availability of requisite safety tests [75]. Melatonin is a radio protective agent because it may neutralise a variety of free radicals and prooxidant enzymes: (NADPH oxidase, xanthine oxidase, or nitric oxide synthase), produced by ionising radiation. Melatonin also has neuroprotective properties, since it protects the brain from the negative effects of adjuvant chemotherapy on cognitive function, sleep quality, and depressive symptoms. As a result, it could be a novel adjuvant therapy to increase the effectiveness of breast cancer treatments [76–78].

Chemotherapy-induced oxidative stress would have a different biofunction mechanism in cancer cells than in normal tissue. Antioxidants may be highly effective in some circumstances, but they may have a negative impact on cells and cause them to degenerate in others. The treatment procedures that a patient should follow to treat cancer are normally prescribed but advise on what foods to eat or whether to take an antioxidant is less precise. Which kind of antioxidant should be given if one is needed or do all antioxidants such as carotenoids, vitamin C, vitamin E, selenium, and others, have the same effect on the body? Additionally, the advantages and disadvantages of antioxidant consumption in cancer patients as well as the relationship between chemotherapies and antioxidants on the immune system should be evaluated and also focusing on the point whether antioxidant uptake is beneficial for individuals receiving chemotherapy, evidence from cellular, animal, and clinical trials. Cognitive impairment is one of the most serious adverse effects of cancer treatment and might last long after the treatment is ended. The chemotherapy-based regimens such anthracyclines, doxorubicin, taxanes, and platinum derivatives, for example, can cause oxidative stress in the blood and brain. Antioxidants have been shown to be effective in treating both oxidative stress and cognitive abnormalities brought on by chemotherapy medications. *N*-acetylcysteine, gamma-glutamyl cysteine ethyl ester, polydatin, caffeic acid phenethyl ester, and sodium 2-mercaptoethane sulfonate were some of these antioxidants.

4.1.6.3 Antioxidants in Conjunction with Radiation Therapy

An essential component of cancer treatment is radiation therapy. In the United States, one-third of cancer patients survived for five years who were treated with radiation therapy [79], and it is anticipated that this number will continue to rise. The most prevalent form of cancer in the world and the main reason why women die from it is breast cancer. In 2018, it was estimated that 0.6 million breast cancer mortality and an estimated 2 million new cases had been observed [80]. The radiation kills cancer cells by generating free radicals. The medicinal moieties are said to be neutralised and maybe eliminated after consumption of dietary antioxidants.

The major target of radiation is DNA; damage to DNA happens directly, but two-thirds of the damage occurs indirectly, as a result of free radicals such as superoxide, hydroxyl radicals, and gas metabolites. Radiation is most damaging to cells during the G_1M phase of the cell cycle; there is evidence that using selective antioxidants after irradiation can counteract some of the side effects. Cancer cells, particularly those in the tumour microenvironment, have a greater baseline level of oxidative stress than normal cells, hence the up-regulated antioxidant system helps to reduce ROS-mediated tumour cell damage. Radiation oncology researchers and practitioners are especially concerned that antioxidants may protect cancer cells from the destructive effects of reactive oxygen species, or oxidants, which are created by radiation and are essential to radiation's ability to kill cancer [81].

Clinical trials have found no indication of tumour protection when synthetic prescription antioxidants such as amifostine, mesna, and dexrazoxane are administered with a range of chemotherapy and radiotherapy regimens [82]. Supplementing with antioxidants may help protect normal cells from the increased damage and negative effects that come with medication. Cancer has been connected to the host system's inability to respond adequately to tumour antigens, which leads to tumour immune evasion [83, 84]. Supplementation during treatment is particularly contentious: no conclusive evidence exists that antioxidant supplements (vitamins, herbs, or herbal compounds) may protect healthy tissues without jeopardising chemotherapeutic drug cytotoxicity. These antioxidant supplements have the ability to preserve healthy tissues without affecting the cytotoxicity of chemotherapeutic medications, however there is no definitive proof to support this claim. Curcumin is a yellow curcuminoid found in turmeric and zingiberaceae that is used as a herbal supplement, food flavouring, and colouring. It also has antioxidant and anti-inflammatory effects, making it useful as an anticancer supplement [85]. Cancer-suppressing polyphenolic substances in the diet have antioxidant effects. Resveratrol suppresses lung cancer metastasis when given in low dosages [86].

Antioxidants have limited benefits and safety during cancer treatment, but their significance in preserving system homeostasis cannot be exaggerated. The decrease of oxidative stress parameters like malondialdehyde and nitric oxide shows that antioxidant multivitamin and mineral supplementation helps to protect cancer patients from oxidative stress caused by radiotherapy or chemotherapy. It also improves oesophageal function and endogenous and exogenous antioxidants (SOD, GPx, vitamin C, and vitamin E) [87]. Furthermore, a high daily intake of selenium is cancer-protective, albeit the outcomes vary depending on the kind of cancer [88]. However, various antioxidant transcription factors may be activated in response to irradiation, resulting in the suppression of radiation-induced ROS-dependent damage and a reduction in treatment effectiveness. Furthermore, the source of ROS is considered to be a two-edged sword, as it plays a vital initiating function in radiation-induced normal tissue damage [89]. Radio-resistance and tumour recurrence after radiotherapy are difficult to overcome issues that might lead to treatment failure and tumour return. In cancer radiation, specific alterations in ROS generation and antioxidant concentrations are important. According to a recent study, reducing oxidative stress may help patients with radiation resistance during radiotherapy [90].

4.1.6.4 Post-treatment Antioxidants

Antioxidants, which are often produced from all-natural sources, are a tempting option to standard medication for many patients seeking to address illnesses like cancer, rheumatoid arthritis, neurological disorders, etc. According to research on β-Carotene, common phytochemicals, and glutathione, there are three key aspects that influence the potential for an antioxidant-containing molecule to cause side effects: the dosage, the patient's specific physiology, and the product's type. It does not appear that the antioxidant activity of these substances is directly responsible for any harmful effects because there are no clear correlations between the negative effects identified for different antioxidants [91].

A meta-analysis based on seven prospective clinical trials, evaluated dietary β-Carotene intake in relation to overall mortality, and showed that high level of β-Carotene level in blood was associated with a significant lower risk of all-cause mortality (RR for highest vs. lowest group = 0.69, 95%CI: 0.59–0.80) with low heterogeneity (I2 = 37.1%, P = 0.145) [92]. A 2015 study compared oral glutathione treatment to sublingual glutathione supplementation. Despite the study's limited sample size, none of the subjects reported any negative side effects regardless of the glutathione (GSH) supplementation method (just 20 participants), when viewed in the light of prior research on the subject, these data show that patients are unlikely to encounter negative side effects from using GSH. Even if they do, the negative effects of this antioxidant-containing molecule are expected to be significantly less severe than those frequently reported for the most commonly prescribed pharmaceutical medications [93]. The safety profile of quercetin, another phytochemical with favourable antioxidant action, was investigated in a 2018 review published in the journal Molecular Nutrition and Food Research. Negative side effects "have rarely been recorded in human research investigations, and any such effects were moderate in nature," according to the researchers [94]. Antioxidant action of glutathione production extends beyond the correction of the original oxidative stressor or performs several tasks other than intracellular maintenance [95]. Finally, free sulfhydryl groups (–SH groups) in glutathione may have antioxidant properties while also binding to chemotherapeutic reactive intermediates and preventing effective tumour cell death [96]. This could explain why glutathione hasn't proven to be as successful in cancer-fighting techniques, as it was once thought that cancers with mutant p53 have high levels of Nrf2 (nuclear factor erythroid 2-related factor 2) activation, which may protect tumour cells against reactive adduct-induced DNA damage [97].

Antioxidant effectiveness and other potential health advantages appear to exceed their long-term negative side effects. If a patient experiences mild gastrointestinal discomfort after increasing their antioxidant intake (either through nutritional supplementation or dietary changes), they may still be able to benefit from antioxidant intake by experimenting with a different dosage or an antioxidant compound that has been shown to play a similar physiological role. Further investigation into the efficacy of these substances may also throw more light on why some individuals have unpleasant effects while others do not. For the time being, patients and practitioners can rest assured that most antioxidants are usually deemed safe and have a low risk of adverse effects, particularly when compared to pharmaceutical medications that might otherwise be used to prevent and cure serious health problems. Supplements made with improved delivery systems should be considered by patients who want to maximise possible benefits while lowering the risk of negative effects.

4.1.7 Conclusion

Excessive levels of ROS can result in oxidative damage to the cell membrane proteins, lipids, and DNA, preventing them from performing their functions normally. When there is a lack of antioxidants, overproduction of ROS causes oxidative stress, which disrupts the equilibrium status of prooxidant/antioxidant processes in living organisms. A few in vitro experiments using polyphenolic compounds showed promising results in terms of antioxidant response to cancer cell growth inhibition. However, mixed outcomes were reported in other laboratory and animal trials in different studies. There have been studies that show the proliferation of cancer cells in response to the administration of antioxidants, and it is dependent on a few parameters such as the type of cancer and the agents used. The first line of antioxidant defence system is achieved by the activities of Catalase (CAT), Superoxide Dismutase (SOD), and Glutathione Peroxidase (GPX). Because oxidative stress has been linked to cancer, it makes sense that antioxidants could help to prevent cancer appearance and progression. Even though several antioxidant therapy techniques have been investigated and some are currently being tested in clinical trials, their efficacy remains unsatisfying. Instead of dietary dosage based on in vitro tests, the majority of studies use pharmacological doses of medication. However, (1) antioxidants may be influenced by complex in vivo environments, (2) antioxidant distribution in various tissues may be unequal, and (3) depending on their amounts, some antioxidants may have antioxidant or prooxidant properties. ROS and oxidative stress are side effects of many chemotherapy drugs. Thus, antioxidant therapy may have a harmful impact on chemotherapeutic drug-induced cell death in cancer patients. The development of innovative therapeutic drugs in the form of antioxidants that may be beneficial in the prevention and treatment of cancer will be aided by a better understanding of their pathways. By lowering OS-induced sperm damage and increasing hormone synthesis, spermatozoa concentration, motility, and quality in males with low-quality sperm, antioxidant supplementation in the diet may assist to enhance overall sperm quality.

Finally, it is unclear how antioxidants affect the development and metastatic phases of carcinogenesis. Future research is intended to clarify the regulation of oscillations between epithelial mesenchymal transition and total mesorectal excision, which will provide more data on the adaptive mechanisms used by different tumour cell types to colonise distant tissues. Further research should be done on the impact of antioxidants on extracellular signal-regulated kinase (ERK) signalling in various tumour forms, as well as the possibility that antioxidants may promote reductive stress in specific tumour types. These issues can be resolved to enhance treatment approaches. To benefit from their combined modes of action, future clinical trials should concentrate on the combination of various antioxidants. The prospect of interdisciplinary collaborations between oncologists, pharmacists, and biochemists to better understand cancer-specific redox signalling events which paves the way towards minimising side effects of prooxidants and antioxidants, antineoplastic therapies.

References

1. Oppenheimer CH, Stern KG (2013) Biological oxidation. Springer
2. Ferreira CA et al (2018) Scavenging of reactive oxygen and nitrogen species with nanomaterials. Nano Res 11(10):4955–4984
3. Phaniendra A, Jestadi DB, Periyasamy L (2015) Free radicals: properties, sources, targets, and their implication in various diseases. Indian J Clin Biochem 30(1):11–26
4. Dumont S, Rivoal J (2019) Consequences of oxidative stress on plant glycolytic and respiratory metabolism. Front Plant Sci 10:166
5. Huang H et al (2019) Mechanisms of ROS regulation of plant development and stress responses. Front Plant Sci 10:800
6. Mishanina TV, Libiad M, Banerjee R (2015) Biogenesis of reactive sulfur species for signaling by hydrogen sulfide oxidation pathways. Nat Chem Biol 11(7):457–464
7. Barnes RP, Fouquerel E, Opresko PL (2019) The impact of oxidative DNA damage and stress on telomere homeostasis. Mech Ageing Dev 177:37–45

8. Chang M-C et al (2015) Effects of camphorquinone on cytotoxicity, cell cycle regulation and prostaglandin E2 production of dental pulp cells: role of ROS, ATM/Chk2, MEK/ERK and hemeoxygenase-1. PLoS ONE 10(12):e0143663
9. Srinivas US et al (2019) ROS and the DNA damage response in cancer. Redox Biol 25:101084
10. Di Meo S et al (2016) Role of ROS and RNS sources in physiological and pathological conditions. Oxid Med Cell Longev
11. Rhee SG, Kil IS (2017) Multiple functions and regulation of mammalian peroxiredoxins. Annu Rev Biochem 86:749–775
12. Brigelius-Flohé R, Flohé L (2020) Regulatory phenomena in the glutathione peroxidase superfamily. Antioxid Redox Signal 33(7):498–516
13. Görlach A et al (2015) Reactive oxygen species, nutrition, hypoxia and diseases: problems solved? Redox Biol 6:372–385
14. Latorre-Pellicer A et al (2016) Mitochondrial and nuclear DNA matching shapes metabolism and healthy ageing. Nature 535(7613):561–565
15. Mills EL et al (2016) Succinate dehydrogenase supports metabolic repurposing of mitochondria to drive inflammatory macrophages. Cell 167(2):457–470, e13
16. Acín-Pérez R et al (2020) Fgr kinase is required for proinflammatory macrophage activation during diet-induced obesity. Nat Metab 2(9):974–988
17. Chouchani ET et al (2016) A unifying mechanism for mitochondrial superoxide production during ischemia-reperfusion injury. Cell Metab 23(2):254–263
18. Harris IS, DeNicola GM (2020) The complex interplay between antioxidants and ROS in cancer. Trends Cell Biol 30(6):440–451
19. Shen X et al (2015) Measurement of H2S in vivo and in vitro by the monobromobimane method. Methods in enzymology. Elsevier, pp 31–45
20. Cakmak KC, Gülçin İ (2019) Anticholinergic and antioxidant activities of USNIC acid—an activity-structure insight. Toxicol Rep 6:1273–1280
21. Shivakumar A, Yogendra Kumar M (2018) Critical review on the analytical mechanistic steps in the evaluation of antioxidant activity. Crit Rev Anal Chem 48(3):214–236
22. Chiang S-C et al (2017) Mitochondrial protein-linked DNA breaks perturb mitochondrial gene transcription and trigger free radical–induced DNA damage. Sci Adv 3(4):e1602506
23. Tsatsakis A et al (2019) A mechanistic and pathophysiological approach for stroke associated with drugs of abuse. J Clin Med 8(9):1295
24. Padureanu R et al (2019) Oxidative stress and inflammation interdependence in multiple sclerosis. J Clin Med 8(11):1815
25. Liu Z-Q (2020) Bridging free radical chemistry with drug discovery: A promising way for finding novel drugs efficiently. Eur J Med Chem 189:112020
26. Akbarirad H et al (2016) An overview on some of important sources of natural antioxidants. Int Food Res J 23(3)
27. Fernandez-Marcos PJ, Nóbrega-Pereira S (2016) NADPH: new oxygen for the ROS theory of aging. Oncotarget 7(32):50814
28. Ighodaro O, Akinloye O (2018) First line defence antioxidants-superoxide dismutase (SOD), catalase (CAT) and glutathione peroxidase (GPX): their fundamental role in the entire antioxidant defence grid. Alex J Med 54(4):287–293
29. Surai PF (2018) Selenium in poultry nutrition and health. Wageningen Academic Publishers
30. Gaucher C et al (2018) Glutathione: antioxidant properties dedicated to nanotechnologies. Antioxidants 7(5):62
31. Borgstahl GE, Oberley-Deegan RE (2018) Superoxide dismutases (SODs) and SOD mimetics. In: MDPI, p 156
32. Liu Y, Liu C, Li J (2020) Comparison of vitamin C and its derivative antioxidant activity: evaluated by using density functional theory. ACS Omega 5(39):25467–25475
33. Meščić Macan AT, Kraljević G, Raić-Malić S (2019) Therapeutic perspective of vitamin C and its derivatives. Antioxidants 8(8):247
34. Kaur G et al (2016) Dietary antioxidants and their indispensable role in periodontal health. J Food Drug Anal 24(2):239–246

35. Li S et al (2014) Research progress of natural antioxidants in foods for the treatment of diseases. Food Sci Human Wellness 3(3–4):110–116
36. Wang EW et al (2017) Vitamin D deficiency, oxidative stress and antioxidant status: only weak association seen in the absence of advanced age, obesity or pre-existing disease. Br J Nutr 118(1):11–16
37. Manosso LM et al (2020) Vitamin E for the management of major depressive disorder: possible role of the anti-inflammatory and antioxidant systems. Nutr Neurosci 1–15
38. Lalkovičová M, Danielisová V (2016) Neuroprotection and antioxidants. Neural Regen Res 11(6):865
39. Petruk G et al (2018) Antioxidants from plants protect against skin photoaging. Oxid Med Cell Longev
40. Liu X et al (2020) Co-encapsulation of vitamin C and β-Carotene in liposomes: storage stability, antioxidant activity, and in vitro gastrointestinal digestion. Food Res Int 136:109587
41. Short SP, Williams CS (2017) Selenoproteins in tumorigenesis and cancer progression. Adv Cancer Res 136:49–83
42. Lahnwong S, Chattipakorn SC, Chattipakorn N (2018) Potential mechanisms responsible for cardioprotective effects of sodium–glucose co-transporter 2 inhibitors. Cardiovasc Diabetol 17(1):1–17
43. Cunha-Oliveira T et al (2020) Oxidative stress in amyotrophic lateral sclerosis: pathophysiology and opportunities for pharmacological intervention. Oxid Med Cell Longev
44. Eratne D et al (2018) Alzheimer's disease: clinical update on epidemiology, pathophysiology and diagnosis. Aust Psychiatry 26(4):347–357
45. Sharma A et al (2021) Reactive oxygen species modulators in pulmonary medicine. Curr Opin Pharmacol 57:157–164
46. Mateen S et al (2016) Increased reactive oxygen species formation and oxidative stress in rheumatoid arthritis. PLoS ONE 11(4):e0152925
47. Liakopoulos V et al (2019) Oxidative stress in hemodialysis: causative mechanisms, clinical implications, and possible therapeutic interventions. In: Seminars in dialysis. Wiley Online Library
48. Bungau S et al (2019) Health benefits of polyphenols and carotenoids in age-related eye diseases. Oxid Med Cell Longev
49. Huang C et al (2018) Is male infertility associated with increased oxidative stress in seminal plasma? A-meta analysis. Oncotarget 9(36):24494
50. Asadi N et al (2017) The impact of oxidative stress on testicular function and the role of antioxidants in improving it: a review. J Clin Diagn Res JCDR 11(5):IE01
51. Dodson M, Castro-Portuguez R, Zhang DD (2019) NRF2 plays a critical role in mitigating lipid peroxidation and ferroptosis. Redox Biol 23:101107
52. Sznarkowska A et al (2017) Inhibition of cancer antioxidant defense by natural compounds. Oncotarget 8(9):15996
53. Ahmed Amar SA et al (2019) Determination of oxidative stress levels and some antioxidant enzyme activities in prostate cancer. Aging Male 22(3):198–206
54. Kangari P et al (2018) Enzymatic antioxidant and lipid peroxidation evaluation in the newly diagnosed breast cancer patients in Iran. Asian Pac J Cancer Prev APJCP 19(12):3511
55. Gulcin İ (2020) Antioxidants and antioxidant methods: an updated overview. Arch Toxicol 94(3):651–715
56. Atta EM, Mohamed NH, Silaev AAA (2017) Antioxidants: an overview on the natural and synthetic types. Eur Chem Bull 6(8):365–375
57. Nogueira V et al (2008) Akt determines replicative senescence and oxidative or oncogenic premature senescence and sensitizes cells to oxidative apoptosis. Cancer Cell 14(6):458–470
58. Hercberg S et al (2005) Alterations of the lipid profile after 7.5 years of low-dose antioxidant supplementation in the SU.VI.MAX study. Lipids 40(4):335–342
59. Gaziano JM et al (2009) Vitamins E and C in the prevention of prostate and total cancer in men: the physicians' health study II randomized controlled trial. JAMA 301(1):52–62

60. Mohammed AA (2020) Evaluation of mastalgia in patients presented to the breast clinic in Duhok city, Iraq: cross sectional study. Ann Med Surg 52:31–35
61. Chen Z et al (2021) Vitamin C intake and cancers: an umbrella review. Front Nutr 8
62. Poschner S et al (2019) Resveratrol and other dietary polyphenols are inhibitors of estrogen metabolism in human breast cancer cells. J Steroid Biochem Mol Biol 190:11–18
63. Yamagiwa Y et al (2019) Fruit and vegetable intake and pancreatic cancer risk in a population-based cohort study in Japan. Int J Cancer 144(8):1858–1866
64. Zhao Z et al (2018) No associations between fruit and vegetable consumption and pancreatic cancer risk: a meta-analysis of prospective studies. Oncotarget 9(63):32250
65. Bastide N et al (2017) Dietary antioxidant capacity and all-cause and cause-specific mortality in the E3N/EPIC cohort study. Eur J Nutr 56(3):1233–1243
66. Kim K et al (2018) Dietary total antioxidant capacity is inversely associated with all-cause and cardiovascular disease death of US adults. Eur J Nutr 57(7):2469–2476
67. Henríquez-Sánchez P et al (2016) Dietary total antioxidant capacity and mortality in the PREDIMED study. Eur J Nutr 55(1):227–236
68. Kashino I et al (2019) Higher dietary non-enzymatic antioxidant capacity is associated with decreased risk of all-cause and cardiovascular disease mortality in Japanese adults. J Nutr 149(11):1967–1976
69. Park S-J et al (2017) Effects of vitamin and antioxidant supplements in prevention of bladder cancer: a meta-analysis of randomized controlled trials. J Korean Med Sci 32(4):628–635
70. Wang J, Lei K, Han F (2018) Tumor microenvironment: recent advances in various cancer treatments. Eur Rev Med Pharmacol Sci 22(12):3855–3864
71. Shomali N et al (2020) A new insight into thymosin β4, a promising therapeutic approach for neurodegenerative disorders. J Cell Physiol 235(4):3270–3279
72. Gaya-Bover A et al (2020) Antioxidant enzymes change in different non-metastatic stages in tumoral and peritumoral tissues of colorectal cancer. Int J Biochem Cell Biol 120:105698
73. Ambrosone CB et al (2020) Dietary supplement use during chemotherapy and survival outcomes of patients with breast cancer enrolled in a cooperative group clinical trial (SWOG S0221). J Clin Oncol 38(8):804
74. Athreya K, Xavier MF (2017) Antioxidants in the treatment of cancer. Nutr Cancer 69(8):1099–1104
75. Kroon P, Williamson G (2005) Polyphenols: dietary components with established benefits to health? J Sci Food Agric 85(8):1239–1240
76. Griffin F, Marignol L (2018) Therapeutic potential of melatonin for breast cancer radiation therapy patients. Int J Radiat Biol 94(5):472–477
77. Kubatka P et al (2018) Melatonin and breast cancer: evidences from preclinical and human studies. Crit Rev Oncol Hematol 122:133–143
78. Palmer ACS et al (2020) Clinical impact of melatonin on breast cancer patients undergoing chemotherapy; effects on cognition, sleep and depressive symptoms: a randomized, double-blind, placebo-controlled trial. PLoS ONE 15(4):e0231379
79. Bryant AK et al (2017) Trends in radiation therapy among cancer survivors in the United States, 2000–2030 radiation therapy in cancer survivors. Cancer Epidemiol Biomark Prev 26(6):963–970
80. Bray F et al (2018) Global cancer statistics 2018: GLOBOCAN estimates of incidence and mortality worldwide for 36 cancers in 185 countries. CA Cancer J Clin 68(6):394–424
81. Yun K-L, Wang ZY (2017) Target/signalling pathways of natural plant-derived radioprotective agents from treatment to potential candidates: a reverse thought on anti-tumour drugs. Biomed Pharmacother 91:1122–1151
82. Jiang Q et al (2015) Continuous IV infusion of MESNA can prevent hemorrhagic cystitis in HSCT and retain MESNA concentration in urine. Bone Marrow Transplant 50(11):1490–1492
83. Yan X et al (2016) Lewis lung cancer cells promote SIGNR1 (CD209b)-mediated macrophages polarization induced by IL-4 to facilitate immune evasion. J Cell Biochem 117(5):1158–1166

84. Vences-Catalán F et al (2015) Tetraspanin CD81 promotes tumor growth and metastasis by modulating the functions of T regulatory and Myeloid-derived suppressor cells CD81 promotes tumor growth and metastasis. Cancer Res 75(21):4517–4526
85. Sahu PK et al (2016) Structure activity relationship, cytotoxicity and evaluation of antioxidant activity of curcumin derivatives. Bioorg Med Chem Lett 26(4):1342–1347
86. Thyagarajan A, Sahu RP (2018) Potential contributions of antioxidants to cancer therapy: immunomodulation and radiosensitization. Integr Cancer Ther 17(2):210–216
87. Patil RY, More HN (2020) Antioxidants with multivitamin and mineral supplementation attenuates chemotherapy or radiotherapy-induced oxidative stress in cancer patients. Indian J Pharm Educ Res 54(2):484–490
88. Kuria A et al (2020) Does dietary intake of selenium protect against cancer? A systematic review and meta-analysis of population-based prospective studies. Crit Rev Food Sci Nutr 60(4):684–694
89. Perillo B et al (2020) ROS in cancer therapy: the bright side of the moon. Exp Mol Med 52(2):192–203
90. Hu J et al (2020) Targeting Epstein-Barr virus oncoprotein LMP1-mediated high oxidative stress suppresses EBV lytic reactivation and sensitizes tumors to radiation therapy. Theranostics 10(26):11921
91. Schmitt B et al (2015) Effects of *N*-acetylcysteine, oral glutathione (GSH) and a novel sublingual form of GSH on oxidative stress markers: a comparative crossover study. Redox Biol 6:198–205
92. Zhao L-G et al (2016) Dietary, circulating beta-carotene and risk of all-cause mortality: a meta-analysis from prospective studies. Sci Rep 6(1):1–10
93. Richie JP et al (2015) Randomized controlled trial of oral glutathione supplementation on body stores of glutathione. Eur J Nutr 54(2):251–263
94. Andres S et al (2018) Safety aspects of the use of quercetin as a dietary supplement. Mol Nutr Food Res 62(1):1700447
95. Holmström KM, Kostov RV, Dinkova-Kostova AT (2016) The multifaceted role of Nrf2 in mitochondrial function. Curr Opin Toxicol 1:80–91
96. Deponte M (2017) The incomplete glutathione puzzle: just guessing at numbers and figures? Antioxid Redox Signal 27(15):1130–1161
97. Tung M-C et al (2015) Mutant p53 confers chemoresistance in non-small cell lung cancer by upregulating Nrf2. Oncotarget 6(39):41692

Micronutrients Importance in Cancer Prevention—Vitamins

5

Rida Fatima Saeed, Shumaila Naz, Uzma Azeem Awan, Sana Gul, Fazli Subhan, and Sidra Saeed

Contents

R. F. Saeed (✉) · S. Naz · U. A. Awan · S. Gul · F. Subhan
Department of Biological Sciences, National University of Medical Sciences (NUMS), Rawalpindi, Pakistan
e-mail: rida.saeed@numspak.edu.pk; rida.saeed@hotmail.co.uk

S. Naz
e-mail: Shumaila.naz@numspak.edu.pk

U. A. Awan
e-mail: uzma.awan@numspak.edu.pk

S. Gul
e-mail: sana.gul@numspak.edu.pk

F. Subhan
e-mail: fazli.subhan@numspak.edu.pk

S. Saeed
University Centre Leeds, Leeds LS3 1AA, UK
e-mail: sidra.saeed@ucleeds.ac.uk

R. F. Saeed and S. ul. Shaheed (eds.), *Nutrition and Dietary Interventions in Cancer*, Cancer Treatment and Research 191, https://doi.org/10.1007/978-3-031-55622-7_5

Abbreviations

BRAF	BRAF is a gene found on chromosome seven that encodes a protein
BC	Breast cancer
CRC	Colorectal cancer
GC	Gastric cancer
HER2	Human epidermal growth factor receptor 2
KRAS	Kirsten rat sarcoma viral oncogene
PCA	Pancreatic cancer
PC	Prostate cancer
RR	Relative risk
RA	Retinoic acid
25(OH)D	Vitamin D (1,25(OH)2D3)
VDR	Vitamin D receptors
WHO	World Health Organization

5.1 Introduction to Micronutrients Importance in Cancer

Ever since 1980s, epidemiological research work has shown an association between lack of micronutrients and the development of tumour processes have been emerging [1]. The World Health Organization (WHO) estimates that cancer will be the main cause of death in 112 out of 183 nations in 2019 [2]. Around 10.0 million cancer deaths and 19.3 million new cancer cases are projected to have occurred globally in 2020. With 935,000 fatalities in 2020, colon and rectum cancer came in second after hepatic (830,000 fatalities) and stomach cancers (769,000 deaths) [3]. For many years, chemotherapy and radiotherapy have been the mainstay treatments for patients with various forms of cancer, either alone or in combination. However, numerous key concerns with traditional chemotherapies, such as increased side effects, limited access to tumour areas may outweigh their therapeutic benefits in some cases [4]. For decades, scientists have speculated that diet had a substantial impact on the probability of developing cancer. A significant percentage of cancers can be prevented with proper nutrition, exercise, and body weight maintenance [5, 6]. It is estimated that approximately 30–40% of different types of cancer can be controlled through diet and lifestyle changes. Cancer prevention diet should include all micronutrients, including antioxidants such carotenoids, folic acid, selenium, vitamin B12 and vitamin D [7]. Interestingly, inadequate levels of micronutrients afflict about two billion people worldwide [8, 9], which lowers immunity to diseases and is a common reason of immunodeficiency in underdeveloped nations [10]. Patients who have micronutrient deficiencies are more vulnerable to many infections and malignancies due to lower immune responses [11]. Administration of micronutrients intravenously and in the form of oral supplements could improve immune functions, which support the body's to fight against pathogens and may also be effective in cancer prevention and therapy [12].

Adjuvant and supplementary oncological treatment now include providing cancer patients with laboratory-validated micronutrients. As a consequence, in adding to energy substrates (such as carbohydrates, fats and proteins), it is vital to ensure that immune-stabilizing micronutrients are supplemented optimally [12]. Micronutrients with immune-modulating and antioxidant properties, as well as vitamins with a lower storage capacity, are crucial for these patients [13–16]. There has been evidence of elevated oxidative stress indicators in cancer patients with low nutritional status due to inadequate antioxidant micronutrient supplementation [17]. According to recent research, nutrients in the tumour microenvironment can affect immunotherapy response and cancer cell metabolic pathways [18, 19]. Vitamin C, for example, can improve immune cell activity by altering the tumour microenvironment via hypoxia-inducible factors [20]. In T cell-dependent way, high amount vitamin C inhibits cancer cell proliferation via modulating immune cell intrusion of the tumour microenvironment and promotes cell growth and maturation of natural killer and T cells [21]. Vitamin D supplementation inhibits the cancer process such as angiogenesis, progression, and metastasis through interacting with tumour microenvironment components [22]. Together, these findings could reaffirm anti-cancer properties of vitamin.

Numerous studies have pointed to the possible relevance of micronutrient supplementation in enhancing cancer patients' life quality and prognosis. Micronutrient consumption has been demonstrated to lower the incidence and progression of malignancies in recent studies [23]. In vitro and in vivo investigations on more than fifty cancerous cell lines have revealed that micronutrient combinations have a good anti-cancer impact. It's also been well established that those nutritional combinations have pleiotropic effects on tumour development, invasion, and metastasis. Few clinicians, on the other hand, are alarmed about putative inhibitory effects of micronutrients on chemotherapy [24]. On the other hand, consistent studies have been done on the advantages of antioxidants and micronutrients for cancer patients receiving cancer treatment [25, 26]. Furthermore, there was no interference when antioxidants were administered alongside chemotherapy in other experiments. Many studies on specific cancer types have also shown beneficial effects of micronutrients. One such study was conducted at the Mayo clinic on patients of lung cancer. This study has shown 26% reduction in cancer-related mortality, prolonged survival, and improved quality of life by using micronutrient supplementation [27]. Immuno-nutrition appears to have the capacity to alter immune system activity using certain foods. It can be combined with immunotherapy to enhance immune function, control the induced immune response, lessen the

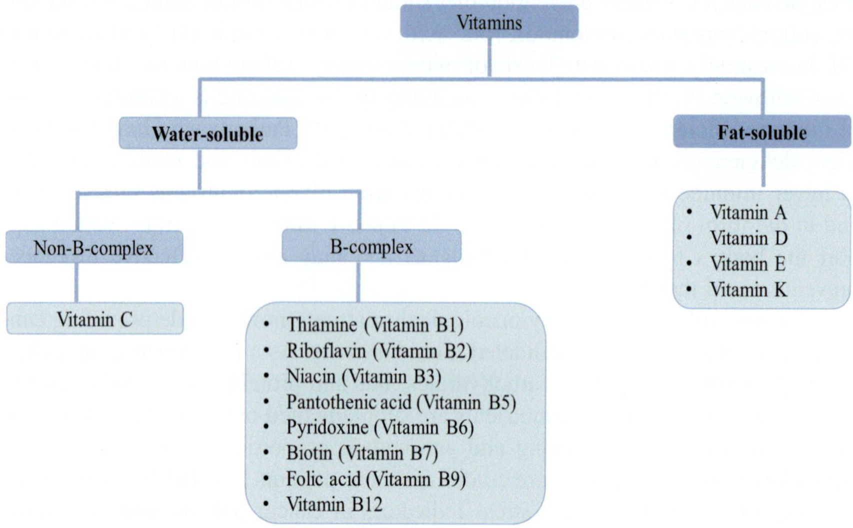

Fig. 5.1 Classification of vitamins

negative effects of treatment, and enhance patient outcomes [28]. However, further research is required to advance a comprehensive and clear understanding of micronutrient dosage and side effects.

5.2 What Are Vitamins?

Vitamins are a collection of substances demanded by the body's biochemical and physiological activities and are necessary for a balanced diet [29]. Vitamins can be split into two groups: fat-soluble and water-soluble as shown in Fig. 5.1. In cancer patients with a poor nutritional state, bleeding has also been linked to severe zinc shortage [30]. In this chapter, we compile a variety of data on a variety of topics: comprising vitamin A, vitamin B, vitamin C, vitamin D, and vitamin E are all promising anti-cancer vitamins. Even though other vitamins are also important, but this chapter is focused only on few vitamins.

5.3 Vitamin C

Vitamin C was originally reported to have cancer-fighting effects in the 1930s and has since been the topic of discussion. It has been suggested around six decades ago that spread of cancer may be linked to a possible deficiency of vitamin C causing a higher incidence of connective tissue deterioration. Maintaining appropriate collagen production levels with vitamin C, therefore, has been linked to preventing the metastatic process. Despite this assumption, the potential value of vitamin C as a therapeutic adjuvant in cancer has been debated because of vitamin C, in eliciting selective cancer cell toxicity in vitro as well as in mice models remains unknown. Linus Pauling, the two-time Nobel Prize laureate, postulated in the early 70 s that ascorbic acid (vitamin C) acting as antioxidant and reduces the risk of cancer if given in 10 g/day intravenous doses of vitamin followed up by oral administration. However, the two big clinical trials conducted at the Mayo Clinic in the late 70s and mid-80s, proved that oral administration of high doses of vitamin C had no efficacy as a form of cancer treatment. Dietary antioxidants have also failed in clinical studies as a possible anti-cancer treatment [31–33]. Based on the above premise, the role of vitamin C in the treatment of cancer, its toxicity limits, and its role as a supplement, in innumerable types of cancers will be discussed here.

5.3.1 Colorectal Cancer

One of the utmost prevalent type of cancer in both sexes and one of the top three in terms of estimated incident cases and mortality is colorectal cancer (CRC) [34]. It is third furthermost commonly diagnosed malignant tumour in the world, CRC causes over 9% of all cancer-related deaths each year [35]. Adenocarcinoma, which develops from healthy glandular colonic and rectum epithelium, accounts for more than 90% of CRCs. Due to the slow growth, there is a window of opportunity for screening precursor lesions and early cancer detection [36]. But by 2035, it is anticipated that the prevalence of the CRC will have more than doubled globally, with the greatest high increase coming in less developed nations as a result of the sharp increase in cases that have been identified in the elderly population [37]. Long noncoding RNA (lncRNA) has been proven to alter genes by epigenetic modifications, RNA–protein interactions, and by functioning as miRNA precursors, regulating cell multiplication, differentiation, invasion, and metastasis, according to a number of studies. It is unknown, however, if the manifestation profile of CRC associated lncRNAs modifies with high dosages of vitamin C. hence, high-dose of vitamin C was found to have a retardation outcome on the growth of tumours in xenograft models [38].The p53, a gene linked to the suppression of tumours by arresting the cell cycle plays a precarious role in the outcome of colon cancer as it progresses from adenoma to carcinoma. There activation of p53 in colon cancer, so, is a probable therapeutic target. In one of the studies, a combination of sulindac and vitamin C was evaluated and has been proved to initiate cell death. Therefore, in the future, this combination treatment of vitamin C with sulindac may show to be an innovative anti-tumour therapeutic approach for colon tumours with p53 wild-type [39]. More than half of all CRC are proven to have mutations that are frequently resistant to therapy. When exposed to high amounts of vitamin C, cultured human CRC cells with mutations are selectively destroyed, as the greater uptake of the oxidized form of vitamin C is responsible for this impact. These conclusions provide a molecular basis for further exploring the therapeutic use of vitamin C in CRCs with mutations [40]. In another study, it has been postulated that there is a significant downregulation of the glucose transporters (GLUT-1) also pyruvate kinase M2 (PKM2)-PTB, resulting in a considerable blocking of the Warburg effect and hence energy strain. Therefore, a mix of standard chemotherapy and metabolic methods, such as vitamin C or other compounds targeting important key actors implicated in the Warburg effect, may represent a new paradigm in anticancer therapies [41]. Recent research on different cancer types has revealed that cells that survive early therapy with targeted drugs are frequently prone to changes in cell metabolism. Vitamin C being an antioxidant in therapeutic doses can paradoxically cause oxidative toxicity. Vitamin C combine cetuximab activates a fatal metabolic cell death chain, significantly limiting the establishment of anti-EGFR antibody resistance, indicating that greater dose vitamin C may be safe in cancer patients [42].

5.3.2 Breast Cancer

Breast cancer (BC) is listed as the second-most prevalent disease worldwide, according to reports from the WHO. The BC incidence is high in the US and Europe, but the condition is quite prevalent in less developed nations as well [43]. Within their lifetime, invasive BC is predicted to affect 1 in 8 women. In 2021, BC was anticipated to account for 30% of all new cancer cases in women. The over-expression of human epidermal growth factor receptor 2 (HER2) and the expression of certain hormone receptors are two molecular characteristics of BC, which is a diverse disease [44]. HER2, Luminal type A and B and basal-like being the four main subtypes of BC that are frequently mentioned [45]. Surgery, radiation, chemotherapy, endocrine therapy, and targeted therapy are currently available treatment options for BC. Although in vivo studies for BC are rare, vitamin C has been regularly stated to promote the retarding effect in human BC cells while exhibiting no effect on normal cells. More information is available about the synergistic effect of vitamin C with chemotherapy medicines, rather than the useful effects of vitamin C in isolation. The probable synergistic effects of vitamin C and several other anti-cancer drugs used in BC treatment, by using 1 M and 100 M ascorbate on BC cell lines, MDA-MB-231 and MCF-7, along with chemotherapeutic drugs doxorubicin, cisplatin, and paclitaxel was studied. It was found that even with normal vitamin C doses, the impact was synergistic with anti-cancer drug doxorubicin at 1 M and 100 M concentrations in both BC cell lines. A high-dose of vitamin C produced inhibitory effects on a variety of anti-cancer drug-resistant breast cell lines, and significantly reduced cell proliferation in some other. Besides, vitamin C had just a minor influence on the normal cells of breast epithelial [46, 47]. Furthermore, when paired with conventional treatments, an additive anti-cancer impact was demonstrated. This has provided a piece of significant evidence that vitamin C in high doses is a likely therapeutic medication, particularly when BC patients with metastatic disease ultimately become resistant to conventional medicines. Achieving a level of 100 μM of vitamin C in the plasma can prevent BC metastases in vivo as well as in vitro. The adding of ascorbic acid to the drinking water has been shown to reduce the growth of the implanted tumour in mice significantly. The same outcome was found when an ascorbic acid and cupric sulphate mixture was either orally or intraperitoneally. But when ascorbic acid and cupric sulphate were administered separately, no effects were observed [48–50]. Vitamin C appears to work by lowering oxidative stress that is individual of the furthermost serious adverse effects of chemo as well as radiotherapy, because tumour cell metabolism, radiation, and chemotherapy all raise the level of reactive oxygen species (ROS), producing oxidative strain in the body. Individuals in advanced stages of disease had lower levels of vitamin C and vice-versa [51]. The effects of vitamin C were noticed in lowering pain, improving quality of life, and improving appetite. Furthermore, some patient survival times were extended, when vitamin C was used as an alternative therapeutic technique with chemotherapy. To determine the benefits of intravenous vitamin C in patients with primary non-metastasized BC being treated with anti-cancer medications, an intriguing study was conducted. Contrary to chemotherapy and radiotherapy, intravenous vitamin C the administration had an effect that was equivalent. As was already mentioned, patients receiving an intravenous vitamin C had better overall health, which may have strengthened their immune systems. Last but not least, vitamin C has a potent anti-inflammatory impact and stimulates the immune system, which prevents tumour growth and treatment resistance [52, 53].

5.3.3 Prostate Cancer

Amongst the most widespread genitourinary cancers and the foremost cause of cancer mortality in male population globally is prostate cancer (PC), which affects 15% of newly diagnosed patients with high-risk localized disease [54, 55]. Treatment of PC cells results in a decrease in cell viability, proportional to vitamin C dose, and duration of treatment. It has also been hypothesized that the cytotoxic outcome of vitamin C is associated with the formation of hydrogen peroxide. In contrast, no significant reduction in tumour growth was noted in a study group of nonresponsive patients with PC to chemotherapy who received weekly intravenous vitamin C injections of 5, 30, or even 60 g [53, 56]. Vitamin C, as a reducing agent that acts as an antioxidant in plasma membranes and inside the cells. On the other hand, there have been limited large population-based studies on PC, with the large data pointing towards an absence of a relationship between the disease outcome and the dose of vitamin C. A population-based case–control research on PC called PROtEuS, conducted in Montreal, Canada, established no link between vitamin C consumption and incidence/grade at the time of diagnosis. The research that is now available suggests that vitamin C intake is not expected to play a role in PC prevention [57].

5.3.4 Lung Cancer

High mortality, low detection rates, and high incidence are all features of lung cancer [58]. Based on the pathological nature, lung cancer can be classified into small cell lung cancer (SCLC) and non-small cell lung cancer (NSCLC). Many studies have shown that intravenous vitamin C infusions are useful in the treatment of lung as well as many other types of cancers. According to Dr. Abram Hoffer, cancer patients who improve the quality of their life, do so by improving the quality of their diet with regular vitamin C supplementation [59]. Dr. Hoffer also revealed that the patients who adhered to the nutrition and supplementation program for prolonged periods, lived longer than the patients who did not. According to numerous case reports, people with lung cancer who receive high doses of vitamin C infusions, go on to live for up to ten years. Greater than 400 mg/dL blood levels of vitamin C, considered hazardous to tumour cells, can be achieved with regular vitamin C infusions, with no negative side effects. In this context, evidence suggests that chemotherapy reduces ascorbic acid levels, in turn reducing the levels of Luo et al. conducted another lung cancer meta-analysis in 2014, analyzing 21 trials involving 8938 participants aged 20 to 89 years. The scientists discovered that increasing vitamin C intake by 100 mg/day reduced the frequency of lung cancer by 7% [60, 61]. In 2021, the relationship between blood vitamin C levels and cancer risk was examined in a single Mendelian randomization trial. This MR investigation statistically evaluated the causal relationships between vitamin C and the occurrence of prostate, lung, rectal and breast cancers as well as the effects of gene variants [9] on vitamin C levels. The incidence of the five forms of cancer mentioned above and blood levels of vitamin C were not linked, according to the researchers. The scientists proposed that antioxidants in fruits and vegetables might be advantageous because past meta-analysis research showed that vitamin C consumption from natural sources is more effective than pills. Overall, vitamin C protects the lungs and BCs, especially when taken orally [62].

5.3.5 Stomach Cancer

In 2020, stomach cancer (also known as gastric cancer (GC)) was the fourth most prevalent cancer death cause, accounting for about 800,000 fatalities [63]. *H. pylori* infection, low socioeconomic standing, a diet high in salty and smoked foods in addition to low in fruits and vegetables, as well as fibre intake, are all risk factors for stomach cancer [64]. Other risk factors include a favourable family history, a hereditary propensity, smoking, drinking, inactivity, obesity, radiation exposure, gastroesophageal reflux illness, and radiation exposure. However, it is still unclear what causes stomach cancer. The reduced form of vitamin C, ascorbic acid, has been shown in follow-up studies on high-risk populations to have a preventive outcome against GC, for which *H. pylori* is a significant risk factor [65]. Most notably, vitamin C can reduce ROS formed in the gastrointestinal tract, minimizing the damage to the gastric epithelium, and can decrease nitrate levels, ultimately decreasing the in vivo generation of carcinogenic compounds. Normal quantities of vitamin C can be found in the stomach mucosa and gastric juice. However, gastric illness impairs the release of vitamin C into gastric juice, lowering the amounts of vitamin C. In fact, vitamin C deficiency in the diet can cause gastric dysplasia to proceed to GC, but vitamin C supplementation can speed the regressive process of gastric pre-cancerous lesions. The link between dietary vitamin C consumption and the risk of GC has also been found to be contrary in some case–control studies. Although the impact of vitamin C intake on the risk of GC may differ based on the location of the cancer in the stomach or its histological subtype. Some recent studies have shown that oral intake of vitamin C has either no association with GC or is inversely linked to sub-sites and subtypes of GC [66].

5.3.6 Pancreatic Cancer

Pancreatic cancer (PAC) has been more common during the past several years. It accounts for around two per cent of all malignancies and contributes to five per cent of cancer-related fatalities [67]. The majority of patients have no overt symptoms until the disease progresses to advanced pancreatic metastasis, when tumour cells are very invasive. Some risk factors for PAC include diabetes, pancreatitis, and family history. There are currently no international standards programs for screening people with a high risk of PAC. In an effort to provide PAC patients a better prognosis, we assessed recent advancements in risk factors, diagnosis, and therapy. In the previous decade, there were three early phase clinical trials that used chemotherapy and vitamin C to treat metastatic PAC. In a pancreatic cancer trial, gemcitabine given in combination with high-dose vitamin C significantly inhibited the tumour development in mice harbouring pancreatic xenografts as compared to control or "gemcitabine-only" groups. In cases of stage IV PAC, patients receiving two-drug chemotherapy with intravenous infusions of vitamin C, 8 out of 9 patients showed tumour reduction after only two months of treatment. Welsh et al. showed similar good outcomes when IVC was paired with a single drug, with 6 out of 9 patients either maintaining or enhancing their overall health status [68]. In both investigations, the median overall survival was 6 and 13 months, respectively. Ten grade-III or higher side effects were documented in the 14 PAC patients involved in the study of Monti et al. [69]. All the documented side effects are common in PAC disease progression and hence are unlikely to be related to associate IVC administration. The Wang et al. trial included 36 patients, of the most serious side effects noted, the most common was neutropenia (five occurrences), most probably caused by the chemotherapy regimen. Similarly, none of the adverse effects observed in the Kawada et al. trial was likely to have been caused by intravenous infusions of vitamin C [69]. It has been demonstrated that vitamin C selectively kills KRAS and BRAF mutant CRC cells by targeting GAPDH, which is why vitamin C appears to be helpful in the treatment of PAC, where KRAS mutations are seen in over 90% of cases [70] (Table 5.1).

Table 5.1 Selected applications of vitamin C and E in various cancers

Vitamins	Cancers	Study type	Outcomes	References
Vitamin C	Colorectal cancer	In vivo	Patient-derived xenografts, vitamin C + cetuximab inhibits the formation of drug persisters, limits CRC organoid growth, and greatly delays acquired resistance	[42]
	Breast cancer	In vivo	Through suppression of EMT, high-dose VC limits cell migration and invasion in BC cell lines	[48]
	Prostate cancer	Clinical trial	Use of intravenous AA outside clinical trials is not recommended as no patient achieved a 50% PSA reduction	[56]
	Lung cancer	Meta-analysis	Has protective effect against lung cancer, but needs further confirmation	[61]
Vitamin E	Colorectal cancer	In vitro	Levels of DNA lesions were much lower in CRC tissues than in non-cancerous tissues surrounding them	[71]
	Breast cancer	Case–control	Vitamin supplementation with zinc in postmenopausal women for 10 or more years may protect women from developing BC	[72]
	Prostate cancer	Clinical trial	Vitamin E significantly improved the risk of PC	[73]
	Lung cancer	Meta-analysis	The consumption of vitamin E is linked to a combined relative risk of lung cancer	[74]

5.4 Vitamin D

Vitamin D is famous for its function in bone metabolism, especially the calcium absorption from the gastrointestinal tract and bone restoration. Most individuals get their vitamin D via exposure to ultraviolet rays of the sunlight, which are converted in the skin to vitamin D, and then hydroxylated to 25-hydroxyvitamin D, a seco-steroid hormone. Vitamin D also regulates cell cycle, cellular proliferation, and cell signalling at the molecular level, thus establishing its role as an agent capable of forming or tending to form tumours or otherwise. The importance of vitamin D treatment, its toxicity limits, supplements, and deficiencies in different types of cancer as shown in Fig. 5.2 will be discussed in the succeeding paragraphs.

5.4.1 Colorectal Cancer

Vitamin D is a low-cost, non-toxic, and easily available therapy having anti-cancer properties against CRCs. The vitamin D Receptors (VDR) are abundantly present

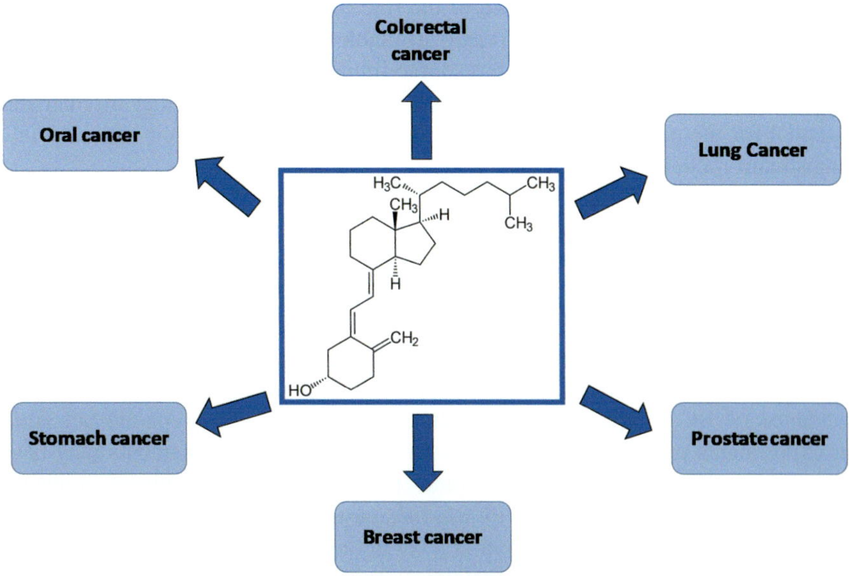

Fig. 5.2 Various cancers caused due to vitamin D deficiency

in colon cancer cells, by binding on which, vitamin D can promote apoptosis. In a mouse model of intestinal carcinogenesis, deletion of the VDR gene increased tumour burden, whereas therapy using vitamin D or else its synthetic equivalent lowered it [75, 76]. Cohort research which involved monitoring the blood levels of 25-hydroxyvitamin D (25(OH)D) before or at the cancer diagnosis consistently revealed vitamin D insufficiency amongst CRC patients. CRC patients with greater levels of 25(OH)D outlived those with lower levels. Subgroup follow-up of a group of 304 CRC patients revealed a stronger correlation of 25(OH)D levels with total survival amongst patients with higher stages of disease as compared to milder forms of the illness. However, in such trials that comprised patients with different levels of severity of the disease, including a small segment of the metastatic variety, insufficient evidence was available to examine the link between vitamin D levels and survival rates [77, 78]. The effect of greater 25(OH)D levels in extending survival has not been established, despite observational studies' significant correlation between blood 25(OH)D levels and average survival in patients with metastatic CRC. Vitamin D deficiency can lead to generalized poor health or be a cause of a more serious condition, which might weaken the underlying relationship between serum levels of vitamin D and the overall survival of a patient suffering from CRC. SUNSHINE, a double-blind randomized clinical study, was thus carried out to investigate whether the administration of high-dose of vitamin D3 (4000 IU/day) in addition to the usual chemo treatment can improve results in patients with metastatic CRC [78, 79]. The change of vitamin D to a possible anti-cancer therapy is a typical case of the role of diet and lifestyle in CRC treatment. Use a safe, economical, and easily available vitamin like it is likely to have a far-reaching global impact, even in resource-limited countries. Strong funding and support are thus required to do additional research on the molecular mechanisms essential for the mode-of-action of vitamin D, in order to ease their inclusion into mainstream models of patient care [79].

5.4.2 Breast Cancer

Observational epidemiology studies have established connections between raised serum levels of vitamin D and BC lower risk. An analysis of twenty-two observational studies showed upper vitamin D consumption was related to a lesser incidence of BC. A quantitative statistical analysis of seven separate but similar experiments published in 2014 showed that vitamin D supplements may have a preventive effect against BC [80]. Some epidemiological data suggest an inverse relationship of vitamin D levels with BC risk, casting a doubt in the use of vitamin D for the prevention of BC. Vitamin D level in the body can be estimated by measuring blood levels of 25(OH)D (calcidiol) and 1,25(OH)2D (calcitriol). Recent population-based studies have verified a strong dose-dependent inverse correlation between serum levels of calcidiol and invasive BC. Previous work has also revealed that the link between vitamin D and BC risk is higher in younger females than in women who had reached the age of menopause. The Iowa Women Health research discovered that women with BC who were negative for oestrogen or progesterone receptor status had a greater protective benefit from vitamin D supplement use [81]. The effective dose of vitamin D3, has its role in calcium and phosphate metabolism by binding to the VDR in target organs like the intestine, kidneys, and bone. However, VDR also express itself in a wide range of other normal and malignant tissues, where it moderates the anti-proliferative, differentiating, and immune-modulatory actions of 1,25(OH)2D3. Randomized Mendelian studies, on the other hand, have found no link between decreased blood levels of 25(OH)D with BC hazard. Still, most randomized controlled clinical trials were failed to show a significant reduction in BC incidence with vitamin D3 treatment. Nonetheless, 1,25(OH)2D3 or its equivalents appear to be more physiologically active and could have greater anti-cancer activity in BC when combined with established cancer medications [82].

5.4.3 Prostate Cancer

Clinical trials in PC patients indicate that vitamin D may slow the course of the disease. A daily dose of 4000 IU for a year has been informed not to lower the blood levels of prostate specific antibodies (PSA) levels. The short duration of follow-up in each of these trials may have contributed to the absence of significant findings:

Therefore, more research using large doses of vitamin D to prevent PC development and to determine the long-term safety of vitamin D usage in these patients [83, 84]. While the biochemical changes linked to vitamin D therapy have been extensively researched in the prostate as well as other cancer types, the complete mechanisms leading to reduced survival and diminished proliferation of cancer cells still remain unknown. Calcitriol, which has received the maximum attention of scientists during in vitro plus in vivo studies, is reported to retard growth of tumours, primarily by inhibition of angiogenesis, and motility, and variation of tumour related factors [85]. Furthermore, there is substantial evidence that vitamin D signalling also plays a role in the betterment of the immunological function of the body, which has been acknowledged as an effective cancer therapeutic and preventative approach.

5.4.4 Lung Cancer

According to research, vitamin D has been associated to the aetiology of multiple diseases, including cancer, with its involvement in a variety of biological pathways. In vitro along with in vivo trials have shown vitamin D to have immunomodulatory and anti-cancer properties. Numerous outlines of proof advocate that vitamin D role in treatment as well as prevention of several infective diseases of the lung including the lung cancer. Proof suggests that seasonal differences and latitudinal gradients influence a vitamin D generation in the skin. It has been discovered that the dose of UV light received by skin varies dramatically from south to north in the UK and Norway. Furthermore, mortality rates from lung cancer varied across these countries due to seasonal differences and latitudinal gradients in UV exposure. In the UK population, there was a substantial difference in vitamin D concentration between the regions as well as between the seasons. In 45,000 lung cancer patients monitored in a large study of the Norwegian population, it was discovered that patients under the age of 50 had a 15% lower risk of death from lung cancer in the hotter seasons compared to the cold seasons during the first 18 months after diagnosis.

A meta-analysis research that incorporated data from 111 people to estimate the relationship between UV contact, and the level of risk of lung cancer, discovered a link between the location of latitude and the lung cancer risk [86, 87]. In vitro research has shown that vitamin D in addition to its analogues can decrease the proliferation of lung cancer cells. In vivo analogues of vitamin D have been shown to be more than 284 times more effective than vitamin D itself in reducing the proliferation of the lung cancer H520 cells by arresting the cell cycle in the phase of G1, thus impeding DNA synthesis and, ultimately, the cell growth. These studies suggest that vitamin D analogues can inhibit the growth of lung cancer cells [88, 89]. However, many observational and meta-analysis studies have not supported the link between serum levels of vitamin D and the danger of lung cancer. Nonetheless, data on the impact of vitamin D on the signalling pathways of lung tumour cells is sparse, as is the information on whether genetic alterations in these genes are implicated in vitamin D action. Furthermore, variations in the vitamin D/VDR signalling pathway, as well as associated molecules, may influence the quality and quantity of vitamin D therapeutic outcomes. The optimum level of vitamin D to act positively in preventing or treating lung cancer with insignificant harm is so far to be determined. Small-sized clinical research done so far, to investigate the positive effects of vitamin D in the prevention and treatment of lung cancer, has shown mixed results at best. In the long run, public health planners should focus on developing adequate amount of vitamin D in the population to identify the useful benefits of vitamin D in the prevention of lung cancer.

5.4.5 Gastric Cancer

Increased serum levels of vitamin D lower the possibility of gastric carcinoma. Paricalcitol, calcitriol and their analogue, inhibits the proliferation of GC cells by altering the cell life cycle and suppressing the inflammatory processes, without lowering the serum calcium levels. Bao et al. discovered that direct use of 1,25(OH)2D3 causes cellular death in GC cells, lending credence to vitamin Ds anti-tumoural effect on GC [90]. Vitamin D inhibits cell survival by inhibiting the expression of multiple target genes, in GC cells via the hedgehog signalling pathway. Vitamin D, significantly increases apoptosis in undifferentiated GC cells. It may also slow the progression of GC via modifying the extracellular milieu, since it is believed to change the action of a variety of various genes involved in extracellular matrix remodelling. By interfering with the interaction between tumour epithelial cells and their surroundings, vitamin D can block Wnt signalling. Vitamin D status is an important predictive aspect in GC patients, and vitamin D insufficiency may be linked to a poor prognosis [91].

5.5 Vitamin A

Vitamin A (retinol, carotene, or retinyl ester), is vital for the body in various cellular processes and can only be got through the diet in these forms. Retinoid are a class of natural and manufactured chemicals with structural and/or functional similarities to vitamin A [92]. Because the processes in which, vitamin A plus retinoids can function at the cellular level are so important, their use in cancer treatment of piqued people's interest right away. Several studies have been developed since the research done by Wolbach and Howe [93], to highlight the crucial involvement of vitamin A in oncogenesis. In cancer cells of BC, the alteration of retinol to retinoic acid is hindered, and these results were confirmed by Williams et al. in ovarian cancer cells [94, 95]. BC is the most studied anti-cancer effect of retinoids, and lung, prostate, and pancreatic cancers reports were also found, though to a lower level. All-trans-RA is the most researched endogenous retinoid, followed by 9-cis-RA and 13-cis-RA, both of which are inactive minor metabolites found in the body. Poor water solubility, teratogenicity, cytotoxicity, tumour resistance, and recurrence have all been documented as side effects of endogenous retinoids. Synthetic retinoids, for example, have recently received a lot of attention. The potential of synthetic retinoids as anti-cancer drugs reveals a new anti-cancer research area in synthetic retinoids medication discovery and development. Synthetic retinoids, which have shown to have higher anti-cancer effects, are therefore highly suggested for use in drug combination strategies, and their effective doses can be found here. Natural retinoids, particularly 13-cis-RA and 9-cis-RA, have been widely explored in recent decades. ALRT1550, a ligand with strong affinity for all three RARs, has been shown in nude mice to have substantial anti-tumour action against xenografts of human oral squamous carcinoma [96]. One of the most promising clinically evaluated retinoids is fenretinide (4-HPR) [97]. 4-HPR has been shown to have strong cytotoxic action against tumour cells by inducing apoptotic and non-apoptotic cell death in a range of cancers, as shown in Table 5.2. Despite various studies has demonstrated to play a prospective role of vitamin A and retinoids in the treatment and prevention of numerous cancers in recent years. However, the mechanisms through which these chemicals exert their anti-carcinogenic actions are still unknown. Elevated amount of certain inhibitory signalling pathways, such as kinase C inhibition or reduction of oncogene expression, is thought to be involved in the processes by which vitamin A in addition retinoids can prevent malignant growth, although further research is needed [98]. Despite the promising preliminary findings, some research indicates that retinoids have little to no impact on the development or spread of solid tumours. Numerous strategies should be researched in order to increase the efficacy of retinoids in the treatment and prevention of cancer. In recent years, an endogenous retinoid called all-trans-RA has been extensively investigated and found to have anti-cancer properties in the CRC. Lee et al. found that all-trans-RA reduced the cell viability of HCT116 (1 M) and SW480 (0.5 M), and further research into the mechanisms of action revealed a decrease in the expression of MED28, cyclin D1, c-MYC, and catenin in the Wnt/-catenin signalling pathway and an increase in e-cadherin and HBP1 [99]. In an 80 M concentration, the same retinoid reduced the migratory ability of RKO cells in a wound healing assay. Its anti-cancer action was similarly regulated by lowering MLCK expression in the ERK1/MAPK signalling pathway [100]. According to epidemiological research, dietary vitamin A intake and the risk of developing cancer are inversely related. Chemically created experimental cancers are less common when vitamin A is administered in pharmaceutical doses [101]. Different types of tumours, including oral cavity, skin, lung, hepatic, gastrointestinal, breast, prostate, and bladder malignancies, have been shown to be inhibited by retinoids [102].

Furthermore, RA or synthetic retinoids may cause nude mice's growth to be stopped, to die, or to differentiate when added to human cancer cell lines or xenografts [101]. Furthermore, various research in animal models shows that retinoids have an inhibitory effect on BC. In mice treated with retinyl acetate, the incidence of BC was reduced by 52% [109]. Retinoids, particularly 9-cis-RA, limit the proliferation of oestrogen receptor-positive (ER) cells in vitro by interrupting the cell cycle [110]. In lung cancer, only endogenous retinoid has been studied in

Table 5.2 Selected studies on synthetic retinoids application in different cancer

Synthetic retinoids	Outcomes	References
ALRT1550	In nude mice, there was potent anti-cancer efficacy against human oral squamous carcinoma xenografts	[96]
Fenretinide	In breast, prostate, colon-rectal small and non-small cell lung malignancies, tumour cells exert cytotoxic action by inducing apoptotic and non-apoptotic cell death	[103–106]
LGD1069 (Targretin)	Prevents BC (animal model)	[107]
ST1926	Inhibited cell proliferation in BC, PC, suppressed tumour development in CRC (stronger than all-*trans*-RA)	[108]

relation to lung cancer in recent years. Using the MTT assay, Zito et al. employed all-trans-RA to lower the cell viability of H1975 cells at 1 and 10 M. The same cell line's apoptosis was seen using an Annexin V-FITC/PI staining test, and its anti-cancer efficacy was demonstrated by down-regulating the expression of EGFR and CTNNB1 in the EGFR and Wnt/-catenin signalling pathways, respectively [111]. These findings demonstrated that all-trans-RA, an endogenous retinoid, is a strong anti-cancer drug that targets the EGFR/MAPK, Wnt/-catenin, and caspase signalling pathways in lung cancer. Lung cancer treatment with all-trans-RA, either alone or in combination, is beneficial. In two separate experiments, the cell viability of an endogenous retinoid, 9-cis-RA [112], and a synthetic retinoid, and ST1926 [113] were tested against PC3 cells at a concentration of 1 M. Both 9-cis-RA and ST1926 had an anti-proliferative effect on PC3 cells, according to these investigations. Furthermore, at the same concentration, 9-cis-RA inhibits cell proliferation in LNCaP cells [112], whereas ST1926 is cytotoxic to DU145 cells [113]. All-trans-RA, on the other hand, had no effect on the viability of DU145 and PC3 cells at 10 M, whereas ST1926 caused a substantial drop at as low as 0.1 M, showing that ST1926 is more cytotoxic than all-trans-RA [113]. The anti-cancer effects of endogenous and synthetic retinoids on PC are equivalent, according to these latest data. As a result, more research on the potency of retinoids is needed, and combination therapy should be investigated by replicating trials done on other types of malignancies. Gemcitabine, a pancreatic cancer chemotherapeutic medication, was coupled with all-trans-RA and found to reduce the growth of AsPC-1 cells by 2.8-fold when compared to gemcitabine [114]. Following that, using the sulforhodamine B assay and the Boyden Chamber assay, this combination therapy inhibited cell proliferation and migration in both MiaPaCa-2 and TB33117 cells [115]. For both cells, the IC50 values were roughly 1.2-fold greater than gemcitabine, showing that gemcitabine has a lower cytotoxicity [115]. Only a small number of synthetic retinoids have been accepted by the FDA or are currently being evaluated in clinical studies, despite the fact that they are thought to be encouraging for the management of cancer. In preclinical studies, synthetic retinoids stop human cancer from spreading.

5.6 Vitamin B Complex

B vitamins are important micronutrients for a variety of metabolic and regulatory activities that are necessary for human health. B1 (thiamin), B2 (riboflavin), B3 (niacin), B5 (pantothenic acid), B6 (pyridoxine), B7 (biotin), B9 (folic acid), and B12 (cobalamin) are all water-soluble vitamins (cobalamin). They serve as cofactors for numerous enzymes that carry out critical tasks including protein and DNA synthesis, energy metabolism, and other key processes. Because of the inconsistent data published thus far, the function of B vitamins in cancer is uncertain. Studies on vitamin B6, B9, and B12 have been shown in order to define their potential function in cancer. Although some writers claim that low vitamin B6, B9, in addition to B12 levels predispose to the development of a variety of malignancies, and have yet to fully explain the part these nutrients play in the progression of cancer. Liu et al. [116] found intriguing relationships between the genes involved in thiamine metabolism and BC oncogenesis. The effects of thiamine supplementation on cancer risk and tumourgenicity have been studied. The findings of the research are variable, with some revealing protective effects and others revealing no significant differences. Thiamine was found to be beneficial in an Italian ORDET cohort of 391BC cases with B vitamin consumption. Thiamine was discovered to be especially protective in HER2-positive patients that lacked both oestrogen and progesterone receptors [117]. When it comes to thiamine's impact on cancer, which can be modest and dependent on cancer subtypes, in vitro plus in vivo study yields contradicting results. More study is needed to clarify apparent differences between findings and investigate thiamine's impact on cancer subtypes, based on existing evidence. Vitamin B2 deficiency has also been linked to cancer risk, however the research on riboflavin and cancer is complicated. Some authors suggested that riboflavin deficiency raises the threat of cancer at specific places, while others suggest that riboflavin may have an anti-carcinogenic effect in the presence of certain carcinogens [118]. Although the data was inconsistent, a meta-analysis of twenty-seven studies studying riboflavin and other B vitamins, which included nearly 50,000 cases in addition of 1.2 million people, revealed that B2 may reduce the incidence of BC [119]. Riboflavin has been shown in several trials to lessen the threat of CRC in women [120], possibly over the FAD-dependent methylenetetrahydrofolate reductase (MTHFR). In case of non-smoking women, higher riboflavin intake has been connected to a decreased risk of lung cancer [121]. Despite how simple it is to make pyridoxine, human cells have a difficult time converting pyridoxin to the associated vitamins. Increased plasma vitamin B6 levels, for example, were linked to a reduced risk of colon cancer development, as discussed here [122]. Numerous epidemiological work has recently underlined the importance of vitamin B6 as a cancer-preventive agent in addition to its well-known role as a cofactor in numerous enzyme activities. Vitamin B6 has been proven to reduce cell growth and improve immune response in vivo tests. At the molecular level, vitamin B6 has the capacity to inhibit the transactivation potential of a number of nuclear receptors. Further study into the mechanism of action and potential clinical applications of vitamin B6 is supported by all of these mechanistic and clinical data.

The water-soluble B vitamin folate, often referred to as folacin, or vitamin B9, is necessary for DNA synthesis, repair, and methylation [123]. Numerous vitamins and meals are fortified with folic acid, a synthetic form of folates because humans are unable to produce them on their own. Due to its importance in DNA repair and modulation of S-adenosyl methionine, a universal methyl donor group for DNA methylation processes, preclinical investigations have demonstrated that folate may have anti-cancer potential. The prevalence of BC was significantly reduced in women who consumed more dietary folate on a daily basis compared to those who consumed less folate, according to a meta-analysis of 16 prospective studies and 26 case–control studies. Surprisingly, circulating folate levels and the incidence of BC were not statistically linked despite this effect [124]. Folic acid, however, has been linked to a significant reduction in the recurrence of colonic adenomas when taken as a supplement, suggesting that it may be a useful chemo-preventive drug for CRC. High blood folate levels were connected to a rise in the incidence of BC in a study of a small group of women with high disease risk (BRCA1/2) [125]. On the other hand, numerous studies have found that women who have the BRCA1 gene mutation can benefit from folic acid supplementation. There was no proof that B6 and B12 were connected [125]. Epidemiological and clinical research has shown an inverse relationship amongst folate intake and blood levels and the risk of CRC. When comparing the greatest and lowest quartiles of folate intake, the risk decrease for CRC is significant and equals a 40% reduction [126]. In males with PC, high serum folate levels have been associated with enhanced cell proliferation [127]. Studies conducted in living organisms allow for a more thorough assessment of specific B vitamins as well as a better understanding of the benefits and drawbacks of B vitamin supplementation in various circumstances. Finally, it is difficult to apply these findings to human intervention research since cancer prevention studies would need long-term compliance in very large cohorts.

5.7 Vitamin E

A family of eight fat-soluble compounds includes vitamin E comprising four types of tocopherols (α, β, γ, and δ) and tocotrienols (α, β, γ, and δ). Alpha-tocopherol is the type of vitamin E that is most frequently detected. It has a number of advantages, including scavenging free radicals, shielding cells, lessening blood clotting, and lowering the risk of several cancers. Numerous research has been conducted over the past 20 years with a focus on the effect of vitamin E in cancer. Major antioxidant vitamins like vitamin E have been suggested as potential CRC preventatives. Their positive effects include a decrease in DNA oxidative damage and the suppression of free radicals [71]. But, some studies established that vitamin E didn't diminish the occurrence of CRC [128]. Hence, the anti-oxidant effects of vitamin supplementation on CRC need further study. Interestingly, vitamin E supplements and food potential role in BC prevention are still unknown [129].

However, dietary vitamin E intake or supplementation did not seem to offer any notable advantages for less than ten years [72]. A greater intake of vitamin E in the food was shown to be significantly related with a lower chance of getting BC in a prior case–control study carried out in the US with 297 BC patients and 311 control subjects. However, taking vitamin E supplements did not make you more likely to have BC [130]. Numerous prospective and case–control studies, however, have not discovered a connection between vitamin E intake from food or supplements and the risk of BC. In a previous large prospective trial, high dietary vitamin E intake did not protect against BC [131]. PC may be prevented by vitamin E, either alone or in conjunction with other nutrients, according to a number of studies undertaken over the past 20 years. Lippman et al. [132] concluded that in the generally healthy, diverse community of men, selenium, vitamin E, or selenium with vitamin E did not prevent PC. Additionally, the medical research community is compelled by these discoveries to keep looking for fresh, efficient PC preventive treatments. In males over 50, taking a daily supplement of selenium and vitamin E for 5.5 years, but did not diminish the risk of prostate or other malignancies [133]. Over the past 20 years, a large body of research has demonstrated that vitamin E, either on its own or in conjunction with other nutrients, may have anti-cancer advantages in PC [73]. Neither the selenium alone nor the selenium + vitamin E groups showed this adverse effect [133]. To summarize the data from epidemiological studies of vitamin E intake and the incidence of lung cancer, a meta-analysis was done. They discovered that the combined RR of lung cancer was 0.858, when vitamin E intake was considered. In the US population and prospective studies (RR = 0.913, 95%), substantial protective relationships were also discovered. Their data suggest that vitamin E supplements may lower lung cancer incidence, notably in the United States.

5.8 Conclusion

Since it has become obvious that vitamins and other micronutrients are essential to the aetiology of many diseases, including cancer, the scientific community has grown more interested in vitamins and other micronutrients. Dietary factors, nutritional state, and the efficacy of anti-cancer therapy are all connected to the prognosis of cancer disease. It has been shown that micronutrients from both dietary and non-dietary sources are negatively correlate with the risk of cancer. They offer a terrific example for cancer clinics in terms of halting the development and spread of disease. Although preliminary, the information on cancer is reassuring. A small number of studies also point to the possibility that micronutrients, particularly antioxidants, can lessen the occurrence of adverse effects brought on by cancer treatments, potentially enhancing the quality of life for cancer patients. From a clinical perspective, the available data are insufficient to make any firm judgments. The various analyses of the data presented by the different research groups were limited and inconsistent. The reported results varied from one to the next, and risk estimations were less precise than if individual data had been supplied. The authors also used a variety of methods to assess the inverse relationship between vitamins and BC or to treat it, which can affect the comparability of different studies due to heterogeneity amongst studies and publication bias, which is difficult to avoid when the number of studies is small. Furthermore, it is critical to optimize cancer patients' nutritional condition and supply them with the necessary levels of micronutrients to escape malnutrition, which might exacerbate the patient's clinical state. In the future, other investigations, such as clinical trials, will be critical in order to corroborate the findings. Despite substantial research into the inverse association between vitamins or pro-vitamins in the cancer development, prevention, and treatment, many questions remain unanswered, necessitating clinical studies.

References

1. Willett WC (1994) Micronutrients and cancer risk. Am J Clin Nutr 59(5 Suppl):1162s-s1165
2. (WHO) WHO Global Health Estimates (2020) Deaths by cause, age, sex, by country and by region, 2000–2019. who.int/data/gho/data/themes/mortality-andglobal-health-estimates/ghe-leadingcauses-of-death Accessed on 11 Dec 2021
3. Sung H, Ferlay J, Siegel RL, Laversanne M, Soerjomataram I, Jemal A, Bray F (2021) Global cancer statistics 2020: GLOBOCAN estimates of incidence and mortality worldwide for 36 cancers in 185 countries. CA Cancer J Clin 71(3):209–249. https://doi.org/10.3322/caac.21660. Epub 2021 Feb 4. PMID: 33538338
4. Senapati S, Mahanta AK, Kumar S, Maiti P (2018) Controlled drug delivery vehicles for cancer treatment and their performance. Signal Transduct Target Ther 3:7–21
5. Brown KF, Rumgay H, Dunlop C, Ryan M, Quartly F, Cox A et al (2018) The fraction of cancer attributable to modifiable risk factors in England, Wales, Scotland, Northern Ireland, and the United Kingdom in 2015. Br J Cancer 118(8):1130–1141
6. Parkin DM, Boyd L, Walker L (2011) The fraction of cancer attributable to lifestyle and environmental factors in the UK in 2010. Br J Cancer 105(2):S77–S81
7. Chakraborty A, Guha S, Chakraborty D (2020) Micronutrients in preventing cancer: a critical review of research. Asian Pacific J Cancer Biol 5(3):119–125
8. Alam W, Ullah H, Santarcangelo C, Di Minno A, Khan H, Daglia M et al (2021) Micronutrient food supplements in patients with gastro-intestinal and hepatic cancers. Int J Mol Sci 22(15):8014
9. Rodgers GM, Becker PS, Blinder M, Cella D, Chanan-Khan A, Cleeland C et al (2012) Cancer-and chemotherapy-induced anemia. J Natl Compr Canc Netw 10(5):628–653
10. Nesher L, Rolston KV (2013) Neutropenic enterocolitis, a growing concern in the era of widespread use of aggressive chemotherapy. Clin Infect Dis 56(5):711–717
11. Gorji A, Ghadiri MK (2021) Potential roles of micronutrient deficiency and immune system dysfunction in the coronavirus disease 2019 (COVID-19) pandemic. Nutrition 82:111047
12. Gröber U, Holzhauer P, Kisters K, Holick MF, Adamietz IA (2016) Micronutrients in oncological intervention. Nutrients 8(3):163
13. Babaknejad N, Sayehmiri F, Sayehmiri K, Rahimifar P, Bahrami S, Delpesheh A et al (2014) The relationship between selenium levels and breast cancer: a systematic review and meta-analysis. Biol Trace Elem Res 159(1):1–7
14. Mayland CR, Bennett MI, Allan K (2005) Vitamin C deficiency in cancer patients. Palliat Med 19(1):17–20

15. Cruciani R, Dvorkin E, Homel P, Culliney B, Malamud S, Shaiova L et al (2004) L-carnitine supplementation for the treatment of fatigue and depressed mood in cancer patients with carnitine deficiency: a preliminary analysis. Ann N Y Acad Sci 1033(1):168–176
16. Churilla TM, Brereton HD, Klem M, Peters CA (2012) Vitamin D deficiency is widespread in cancer patients and correlates with advanced stage disease: a community oncology experience. Nutr Cancer 64(4):521–525
17. Bhagat SS, Ghone RA, Suryakar AN, Hundekar PS (2011) Lipid peroxidation and antioxidant vitamin status in colorectal cancer patients. Indian J Physiol Pharmacol 55(1):72–76
18. Comito G, Ippolito L, Chiarugi P, Cirri P (2020) Nutritional exchanges within tumor microenvironment: impact for cancer aggressiveness. Front Oncol 10:396
19. Muir A, Vander Heiden MG (2018) The nutrient environment affects therapy. Science 360(6392):962–963
20. Van Gorkom GN, Klein Wolterink RG, Van Elssen CH, Wieten L, Germeraad WT, Bos GM (2018) Influence of vitamin C on lymphocytes: an overview. Antioxidants 7(3):41
21. Ang A, Pullar JM, Currie MJ, Vissers MC (2018) Vitamin C and immune cell function in inflammation and cancer. Biochem Soc Trans 46(5):1147–1159
22. Wu X, Hu W, Lu L, Zhao Y, Zhou Y, Xiao Z et al (2019) Repurposing vitamin D for treatment of human malignancies via targeting tumor microenvironment. Acta Pharmaceutica Sinica B 9(2):203–219
23. Cuenca-Micó O, Aceves C (2020) Micronutrients and breast cancer progression: a systematic review. Nutrients 12(12):3613
24. Ambrosone CB, Zirpoli GR, Hutson AD, McCann WE, McCann SE, Barlow WE et al (2020) Dietary supplement use during chemotherapy and survival outcomes of patients with breast cancer enrolled in a cooperative group clinical trial (SWOG S0221). J Clin Oncol 38(8):804
25. Moss RW (2007) Do antioxidants interfere with radiation therapy for cancer? Integr Cancer Ther 6(3):281–292
26. Yasueda A, Urushima H, Ito T (2016) Efficacy and interaction of antioxidant supplements as adjuvant therapy in cancer treatment: a systematic review. Integr Cancer Ther 15(1):17–39
27. Jatoi A, Williams B, Nichols F, Marks R, Aubry M-C, Wampfler J et al (2005) Is voluntary vitamin and mineral supplementation associated with better outcome in non-small cell lung cancer patients?: results from the Mayo Clinic lung cancer cohort. Lung Cancer 49(1):77–84
28. Wang F, Li R (2017) Cancer immunotherapy and immunonutrition. MOJ Anat Physiol 3:00104
29. Young VR, Newberne PM (1981) Vitamins and cancer prevention: issues and dilemmas. Cancer 47(S5):1226–1240
30. Stefanini M (1999) Cutaneous bleeding related to zinc deficiency in two cases of advanced cancer. Cancer Interdisciplin Int J Am Cancer Soc 86(5):866–870
31. Reczek CR, Chandel NS (2015) Cancer revisiting vitamin c and cancer. Science 350(6266):1317–1318
32. van der Reest J, Gottlieb E (2016) Anti-cancer effects of vitamin C revisited. Cell Res 26(3):269–270
33. Roa FJ, Peña E, Gatica M, Escobar-Acuña K, Saavedra P, Maldonado M et al (2020) Therapeutic use of vitamin c in cancer: physiological considerations. 11
34. Siegel RL, Miller KD, Fuchs HE, Jemal A (2021) Cancer statistics 71(1):7–33
35. Bray F, Ferlay J, Soerjomataram I, Siegel RL, Torre LA, Jemal AJ (2018) Global cancer statistics 2018: GLOBOCAN estimates of incidence and mortality worldwide for 36 cancers in 185 countries. 68(6):394–424
36. CDC Division of cancer prevention and control CfDCaP. Colorectal cancer statistics (CDC)
37. Papamichael D, Audisio R, Glimelius B, de Gramont A, Glynne-Jones R, Haller D et al (2015) Treatment of colorectal cancer in older patients: international society of geriatric oncology (SIOG) consensus recommendations 2013. 26(3):463–476
38. Chen J, Qin F, Li Y, Mo S, Deng K, Huang Y et al (2020) High-dose vitamin c tends to kill colorectal cancer with high MALAT1 expression. J Oncol 2020:2621308

39. Gong E-Y, Shin YJ, Hwang I-Y, Kim JH, Kim S-M, Moon J-H et al (2016) Combined treatment with vitamin C and sulindac synergistically induces p53- and ROS-dependent apoptosis in human colon cancer cells. Toxicol Lett 258:126–133
40. Yun J, Mullarky E, Lu C, Bosch KN, Kavalier A, Rivera K et al (2015) Vitamin C selectively kills KRAS and BRAF mutant colorectal cancer cells by targeting GAPDH. Science 350(6266):1391–1396
41. Aguilera O, Muñoz-Sagastibelza M, Torrejón B, Borrero-Palacios A, Del Puerto-Nevado L, Martínez-Useros J et al (2016) Vitamin C uncouples the Warburg metabolic switch in KRAS mutant colon cancer. Oncotarget 7(30):47954–47965
42. Lorenzato A, Magrì A, Matafora V, Audrito V, Arcella P, Lazzari L et al (2020) Vitamin C restricts the emergence of acquired resistance to EGFR-targeted therapies in colorectal cancer. Cancers 12(3):685. https://doi.org/10.3390/cancers12030685. PMID: 32183295; PMCID: PMC7140052
43. Suleman M, Tahir Ul Qamar M, Saleem S, Ahmad S, Ali SS, Khan H et al (2021) Mutational landscape of pirin and elucidation of the impact of most detrimental missense variants that accelerate the breast cancer pathways: a computational modelling study. Front Mol Biosci 8:692835
44. Li C, Fan Z, Lin X, Cao M, Song F, Song F (2021) Parity and risk of developing breast cancer according to tumor subtype: a systematic review and meta-analysis. Cancer Epidemiol 75:102050
45. Carey LA, Perou CM, Livasy CA, Dressler LG, Cowan D, Conway K et al (2006) Race, breast cancer subtypes, and survival in the Carolina breast cancer study. JAMA 295(21):2492–2502
46. Lee SJ, Jeong JH, Lee IH, Lee J, Jung JH, Park HY et al (2019) Effect of high-dose vitamin c combined with anti-cancer treatment on breast cancer cells. Anticancer Res 39(2):751–758
47. Hatem E, Azzi S, El Banna N, He T, Heneman-Masurel A, Vernis L et al (2019) Auranofin/vitamin C: a novel drug combination targeting triple-negative breast cancer. J Cancer Inst 111(6):597–608
48. Zeng L-H, Wang Q-M, Feng L-Y, Ke Y-D, Xu Q-Z, Wei A-Y et al (2019) High-dose vitamin C suppresses the invasion and metastasis of breast cancer cells via inhibiting epithelial-mesenchymal transition. Cancer 12:7405
49. Gan L, Camarena V, Mustafi S, Wang GJN (2019) Vitamin C inhibits triple-negative breast cancer metastasis by affecting the expression of YAP1 and synaptopodin. 11(12):2997
50. Hsu C-H, Peng K-L, Kang M-L, Chen Y-R, Yang Y-C, Tsai C-H, et al TET1 suppresses cancer invasion by activating the tissue inhibitors of metalloproteinases. 2(3):568–579
51. Vollbracht C, Schneider B, Leendert V, Weiss G, Auerbach L (2011) Intravenous vitamin C administration improves quality of life in breast cancer patients during chemo-/radiotherapy and aftercare: results of a retrospective, multicentre, epidemiological cohort study in Germany. Cancer 25(6):983–990
52. Ma Y, Chapman J, Levine M, Polireddy K, Drisko J, Chen QJ (2014) High-dose parenteral ascorbate enhanced chemosensitivity of ovarian cancer and reduced toxicity of chemotherapy. 6(222):222ra18-ra18
53. Carr AC, Maggini SJN (2017) Vitamin C and immune function 9(11):1211
54. Siegel RL, Miller KD, Fuchs HE, Jemal A (2022) Cancer statistics, 2022. CA: a cancer journal for clinicians. 72(1):7–33
55. Devos G, Devlies W, De Meerleer G, Baldewijns M, Gevaert T, Moris L et al (2021) Neoadjuvant hormonal therapy before radical prostatectomy in high-risk prostate cancer. Nat Rev Urol 18(12):739–762
56. Nielsen TK, Højgaard M, Andersen JT, Jørgensen NR, Zerahn B, Kristensen B et al (2017) Weekly ascorbic acid infusion in castration-resistant prostate cancer patients: a single-arm phase II trial. Trans Androl Urol 6(3):517
57. Parent M-E, Richard H, Rousseau M-C (2018) Vitamin C intake and risk of prostate cancer: the Montreal PROtEuS study. Cancer 9:1218
58. Bade BC, Cruz CSDJCICM (2020) Lung cancer 2020: epidemiology, etiology, and prevention. 41(1):1–24

59. A H (2015) Antioxidant nutrients and cancer. J Orthomolec Med 15:193–200
60. Cho E, Hunter DJ, Spiegelman D, Albanes D, Beeson WL, Van Den Brandt PA et al (2006) Intakes of vitamins A, C and E and folate and multivitamins and lung cancer: a pooled analysis of 8 prospective studies. 118(4):970–978
61. Luo J, Shen L, Zheng DJSR (2014) Association between vitamin C intake and lung cancer: a dose-response meta-analysis. Biomed 4(1):1–7
62. Fu Y, Xu F, Jiang L, Miao Z, Liang X, Yang J et al (2021) Circulating vitamin C concentration and risk of cancers: a Mendelian randomization study. BMC Med 19(1):1–14
63. Ferlay J, Colombet M, Soerjomataram I, Parkin DM, Piñeros M, Znaor A et al (2021) Cancer statistics for the year 2020: an overview. Int J Cancer
64. Karimi P, Islami F, Anandasabapathy S, Freedman ND, Kamangar F (2014) Gastric cancer: descriptive epidemiology, risk factors, screening, and prevention. Cancer Epidemiol Biomark Prevent Publ Am Assoc Cancer Res Cospon Am Soc Prevent Oncol 23(5):700–713
65. Feiz HR, Mobarhan SJNR (2002) Does vitamin C intake slow the progression of gastric cancer in Helicobacter pylori-infected populations? 60(1):34
66. Jenab M, Riboli E, Ferrari P, Sabate J, Slimani N, Norat T et al (2006) Plasma and dietary vitamin C levels and risk of gastric cancer in the european prospective investigation into cancer and nutrition (EPIC-EURGAST). 27(11):2250–2257
67. Gillen S, Schuster T, MeyarzumBuschenfelde C, Friess H, Kleeff T (2010) Preoperative/neoadjuvant therapy in pancreatic cancer: a systematic review and meta-analysis of response and resection percentages. Bio Med 7(4):e1000267
68. Welsh JL, Wagner BA, van't Erve TJ, Zehr PS, Berg DJ, Halfdanarson TR et al (2013) Pharmacological ascorbate with gemcitabine for the control of metastatic and node-positive pancreatic cancer (PACMAN): results from a phase I clinical trial. Cancer Chemother Pharmacol 71(3):765–775
69. Monti DA, Mitchell E, Bazzan AJ, Littman S, Zabrecky G, Yeo CJ et al (2012) Phase I evaluation of intravenous ascorbic acid in combination with gemcitabine and erlotinib in patients with metastatic pancreatic cancer. PLoS ONE 7(1):e29794
70. Bryant KL, Mancias JD, Kimmelman AC, Der CJJTIBS (2014) KRAS: feeding pancreatic cancer proliferation. 39(2):91–100
71. Kirkali G, Keles D, Canda AE, Terzi C, Reddy PT, Jaruga P et al (2011) Evidence for upregulated repair of oxidatively induced DNA damage in human colorectal cancer. DNA Rep 10(11):1114–1120
72. Pan SY, Zhou J, Gibbons L, Morrison H, Wen SW (2011) The Canadian cancer registries epidemiology research G: antioxidants and breast cancer risk- a population-based case-control study in Canada. BMC Cancer 11(1):372
73. Klein EA, Thompson IM Jr, Tangen CM, Crowley JJ, Lucia MS, Goodman PJ et al (2011) Vitamin E and the risk of prostate cancer: the Selenium and Vitamin E cancer prevention trial (SELECT). JAMA 306(14):1549–1556
74. Chen G, Wang J, Hong X, Chai Z, Li Q (2015) Dietary vitamin E intake could reduce the risk of lung cancer: evidence from a meta-analysis. Int J Clin Exp Med 8(4):6631–6637
75. Meggouh F, Lointier P, Saez SJCR (1991) Sex steroid and 1, 25-dihydroxyvitamin D3 receptors in human colorectal adenocarcinoma and normal mucosa 51(4):1227–1233
76. Dou R, Ng K, Giovannucci EL, Manson JE, Qian ZR, Ogino SJBJON (2016) Vitamin D and colorectal cancer: molecular, epidemiological and clinical evidence. Bio Med 115(9):1643–1660
77. Maalmi H, Walter V, Jansen L, Boakye D, Schöttker B, Hoffmeister M et al (2018) Association between blood 25-hydroxyvitamin D levels and survival in colorectal cancer patients: an updated systematic review and meta-analysis. 10(7):896
78. Ng K, Meyerhardt JA, Wu K, Feskanich D, Hollis BW, Giovannucci EL et al (2008) Circulating 25-hydroxyvitamin d levels and survival in patients with colorectal cancer. 26(18):2984–2991

79. Yuan C, Sato K, Hollis BW, Zhang S, Niedzwiecki D, Ou F-S et al (2019) Plasma 25-hydroxyvitamin d levels and survival in patients with advanced or metastatic colorectal cancer: findings from CALGB/SWOG 80405 (Alliance) Vitamin D and advanced/metastatic colorectal cancer survival. 25(24):7497–7505
80. Li Z, Wu L, Zhang J, Huang X, Thabane L, Li GJFIN (2021) Effect of vitamin D supplementation on risk of breast cancer: a systematic review and meta-analysis of randomized controlled trials. Bio Med 8:655727
81. Crew KDJISRN (2013) Vitamin d: are we ready to supplement for breast cancer prevention and treatment?
82. Vanhevel J, Verlinden L, Doms S, Wildiers H (2022) The role of vitamin D in breast cancer risk and progression. Cancer 29(2):R33–R55
83. Marshall DT, Savage SJ, Garrett-Mayer E, Keane TE, Hollis BW, Horst RL et al (2012) Vitamin D3 supplementation at 4000 international units per day for one year results in a decrease of positive cores at repeat biopsy in subjects with low-risk prostate cancer under active surveillance. 97(7):2315–2324
84. Wagner D, Trudel D, Van der Kwast T, Nonn L, Giangreco AA, Li D et al (2013) Randomized clinical trial of vitamin D3 doses on prostatic vitamin D metabolite levels and ki67 labeling in prostate cancer patients. 98(4):1498–1507
85. Trump D, Aragon-Ching J (2018) Vitamin D in prostate cancer. Cancer 20(3):244–252
86. Mavroeidi A, O'neill F, Lee P, Darling A, Fraser W, Berry J et al (2010) Seasonal 25-hydroxyvitamin D changes in British postmenopausal women at 57 N and 51 N: A longitudinal study. 121(1–2):459–461
87. Porojnicu AC, Robsahm TE, Dahlback A, Berg JP, Christiani D, Bruland ØS et al (2007) Seasonal and geographical variations in lung cancer prognosis in Norway: does vitamin D from the sun play a role? 55(3):263–270
88. Samuel S, Sitrin MD (2008) Vitamin D's role in cell proliferation and differentiation. Nutr Rev 66(10 Suppl 2):S116–S124
89. Maj E, Filip-Psurska B, Milczarek M, Psurski M, Kutner A, Wietrzyk JJIJOO (2018) Vitamin D derivatives potentiate the anticancer and anti-angiogenic activity of tyrosine kinase inhibitors in combination with cytostatic drugs in an A549 non-small cell lung cancer model. 52(2):337–366
90. Bao A, Li Y, Tong Y, Zheng H, Wu W, Wei C (2013) Tumor-suppressive effects of 1, 25-dihydroxyvitamin D3 in gastric cancer cells. Hepatogastroenterology 60(124):943–948
91. Mahendra A, Karishma, Choudhury BK, Sharma T, Bansal N, Bansal R et al (2018) Vitamin D and gastrointestinal cancer. Journal of laboratory physicians. 10(1):1–5
92. Smith W, Saba NJCRIOH (2005) Retinoids as chemoprevention for head and neck cancer: where do we go from here? 55(2):143–152
93. Wolbach SB (1925) Howe PRJTJoem tissue changes following deprivation of fat-soluble A vitamin. Med Cos 42(6):753–777
94. Mira-Y-Lopez R, Zheng WL, Kuppumbatti YS, Rexer B, Jing Y, Dejjocp ONG (2000) Retinol conversion to retinoic acid is impaired in breast cancer cell lines relative to normal cells. Breast 185(2):302–309
95. Williams SJ, Cvetkovic D, Hamilton TCJGO (2009) Vitamin A metabolism is impaired in human ovarian cancer. Bio Med 112(3):637–645
96. Shalinsky DR, Bischoff ED, Lamph WW, Zhang L, Boehm MF, Davies PJ et al (1997) A novel retinoic acid receptor-selective retinoid, ALRT1550, has potent antitumor activity against human oral squamous carcinoma xenografts in nude mice. 57(1):162–168
97. Cooper JP, Reynolds CP, Cho H, Kang MH (2017) Clinical development of fenretinide as an antineoplastic drug: Pharmacology perspectives. Exp Biol Med (Maywood) 242(11):1178–1184
98. Prasad KN, Cole WC, Kumar B, Prasad KCJ (2001) Scientific rationale for using high-dose multiple micronutrients as an adjunct to standard and experimental cancer therapies. Biomed 20(sup5):450S-S463

99. Lee MF, Hsieh NT, Huang CY, Li CI (2016) All trans-retinoic acid mediates MED28/HMG Box-containing protein 1 (HBP1)/β-catenin signaling in human colorectal cancer cells. J Cell Physiol 231(8):1796–1803
100. Zuo L, Yang X, Lu M, Hu R, Zhu H, Zhang S et al (2016) All-trans retinoic acid inhibits human colorectal cancer cells RKO migration via downregulating myosin light chain kinase expression through mapk signaling pathway. Nutr Cancer 68(7):1225–1233
101. Niles RM (2004) Signaling pathways in retinoid chemoprevention and treatment of cancer. Mutat Res 555(1–2):81–96
102. Altucci L, Gronemeyer H (2001) The promise of retinoids to fight against cancer. Nat Rev Cancer 1(3):181–193
103. Kazmi SM, Plante RK, Visconti V, Lau CY (1996) Comparison of N-(4-hydroxyphenyl)retinamide and all-trans-retinoic acid in the regulation of retinoid receptor-mediated gene expression in human breast cancer cell lines. Can Res 56(5):1056–1062
104. Pollard M, Luckert PH, Sporn MB (1991) Prevention of primary prostate cancer in Lobund-Wistar rats by N-(4-hydroxyphenyl)retinamide. Can Res 51(13):3610–3611
105. Ziv Y, Gupta MK, Milsom JW, Vladisavljevic A, Brand M, Fazio VW (1994) The effect of tamoxifen and fenretinimide on human colorectal cancer cell lines in vitro. Anticancer Res 14(5a):2005–2009
106. Kalemkerian GP, Slusher R, Ramalingam S, Gadgeel S, Mabry M (1995) Growth inhibition and induction of apoptosis by fenretinide in small-cell lung cancer cell lines. J Natl Cancer Inst 87(22):1674–1680
107. Gottardis MM, Bischoff ED, Shirley MA, Wagoner MA, Lamph WW, Heyman RA (1996) Chemoprevention of mammary carcinoma by LGD1069 (Targretin): an RXR-selective ligand. Can Res 56(24):5566–5570
108. Aouad P, Saikali M, Abdel-Samad R, Fostok S, El-Houjeiri L, Pisano C et al (2017) Anti-tumor activities of the synthetic retinoid ST1926 in two-dimensional and three-dimensional human breast cancer models. Anti-Cancer Drugs 28(7)
109. Moon RC, Grubbs CJ, Sporn MB (1976) Inhibition of 7,12-dimethylbenz(a)anthracene-induced mammary carcinogenesis by retinyl acetate. Can Res 36(7 pt 2):2626–2630
110. Zhao Z, Zhang ZP, Soprano DR, Soprano KJ (1995) Effect of 9-cis-retinoic acid on growth and RXR expression in human breast cancer cells. Exp Cell Res 219(2):555–561
111. Zito G, Naselli F, Saieva L, Raimondo S, Calabrese G, Guzzardo C et al (2017) Retinoic Acid affects Lung Adenocarcinoma growth by inducing differentiation via GATA6 activation and EGFR and Wnt inhibition. Sci Rep 7(1):4770
112. Eskra JN, Kuiper JW, Walden PD, Bosland MC, Özten N (2017) Interactive effects of 9-cis-retinoic acid and androgen on proliferation, differentiation, and apoptosis of LNCaP prostate cancer cells. Euro J Cancer Prevent Offic J Euro Cancer Prevent Organisation (ECP) 26(1):71–77
113. Bahmad HF, Samman H, Monzer A, Hadadeh O, Cheaito K, Abdel-Samad R et al (2019) The synthetic retinoid ST1926 attenuates prostate cancer growth and potentially targets prostate cancer stem-like cells. Mol Carcinog 58(7):1208–1220
114. Kuroda H, Tachikawa M, Uchida Y, Inoue K, Ohtsuka H, Ohtsuki S et al (2017) All-trans retinoic acid enhances gemcitabine cytotoxicity in human pancreatic cancer cell line AsPC-1 by up-regulating protein expression of deoxycytidine kinase. Euro J Pharmaceutic Sci Offic J Euro Fed Pharmaceutic Sci 103:116–121
115. Wang K, Baldwin GS, Nikfarjam M, He H (2019) Antitumor effects of all-trans retinoic acid and its synergism with gemcitabine are associated with downregulation of p21-activated kinases in pancreatic cancer. Am J Physiol Gastrointest Liver Physiol 316(5):G632–G640
116. Liu S, Stromberg A, Tai HH, Moscow JA (2004) Thiamine transporter gene expression and exogenous thiamine modulate the expression of genes involved in drug and prostaglandin metabolism in breast cancer cells. Mol Cancer Res MCR 2(8):477–487

117. Cancarini I, Krogh V, Agnoli C, Grioni S, Matullo G, Pala V et al (2015) Micronutrients involved in one-carbon metabolism and risk of breast cancer subtypes. PLoS ONE 10(9):e0138318
118. Rivlin RS (1973) Riboflavin and cancer: a review. Can Res 33(9):1977–1986
119. Zeng J, Gu Y, Fu H, Liu C, Zou Y, Chang H (2020) Association between one-carbon metabolism-related vitamins and risk of breast cancer: a systematic review and meta-analysis of prospective studies. Clin Breast Cancer 20(4):e469–e480
120. de Vogel S, Dindore V, van Engeland M, Goldbohm RA, van den Brandt PA, Weijenberg MP (2008) Dietary folate, methionine, riboflavin, and vitamin B-6 and risk of sporadic colorectal cancer. J Nutr 138(12):2372–2378
121. Takata Y, Cai Q, Beeghly-Fadiel A, Li H, Shrubsole MJ, Ji BT et al (2012) Dietary B vitamin and methionine intakes and lung cancer risk among female never smokers in China. Cancer Causes Control: CCC 23(12):1965–1975
122. Sujol G, Docquier A, Boulahtouf A, Castet-Nicolas A, Cavaillès V (2011) Vitamin B6 and cancer: from clinical data to molecularly mechanisms. Bull Cancer 98(10):1201–1208
123. Bailey LB, Gregory JF 3rd (1999) Folate metabolism and requirements. J Nutr 129(4):779–782
124. Chen P, Li C, Li X, Li J, Chu R, Wang H (2014) Higher dietary folate intake reduces the breast cancer risk: a systematic review and meta-analysis. Br J Cancer 110(9):2327–2338
125. Kim SJ, Zhang CXW, Demsky R, Armel S, Kim Y-I, Narod SA et al (2019) Folic acid supplement use and breast cancer risk in BRCA1 and BRCA2 mutation carriers: a case-control study. Breast Cancer Res Treat 174(3):741–748
126. Fardous AM, Beydoun S, James AA, Ma H, Cabelof DC, Unnikrishnan A et al (2021) The timing and duration of folate restriction differentially impacts colon carcinogenesis. Nutrients 14(1):16
127. Tomaszewski JJ, Cummings JL, Parwani AV, Dhir R, Mason JB, Nelson JB et al (2011) Increased cancer cell proliferation in prostate cancer patients with high levels of serum folate. Prostate 71(12):1287–1293
128. Bjelakovic G, Nikolova D, Simonetti RG, Gluud C (2004) Antioxidant supplements for prevention of gastrointestinal cancers: a systematic review and meta-analysis. Lancet 364(9441):1219–1228
129. Kimmick GG, Bell RA, Bostick RM (1997) Vitamin E and breast cancer: a review. Nutr Cancer 27(2):109–117
130. Freudenheim JL, Marshall JR, Vena JE, Laughlin R, Brasure JR, Swanson MK et al (1996) Premenopausal breast cancer risk and intake of vegetables, fruits, and related nutrients. J Natl Cancer Inst 88(6):340–348
131. Hunter DJ, Manson JE, Colditz GA, Stampfer MJ, Rosner B, Hennekens CH et al (1993) A prospective study of the intake of vitamins C, E, and A and the risk of breast cancer. N Engl J Med 329(4):234–240
132. Lippman SM, Klein EA, Goodman PJ, Lucia MS, Thompson IM, Ford LG et al (2009) Effect of selenium and vitamin E on risk of prostate cancer and other cancers: the Selenium and Vitamin E Cancer Prevention Trial (SELECT). JAMA 301(1):39–51
133. Ezzedine K, Latreille J, Kesse-Guyot E, Galan P, Hercberg S, Guinot C et al (2010) Incidence of skin cancers during 5-year follow-up after stopping antioxidant vitamins and mineral supplementation. Euro J Cancer 46(18):3316–3322

Micronutrients Importance in Cancer Prevention—Minerals

6

Rida Fatima Saeed, Uzma Azeem Awan, Shaista Aslam, Asma Saleem Qazi, Muhammad Zeeshan Bhatti, and Nosheen Akhtar

Contents

R. F. Saeed (✉) · U. A. Awan · S. Aslam · A. S. Qazi · M. Z. Bhatti · N. Akhtar
Department of Biological Sciences, National University of Medical Sciences (NUMS), Rawalpindi, Pakistan
e-mail: rida.saeed@numspak.edu.pk; rida.saeed@hotmail.co.uk

U. A. Awan
e-mail: uzma.awan@numspak.edu.pk

S. Aslam
e-mail: shaista.aslam@numspak.edu.pk

A. S. Qazi
e-mail: asma.qazi@numspak.edu.pk

M. Z. Bhatti
e-mail: zeeshan.bhatti@numspak.edu.pk

N. Akhtar
e-mail: nosheenakhtar@numspak.edu.pk

R. F. Saeed and S. ul. Shaheed (eds.), *Nutrition and Dietary Interventions in Cancer*, Cancer Treatment and Research 191, https://doi.org/10.1007/978-3-031-55622-7_6

Abbreviations

4E-BP1	4E binding protein 1
AKT	Ak strain transforming
ATP7A	Atpase copper transporter 7A
CNX	Calnexin
CRT	Calreticulin
CTR1	Copper transporter 1
ER	Endoplasmic reticulum
ERp72	Endoplasmic reticulum resident protein 72
HO•	Hydroxyl radical
IP3	Inositol 1,4,5-trisphosphate
IP3R	Inositol trisphosphate receptor
LOX	Lysyl oxidase
MTORC1	Mammalian target of rapamycin complex 1
MAPK	Mitogen-activated protein-kinase
NADH	Nicotinamide adenine dinucleotide hydride
NF-kB	Nuclear factor kappa B
PI3K	Phosphoinositide 3-kinases
QL	Quality of life
RO	Reactive oxygen species
RDA	Recommended daily allowance
SERCA	Sarco/endoplasmic reticulum calcium atpases
SPARC	Secreted protein acidic and rich in cysteine
SOD3	Super-oxide dismutase isoform 3
MURR1	U2af1-Rs1 region 1 protein
ULK	Unc-51-Like autophagy activating kinase
XIAP	X-linked inhibitors of apoptosis

6.1 Minerals

Globally, cancers represent a significant portion of the burden of disease, and predictions indicate that this problem will increase for at least the next two decades [1]. Apart from the treatment and diagnosis of the disease, its prevention strategy does play an important role. The growing area of chrono-nutrition has likewise stressed the importance of a food's composition, quantity, and timing for preserving health [2]. An increasing number of animal and human research models have shown that the time of energy and macronutrient intake had an impact on the internal biological clocks and circadian patterns, which were related to the development of cancer [3, 4]. Minerals are crucial micronutrients for people since they not only build human tissues, but also support the body's normal physiological processes [5]. Over the past 50 years, certain elements have become less abundant in food, most notably zinc, copper, and iron [6, 7]. This phenomenon is reflected in the widespread incidence of "hidden hunger," which is characterised as a protracted absence of vitamin or mineral consumption (together referred to as micronutrients) [8].

The onset of different cancers may be influenced by dietary intake of certain minerals, according to numerous population studies. The incidence of colorectal cancer in women was dramatically decreased by eating a diet heavy in salt and potassium [9]. According to the Muka et al., eating foods high in zinc and iron lower the risk of developing lung cancer [10]. Greater consumption of magnesium, calcium, and potassium could help lower the risk of colon cancer; however, greater consumption of iron may raise that risk of disease [11].

Minerals are abundant in natural food sources and frequently included in dietary supplements; however, they are frequently reduced or altered highly processed industrial food. Mineral deficiency delays the process of destroying tumours [12]. It also impairs immune-competence, increases the complications, and effects the patient's physical and mental quality of life. Since micronutrient build up and/or shortages are harmful regulators of the development of malignant disease and the anti-tumour efficacy of treatment, research on micronutrient supplementation and anti-cancer therapy is now equally focused on. Some minerals have the ability to scavenge free radicals and also play other crucial metabolic roles like immunomodulation, inducing apoptosis, and controlling cell division and proliferation. We sought to discuss the probable role of particular minerals in cancer in this chapter. The main molecular processes connecting minerals to oncogenesis will be highlighted in this chapter first, afterwards, a report on clinical evidence with a focus on recent findings is presented linking mineral intake and risk of cancer. Table 6.1 provides a summary of the most popular minerals' recommended daily intakes and sources.

Table 6.1 Lists some of the common minerals mentioned in this chapter, along with the recommended daily intakes and sources for each

Mineral	Source	Recommended daily allowance (RDA) (μg/Day)	References
Zinc	Legumes, eggs, fish, grains, red meat, beans, nuts, crab, lobster, whole grains, cereals, and dairy products	8000–11,000	[13]
Copper	Seeds, nuts, shellfish, meats, whole-grain products, cereals, and chocolate	900	[14]
Selenium	Brazil nuts, meats, cereals, seafoods, grains, and dairy products	30–70	[15]
Iron	Lean meat, poultry, seafood, beans, iron-fortified breakfast cereals, and breads	8000	[16]
Calcium	Yogurt, milk, cheese, vegetables like Chinese cabbage, kale, broccoli, and canned salmon and sardines	1,000,000	[17]
Phosphorus	Dairy products	700,000	[18]

6.2 Zinc

Zinc is an essential trace element that functions for over 300 enzymes and required by more than 2000 transcription factors for gene regulation, enzyme activity, and protein structure. Zinc controls important physiological and biochemical functions including cellular response to oxidative stress, cell cycle progression, DNA replication and damage repair, and apoptosis [19–21]. A significant zinc-containing transcription factor like p53, for instance, is linked to the cellular response to DNA damage.

Numerous epidemiological studies show that a zinc deficiency raises the likelihood of developing cancer [21–23]. Severe zinc deficiency is linked to protein-energy malnutrition and effects in lower immune function in both tissue mediated and humoral responses [24, 25]. However, there is still some debate over the optimal way to manage zinc concentration in cancer prevention and treatment. Only few studies have provided evidence indicating exposure to zinc and cancer risk. According to Stocks et al., zinc and copper abundance linked with cancer mortality and found that high levels of zinc and copper were found to be related with gastric cancer mortality [26]. However, it was also noted that zinc levels were more important than the copper levels. Another study carried out by Strain et al. [27] also compared the zinc and copper levels in bronchogenic carcinoma patient serum. They found a higher ratio of both micronutrients among cancer patients [27].

Zinc intake is also interrelated with age adjusted mortality in breast, prostate, intestine, leukaemia, and skin cancers [28, 29]. It was found that these cancers are interconnected with zinc and selenium proportions that are antagonist to each other. Additionally, it was discovered that the median levels of zinc in healthy people's blood were directly associated with the corresponding mortality rates for bowel, ovarian, breast, bladder, oral, and lung cancers [28, 29]. Similarly, in another study by Van Rensburg et al. [30] found that a wheat and corn diet containing little levels of zinc, nicotinic acid, riboflavin, and magnesium and deficiency of any of these micronutrients is relates to oesophageal cancer [24]. Gyorkey et al. found lower levels of zinc in malignant prostatic patient's tissue, whereas higher zinc levels were found in benign prostatic tissues. In above-mentioned studies altered zinc levels were followed and studied at different stages of cancers. It is also thought that tumours have low zinc levels because developing tumour cells needs more zinc for DNA synthesis, which is necessary for cell proliferation and synthesis [31]. This could be one of the possible explanations for getting variable results.

Although the relationship between zinc and cancer is not fully understood, it is known that this mineral is connected to both cellular growth and immune response. The control of numerous factors in the cell signalling pathways, such as protein kinase C, cAMP-dependent protein kinase A, phophodiesterase, and nuclear factor kappa-light-chain-enhancer of activated B cells (NF-B), is specifically affected by zinc [32]. Fong and his colleagues conducted a number of in vivo tests to demonstrate that dietary zinc deficit (ZD) raises the risk of oesophageal cancer development in rats lacking the miR-31 gene [33]. Squamous cell carcinoma of the oral cavity patients' blood zinc levels was around half as high as those of healthy controls (p-value 0.001) [34]. Zinc supplementation has been shown to alter the immune response like reduce angiogenesis and inflammatory cytokines, as well as inducing apoptosis [35] and the normalization impact of zinc on the anti-oxidant and histoarchitecture status in experimentally induced colon carcinogenesis [36]. Zinc can potentially modulate T cell dependent immune response, in addition attenuating the carcinogenesis response from nuclear factor kappa B (NF-kB) activation [37]. Prasad et al. advocated that zinc supplementation aids in the prevention of carcinogenesis and the sensitization of chemotherapeutic responses to traditional anti-cancer treatments [37]. Interestingly, 100 mg/d zinc consumption was linked to a 2.9-fold increased risk of metastatic prostate cancer [38]. According to widespread consensus, zinc has anti-oxidant and pro-apoptotic qualities that work to protect against the development of cancer by reducing oxidative stress and enhancing immunological function.

6.3 Copper

It has been established that trace metals like copper, are involved in numerous physiological processes, which cause structural abnormalities or the loss of some crucial physiological activities. Copper is essential for oxidation reactions and found in numerous enzymes, including mono- and dioxygenases, oxidases, reductases, and dehydrogenases [44]. Copper transporter known as copper transporter 1 (CTR1) involves in the dietary copper (Cu^+) uptake into the epithelial cells that are located in the small intestine. The majority of the copper in the blood is transported in serum that bound to ceruloplasmin, with smaller amounts also being carried by albumin and transcuprein. Copper builds up in hepatocytes before either being circulated to other cells or being eliminated in the bile. The CTR1 on the cell surface absorbs copper and stores it with metallothioneins [45]. Recently, it was discovered that inhibiting the CTR1–copper interaction reduced the AKT signalling pathway and, consequently, reduces tumorigenesis in AKT-driven cancers [46].

The expression of CTR1 in a suitable complex was considered that the creation of free radicals was the cause of its promise as a therapeutic target for cancer therapy. However, there are issues of poor solubility in physiological buffer systems and occasionally unpredictable methods of action. Furthermore, X-linked inhibitors of apoptosis (XIAP) target the mouse U2af1-rs1 region 1 protein (MURR1), which also controls the quantity of copper in cells [47–49]. The cell cycle is affected at specific points by some non-transporter copper proteins. In order to preserve homeostasis, defective biological elements produced by reactive oxygen species (ROS) activity are confiscated inside vesicles during the autophagic process, which is influenced by copper. Damaged biological molecules must be removed from the cellular environment in order to prevent apoptosis and effectively prolong tumour viability. The activity of the Unc-51-like autophagy activating kinase (ULK) complexes 1 and 2, which are involved in the creation of autophagosomes, is increased by copper, supporting the development of cancers [50–53].

Since copper is an element and cannot be produced by metabolic processes, its distinct chemistry enables it to be extracted from food sources with great precision using copper chelators. Hence, promising chemicals for the therapy of cancer include chelators that decrease cellular copper bioavailability or ionophores that improve cellular copper bioavailability [54].When copper concentrations within resected tumours of cancer patients were consistently discovered to be raised relative to normal tissue, and serum copper concentrations followed a similar trend, the idea that tumour cells might have a higher copper need than normal tissues gained popularity [54–63].

Interestingly, copper inhalation was thought to cause hepatic angiosarcoma, pulmonary adenocarcinoma and alveolar cell carcinoma among the working class who sprays fungicides (such as Bordeaux mixture that is a mixture of copper sulphate plus lime) and work in mines especially copper mines [26, 44, 45, 64]. The available evidence is still insufficient to draw a conclusion on specific roles regarding mechanisms involved in carcinogenesis by copper. Hence, higher copper concentration in tissues is proposed as a predictive marker for brain tumours, pancreatic cancer, and hepatocellular carcinoma [42, 65, 66].

Squamous cell carcinoma patients' blood copper levels were almost 45.5% higher than those of healthy controls (*t*-test, *p*-value 0.001) [34]. According to spectroscopic analysis of brain sections, tumoural masses had significantly more copper than the healthy tissues around them (0.0079 and 0.037 g/cm^2, respectively) [42]. In a meta-analysis of cancer, elevated copper levels and decreased Zn levels were found to be related in bladder [60] and colorectal cancers [67].

There have been seven oral tetrathiomolybdate clinical trials in cancer patients to date, all of which followed a very similar protocol that involved taking the copper chelator up to four times daily with meals [68]. TTM binds to dietary copper in the small intestine and prevents its transit into the body. The dose of TTM is carefully titrated to lower blood ceruloplasmin levels to 20% of baseline (5–15 mg/dL) because excessive copper deficit might be detrimental [69, 68]. Unfortunately, individuals with metastatic prostate and kidney cancer did not benefit from the early clinical studies of TTM [69]. Nevertheless, it was suggested that TTM may be more effective when used as an adjuvant to primary therapy or when taken at early stages of disease because therapeutic levels of copper deficiency may take months to acquire [68]. In a more recent Phase II clinical trial, breast cancer patients who had undergone chemotherapy and showed no signs of the disease, but were at high risk of recurrence were evaluated for the therapeutic effectiveness of adjuvant TTM [70]. Overall, it is evident that copper plays a crucial role in the progression of cancer at every stage, from carcinogenesis to metastasis. Copper metabolism is also impacted by the metabolism of cancer cells. As a result, it is anticipated that copper-related prognostic and diagnostic indicators for cancer can be found.

6.4 Selenium

Selenium is involved in cellular metabolism and also acts as an integral part of many enzymes, especially those enzymes which scavenge reactive oxygen species. There are certain studies that have revealed the role and importance of selenium in cancer inhibition, prevention, and retardation [65]. Some ecological studies have revealed that selenium amount in the tissue or blood is inversely correlated to cancer mortality [64]. Yet, there are studies that didn't prove the protective role of selenium in cancer development. It has a protective role in lung cancers [71], still the data are inconclusive and further research data is required to reveal the true picture. The anti-carcinogenic role is related to the anti-oxidant properties of selenium, which enhances the immune response in the body by altering the metabolism of carcinogens to make it less toxic compounds [72, 42].

It is proposed that selenium directly triggers the death of tumour cells and works as a scavenger for by products of oxidation reactions (through glutathione peroxidase activity) produced during standard cancer treatments. Studies on animals and in humans have emphasized the significance of getting enough selenium in order to protect against hepatocytes and lower the chance of developing primary hepatic malignancies [73]. The inverse relationship of selenium and cancer was found in leukaemia, gastrointestinal and gastro urinary tracts, colon, rectum, bladder, breast, ovary, lungs (only in males) pancreases, prostate, and skin [74]. In another study, a direct correlation was observed in the selenium level in drinking water and mortality rates from colorectal cancer [28, 29]. The mechanism underlying the protective role of selenium is still not clearly understood.

The work by Callejón-Leblic et al. showed that the serum selenium levels were higher in lung cancer patients ($n = 48$) than in healthy controls ($n = 39$), at 166.0 and 144.7 ng per gram of serum, respectively [75]. However, the difference was not statistically significant. In prostate cancer, with mean concentrations of 191 and 168 g/kg, respectively, the amount of selenium in prostate tissues was not significantly different between cancer patients ($n = 49$) and healthy controls ($n = 49$) (p-value $= 0.347$) [41]. The remarkable discrepancy in dose-dependent responses is due to endogenous mechanisms, such as the selenoprotein's production rates plateauing at sufficiently high selenium consumption [73].

6.5 Iron

Iron is also a component of several enzymes involved in DNA replication (polymerases, primase, and helicase) and repair (DNA glycosylase, polymerase, helicase) [76] and cellular iron is directly correlated with cellular proliferation [77]. Additionally, iron can stimulate cellular growth by turning on the Wnt signalling pathway when adenomatous polyposis coli mutations are present, raising the risk of colorectal cancer [78]. Iron can generate the ROS-related hydroxyl radical (HO•) through the Fenton reaction [64]. Particularly, lipid peroxidation increases the amount of radicals present inside the cell, changes cellular permeability, and triggers an inflammatory response [79]. When large amounts of iron are present, vitamin C, in the form of ascorbate (AscH-), increases the Fenton reaction by giving more ferrous iron. This helps to recover leaky ferrous iron by changing ferric iron to Fe2+ that can be taken up by ferritin. The ascorbic radical (Asc•) similarly impacts mitochondrial respiration, resulting in a burst of ROS that worsened already-damaged cells [64]. Because these free radicals are also a part of several signal pathways like NF-B, PI3K, and MAPK, high levels of them encourage irregularities in cellular growth and inflammation [80, 81].

Iron is specifically associated with cancer because it affects the cell's oxidative state [77]. Excess cellular iron has been associated to the oncogenesis of hepatocellular and colorectal carcinoma [82, 83]. It was revealed that iron deficiency was found leading to gastric cancer by development of conditions hypochlorhydria and achlorhydria and allowing bacterial colonization in the stomach [84]. These bacteria reduce ingested nitrate to nitrite forming carcinogenic nitosamines in the stomach [82]. However, evidence is required to associate levels of iron to cancer development [73, 85]. The excess amount of iron has been implicated in cancer risk, such as a multicentre randomised controlled, single-blinded clinical trial showed that reduced iron intake subjects ($n = 60$) had a decreased risk of acquiring any cancer than subjects on a typical diet ($n = 38$) [86]. Whereas on the other hand, the risk of cancer rose at high blood iron levels (above 80 g/dL) and low levels (below 60 g/dL), according to an interesting study on cancer patients [87]. Such divergent results highlight the knowledge gap regarding the function of iron in oncogenesis and the requirement for further investigation.

6.6 Calcium

Calcium is important in signalling pathways, cell to cell adhesion and proliferation. Impairment in calcium levels may lead to resistance to apoptosis, profound effect on cell cycle and metastasis [64, 88]. The enzyme Calnexin (CNX) that is embedded in endoplasmic reticulum (ER) and is involved in protein modification and maturation, which performs its function in a calcium dependent manner [89]. Altered expression of these enzymes are directly related to cancer development both these enzymes are found involved in the cancer development in the case of any altered expression [90].

Calcium depletion significantly affects the cell cycle, proliferation, apoptosis, and metastasis because calcium plays a direct role in cell-to-cell adhesion and functions as a second messenger in many signalling pathways [91, 92]. Sarco/endoplasmic reticulum calcium ATPases (SERCA), a particular membrane bounded enzyme, uptake calcium inside the ER, while IP3 receptors (IP3R) release calcium into the cytoplasm in response to IP3 stimulation [93]. The altered expression of SERCA has been suggested as biomarker in colorectal cancer [94].

The ER's lumen contains CRT, which controls calcium absorption and release [90]. Overexpression of ERp72 has been linked to cellular proliferation and has been found to be involved in several processes, including the quick internalization and nuclear translocation of vitamin D3 (as calcitriol), the activation of numerous transcription factors, such as eukaryotic translation initiation factor 4E-binding protein 1 (4E-BP1) and mammalian target of rapamycin complex 1 (mTORC1), as well as being a component of the CNX/CRT complex for the maturation of glycoprotein and DNA repair [95].

In one research study, it was found that calcium levels are directly linked to the development of prostate cancer [41]. Serum calcium levels were also found the same in ovarian cancer subjects. On the contrary, higher levels of serum calcium reduce the risk of breast cancer [96].

Calcium levels in the body also indicate the tendency of an individual to develop cancers [97]. With a sensitivity of 32% and specificity of 94%, calcium levels as high as 2.5 mmol/L can detect bone metastases in bladder cancer patients, increasing the risk of metastasis, and in hepatocellular carcinoma patients, increasing the risk of ocular metastasis with a sensitivity of 19% and specificity of 97% [98, 99].

6.7 Phosphorous

After oxygen, hydrogen, calcium and nitrogen, phosphorus is the most abundant in the body and a major component of bones. Dietary phosphorus is usually present as phospholipids, nucleic acids and proteins [100]. However, phosphorus is found in almost all types of food. Particularly, as an inorganic phosphorus, it is present in soft drinks and here it can be absorbed in the body rapidly with 100% efficacy [101]. It is present in many fast food items, and more and more consumption of it doubles the daily intake of phosphorus in the body. However, calcium chelates the phosphates and thus reduces the phosphorus level in serum [102]. If a patient is suffering from chronic hyperphosphatemia then its risk of developing cancer will double due to the destruction or obliteration of vitamin D protective role [103]. Usually, the samples taken from patients suffering from different types of cancer showed consistent hyperphosphatemia [104]. In lung cancers, higher levels of phosphorus activate the PI3K/AKT signalling pathway by activating 1,4,5-trisphosphate aberrantly [105]. The same pattern was also observed in colorectal, brain, prostate, and bladder cancers [106, 107].

The increased intake of phosphorus was reported in patients with oral squamous cell carcinoma [43] and a considerable no significant greater threat of bladder cancer [108] and prostate cancer [109]. In vitro studies revealed that phosphate can directly activate the protein kinase B (Ak strain transforming (AKT), in contrast to experiments on mice that demonstrated how a high phosphorus diet raises the risk of lung cancer through stimulating the PI3K signalling pathway [105]. The link between hyperphosphatemia and various cancers can be explained by the abnormal activation of the inositol 1,4,5-trisphosphate (IP3)/AKT signalling pathway caused by an excess of cellular phosphate [103].

6.8 Other Minerals Role in Cancer

Molybdenum cofactor deficiency is correlated with cancer. However, in one study it was observed that low levels of molybdenum are linked with high levels of oesophageal cancers [110]. In another study done in China, it was observed that adding supplements to the soil with aluminium molybdate will increase the micronutrient molybdenum and ascorbic acid in vegetables and grains grown in this area while decreasing the nitrate and nitrite contents in it. This proportion was found supportive in the declining incidence of oesophageal cancer in that area [111]. Also the high content of molybdenum in the form of molybdenum oxide is found as one of the causes for lung adenomas [112]. Still, some recent research work is required in this domain to increase the clarity of micronutrients' role in the development of cancers. We are still lacking in recent updates research work in this domain.

Cadmium, lead, and related compounds have been categorized as group 1 carcinogens by [113]. Lead and cadmium also interfere with the expression of inflammatory mediators and indicators and have negative effects on the immune system [114, 115]. Cadmium does perform many physiological functions and in correlation analysis for cadmium level with cancer mortality it was noted that it has direct associations with myeloma, oral cancer, lymphoma, oesophageal, breast, lung, larynx, pharynx, large intestine, and bladder cancers [116]. The significant association was found among breast, ovaries, prostate, intestine, skin cancers, and inverse association was observed in liver cancers [64]. Still, the available data do not provide conclusions about dietary exposure to cadmium.

Research into and evidence for nutrition's contribution to oncogenesis is growing. As a result, research into how micronutrients affect immune response, DNA stability, epigenetic control, and how they function as biomarkers is gaining attention among research community. The risk of developing cancer was specifically linked to greater levels of copper and iron, although the link between zinc, selenium, calcium, and phosphorus was less clear. Higher levels of zinc and copper were most significantly associated with liver cancer than were lower levels of selenium. Table 6.2 summarizes the correlation between minerals and cancer risk from several research.

6.9 Conclusions and Future Prospective

An obvious and present threat, is an unbalanced diet, which is frequently linked to the development of cancer. It was shown that some minerals such as copper, iron, and zinc has a direct correlation with developing cancer, whereas minerals like selenium has an inverse relationship with cancer risk. However, more information is required to determine the efficacy of these minerals and whether they are just appropriate for particular cancer types. The development of sufficient micronutrient panels with diagnostic value to predict a person's risk of acquiring cancer as well as to facilitate prognostic predictions for particular cancer types may be aided

Table 6.2 Associated between selected minerals cancer in tissue samples

Mineral	Cancer	Outcome	Number of samples of cancer patients	References
Zinc	Breast	Zinc accumulated in malignant tissue. Triple-positive and triple-negative breast tumours had the highest levels of zinc	26	[39]
Copper	Glioblastoma	Copper level was increased in a peritumoural zone corresponding to the region of elevated A(1)AR density	6	[40]
Selenium	Prostate	No statistically significant change in the selenium concentration between malignant and healthy prostatic tissues	49	[41]
Iron	Glioblastoma	Decrease in iron concentrations in brain tumour tissue	11	[42]
Calcium	Prostate	Calcium levels were shown to be statistically lower in malignant tissue than in healthy tissues	50	[41]
Phosphorus	Oral Squamous Cell carcinoma	Significant association between red meat, fat, daily energy, phosphorous, vitamin B5, vitamin E, and selenium intake and OSCC presence	27	[43]

by clustered micronutrient studies. Additionally, the necessity of consuming extra food, especially micronutrients, should always be thoroughly questioned if there isn't a clear shortfall.

References

1. Bray F, Jemal A, Grey N, Ferlay J, Forman DJTIO (2012) Global cancer transitions according to the human development index (2008–2030): a population-based study. 13(8):790–801
2. Almoosawi S, Vingeliene S, Karagounis LG, Pot GK (2016) Chrono-nutrition: a review of current evidence from observational studies on global trends in time-of-day of energy intake and its association with obesity. Proc Nutr Soc 75(4):487–500
3. Rothschild J, Hoddy KK, Jambazian P, Varady KA (2014) Time-restricted feeding and risk of metabolic disease: a review of human and animal studies. Nutr Rev 72(5):3–318
4. Srour B, Plancoulaine S, Andreeva VA, Fassier P, Julia C, Galan P, Hercberg S, Deschasaux M, Latino-Martel P, Touvier M (2018) Circadian nutritional behaviours and cancer risk: new insights from the NutriNet-sante prospective cohort study: disclaimers. Int J Cancer 143(10):2369–2379
5. Prentice A, Bates CJ (1994) Adequacy of dietary mineral supply for human bone growth and mineralisatio. Eur J Clin Nutr 48 Suppl 1:S161–176; discussion S177

6. Mayer AMB, Trenchard LF, Rayns and Nutrition JIOOF (2022) Historical changes in the mineral content of fruit and vegetables in the UK from 1940 to 2019: a concern for human nutrition and agriculture. 73(3):315–326
7. Thomas DJN Health (2003) A study on the mineral depletion of the foods available to us as a nation over the period 1940 to 1991. 17(2):85–115
8. Muthayya S, Rah JH, Sugimoto JD, Roos FF, Kraemer K, Black REJP (2013) The global hidden hunger indices and maps: an advocacy tool for action. 8(6):e67860
9. Kune GA, Kune S, Watson LF (1989) Dietary sodium and potassium intake and colorectal cancer risk. Nutr Cancer 12(4):351–359
10. Muka T, Kraja B, Ruiter R, Lahousse L, de Keyser CE, Hofman A, Franco OH, Brusselle G, Stricker BH, Kiefte-de Jong JC (2017) Dietary mineral intake and lung cancer risk: the Rotterdam Study. Eur J Nutr 56(4):1637–1646
11. Meng Y, Sun J, Yu J, Wang C, Su J (2019) Dietary intakes of calcium, iron, magnesium, and potassium elements and the risk of colorectal cancer: a meta-analysis. Biol Trace Elem Res 189(2):325–335
12. Thomas D (2007) The mineral depletion of foods available to us as a nation (1940–2002)--a review of the 6th Edition of McCance and Widdowson. Nutr Health 19(1–2):21–55
13. Zinc (2021) Fact sheet for health professionals. https://ods.od.nih.gov/factsheets/Zinc-HealthProfessional/
14. Copper (2021) Fact sheet for health professionals. https://ods.od.nih.gov/factsheets/Copper-HealthProfessional/
15. Selenium (2021) fact sheet for health professionals. https://ods.od.nih.gov/factsheets/Selenium-HealthProfessional/
16. Iron (2022) Fact sheet for health professionals. https://ods.od.nih.gov/factsheets/Iron-HealthProfessional/
17. Calcium (2022) Fact sheet for health professionals. https://ods.od.nih.gov/factsheets/Calcium-HealthProfessional/
18. Phosphorus (2021) Fact sheet for health professionals. https://ods.od.nih.gov/factsheets/Phosphorus-HealthProfessional/
19. Dhawan D, Chadha VDJ (2010) Zinc: a promising agent in dietary chemoprevention of cancer. 132(6):676
20. Poswillo DE, Cohen B (1971) Inhibition of carcinogenesis by dietary zinc. Nature 231(5303):447–448
21. Wang J, Zhao H, Xu Z, Cheng X (2020) Zinc dysregulation in cancers and its potential as a therapeutic target. Cancer Biol Med 17(3):612–625
22. Hrabeta J, Eckschlager T, Stiborova M, Heger Z, Krizkova S, Adam VJJOMM (2016) Zinc and zinc-containing biomolecules in childhood brain tumors. 94(11):1199–1215
23. Skrajnowska D, Bobrowska-Korczak B (2019) Role of zinc in immune system and anti-cancer defense mechanisms. Nutrients 11(10)
24. Corbo MD, Lam J (2013) Zinc deficiency and its management in the pediatric population: a literature review and proposed etiologic classification. J Am Acad Dermatol 69(4):616–624
25. Golden MH, Harland PS, Golden BE, Jackson AA (1978) Zinc and immunocompetence in protein-energy malnutrition. Lancet 311(8076):1226–1228
26. Stocks P, Davies RI (1964) Zinc and copper content of soils associated with the incidence of cancer of the stomach and other organs. Br J Cancer 18:14–24
27. Strain WH, Mansour EG, Flynn A, Pories WJ, Tomaro AJ, Hill OA Jr (1972) Plasma-zinc concentration in patients with bronchogenic cancer. Lancet 1(7758):1021–1022
28. Schrauzer GN, White DA, Schneider CJ (1977) Cancer mortality correlation studies-III: statistical associations with dietary selenium intakes. Bioinorg Chem 7(1):23–34
29. Schrauzer GN, White DA, Schneider CJ (1977) Cancer mortality correlation studies-IV: associations with dietary intakes and blood levels of certain trace elements, notably se-antagonists. Bioinorg Chem 7(1):35–56
30. van Rensburg SJ (1981) Epidemiologic and dietary evidence for a specific nutritional predisposition to esophageal cancer. J Natl Cancer Inst 67(2):243–251

31. Györkey F, Min KW, Huff JA, Györkey P (1967) Zinc and magnesium in human prostate gland: normal, hyperplastic, and neoplastic. Cancer Res 27(8):1348–1353
32. Jarosz M, Olbert M, Wyszogrodzka G, Młyniec K, Librowski T (2017) Antioxidant and anti-inflammatory effects of zinc. Zinc-dependent NF-κB signaling. Inflammopharmacology 25(1):11–24
33. Fong LY, Taccioli C, Palamarchuk A, Tagliazucchi GM, Jing R, Smalley KJ, Fan S, Altemus J, Fiehn O, Huebner K, Farber JL, Croce CM (2020) Abrogation of esophageal carcinoma development in miR-31 knockout rats. Proc Natl Acad Sci U S A 117(11):6075–6085
34. Elango S, Samuel S, Khashim Z, Subbiah U (2018) Selenium influences trace elements homeostasis, cancer biomarkers in squamous cell carcinoma patients administered with cancerocidal radiotherapy. Asian Pac J Cancer Prev 19(7):1785–1792
35. Prasad AS, Kucuk OJC, Reviews M (2002) Zinc in cancer prevention. 21(3):291–295
36. Chadha VD, Vaiphei K, Dhawan DJM, Biochemistry C (2007) Zinc mediated normalization of histoarchitecture and antioxidant status offers protection against initiation of experimental carcinogenesis. 304(1):101–108
37. Prasad AS, Beck FW, Snell DC, Kucuk O (2009) Zinc in cancer prevention. Nutr Cancer 61(6):879–887
38. Becker NP, Martitz J, Renko K, Stoedter M, Hybsier S, Cramer J, Schomburg LJM (2014) Hypoxia reduces and redirects selenoprotein biosynthesis. 6(5):1079–1086
39. Rusch P, Hirner AV, Schmitz O, Kimmig R, Hoffmann O, Diel and Obstetrics MJOA (2021) Zinc distribution within breast cancer tissue of different intrinsic subtypes. 303(1):195–205
40. Dehnhardt M, Zoriy MV, Khan Z, Reifenberger G, Ekstrom TJ, Sabine Becker J, Zilles K, Bauer A (2008) Element distribution is altered in a zone surrounding human glioblastoma multiforme. J Trace Elem Med Biol 22(1):17–23
41. Çelen İ, Müezzinoğlu T, Ataman OY, Bakırdere S, Korkmaz M, Neşe N, Şenol F, Lekili M (2015) Selenium, nickel, and calcium levels in cancerous and non-cancerous prostate tissue samples and their relation with some parameters. Environ Sci Pollut Res Int 22(17):13070–13076
42. Wandzilak A, Czyzycki M, Radwanska E, Adamek D, Geraki K, Lankosz M (2015) X-ray fluorescence study of the concentration of selected trace and minor elements in human brain tumours. Spectrochim Acta Part B 114:52–57
43. Secchi DG, Aballay LR, Galíndez MF, Piccini D, Lanfranchi H, Brunotto M (2015) Red meat, micronutrients and oral squamous cell carcinoma of argentine adult patients. Nutr Hosp 32(3):1214–1221
44. Blockhuys S, Wittung-Stafshede P (2017) Roles of copper-binding proteins in breast cancer. Int J Mol Sci 18(4)
45. Michalczyk K, Cymbaluk-Ploska A (2020) The role of zinc and copper in gynecological malignancies. Nutrients 12(12)
46. Guo J, Cheng J, Zheng N, Zhang X, Dai X, Zhang L, Hu C, Wu X, Jiang Q, Wu D, Okada H, Pandolfi PP, Wei W (2021) Copper promotes tumorigenesis by activating the pdk1-akt oncogenic pathway in a copper transporter 1 dependent manner. Adv Sci 8(18):e2004303
47. Burstein E, Ganesh L, Dick RD, van De Sluis B, Wilkinson JC, Klomp LW, Wijmenga C, Brewer GJ, Nabel GJ, Duckett CS (2004) A novel role for XIAP in copper homeostasis through regulation of MURR1. EMBO J 23(1):244–254
48. da Silva DA, De Luca A, Squitti R, Rongioletti M, Rossi L, Machado CML, Cerchiaro G (2022) Copper in tumors and the use of copper-based compounds in cancer treatment. J Inorg Biochem 226:111634
49. van De Sluis B, Rothuizen J, Pearson PL, van Oost BA, Wijmenga C (2002) Identification of a new copper metabolism gene by positional cloning in a purebred dog population. Hum Mol Genet 11(2):165–173
50. Redza-Dutordoir M, Averill-Bates DA (2021) Interactions between reactive oxygen species and autophagy: Special issue: Death mechanisms in cellular homeostasis. Biochim Biophys Acta Mol Cell Res 1868(8):119041

51. Tsang T, Posimo JM, Gudiel AA, Cicchini M, Feldser DM, Brady DC (2020) Copper is an essential regulator of the autophagic kinases ULK1/2 to drive lung adenocarcinoma. Nat Cell Biol 22(4):412–424
52. Wang X, Lee J, Xie C (2022) Autophagy regulation on cancer stem cell maintenance, metastasis, and therapy resistance. Cancers (Basel) 14(2)
53. Zischka H, Kroemer G (2020) Copper—a novel stimulator of autophagy. Cell Stress 4(5):92–94
54. Li Y (2020) Copper homeostasis: emerging target for cancer treatment. IUBMB Life 72(9):1900–1908
55. Baharvand M, Manifar S, Akkafan R, Mortazavi H, Sabour S (2014) Serum levels of ferritin, copper, and zinc in patients with oral cancer. Biomed J 37(5):331–336
56. Dragutinović VV, Tatić SB, Nikolić-Mandić SD, Tripković TM, Dunđerović DM, Paunović IR (2014) Copper as ancillary diagnostic tool in preoperative evaluation of possible papillary thyroid carcinoma in patients with benign thyroid disease. Biol Trace Elem Res 160(3):311–315
57. Gupte A, Mumper RJ (2009) Elevated copper and oxidative stress in cancer cells as a target for cancer treatment. Cancer Treat Rev 35(1):32–46
58. Kaba M, Pirincci N, Yuksel MB, Gecit I, Gunes M, Ozveren H, Eren H, Demir H (2014) Serum levels of trace elements in patients with prostate cancer. Asian Pac J Cancer Prev 15(6):2625–2629
59. Lelièvre P, Sancey L, Coll JL, Deniaud A, Busser B (2020) The multifaceted roles of copper in cancer: a trace metal element with dysregulated metabolism, but also a target or a bullet for therapy. Cancers (Basel) 12(12)
60. Mao S, Huang S (2013) Zinc and copper levels in bladder cancer: a systematic review and meta-analysis. Biol Trace Elem Res 153(1–3):5–10
61. Peng F, Lu X, Janisse J, Muzik O, Shields AF (2006) PET of human prostate cancer xenografts in mice with increased uptake of 64CuCl2. J Nucl Med 47(10):1649–1652
62. Shanbhag VC, Gudekar N, Jasmer K, Papageorgiou C, Singh K, Petris MJ (2021) Copper metabolism as a unique vulnerability in cancer. Biochimica et Biophysica Acta (BBA) - Mol Cell Res 1868(2):118893
63. Vaidya SM, Kamalakar PL (1998) Copper and ceruloplasmin levels in serum of women with breast cancer. Indian J Med Sci 52(5):184–187
64. Venturelli S, Leischner C, Helling T, Renner O, Burkard M, Marongiu L (2022) Minerals and cancer: overview of the possible diagnostic value. Cancers (Basel) 14(5)
65. Lener MR, Scott RJ, Wiechowska-Kozłowska A, Serrano-Fernández P, Baszuk P, Jaworska-Bieniek K, Sukiennicki G, Marciniak W, Muszyńska M, Kładny J, Gromowski T, Kaczmarek K, Jakubowska A, Lubiński J (2016) Serum concentrations of selenium and copper in patients diagnosed with pancreatic cancer. Cancer Res Treat 48(3):1056–1064
66. Tamai Y, Iwasa M, Eguchi A, Shigefuku R, Sugimoto K, Hasegawa H, Takei Y (2020) Serum copper, zinc and metallothionein serve as potential biomarkers for hepatocellular carcinoma. PLoS ONE 15(8):e0237370
67. Juloski JT, Rakic A, Ćuk VV, Ćuk VM, Stefanović S, Nikolić D, Janković S, Trbovich AM, De Luka SR (2020) Colorectal cancer and trace elements alteration. J Trace Elem Med Biol 59:126451
68. Lopez J, Ramchandani D, Vahdat L (2019) Copper depletion as a therapeutic strategy in cancer. Met Ions Life Sci 19
69. Lin J, Zahurak M, Beer TM, Ryan CJ, Wilding G, Mathew P, Morris M, Callahan JA, Gordon G, Reich SD, Carducci MA, Antonarakis ES (2013) A non-comparative randomized phase II study of 2 doses of ATN-224, a copper/zinc superoxide dismutase inhibitor, in patients with biochemically recurrent hormone-naïve prostate cancer. Urol Oncol 31(5):581–588
70. Chan N, Willis A, Kornhauser N, Ward MM, Lee SB, Nackos E, Seo BR, Chuang E, Cigler T, Moore A, Donovan D, Vallee Cobham M, Fitzpatrick V, Schneider S, Wiener A, Guillaume-Abraham J, Aljom E, Zelkowitz R, Warren JD, Lane ME, Fischbach C, Mittal V, Vahdat L (2017) Influencing the tumor microenvironment: a phase ii study of copper depletion using

tetrathiomolybdate in patients with breast cancer at high risk for recurrence and in preclinical models of lung metastases. Clin Cancer Res 23(3):666–676
71. Razaghi A, Poorebrahim M, Sarhan D, Bjornstedt M (2021) Selenium stimulates the antitumour immunity: Insights to future research. Eur J Cancer 155:256–267
72. Gilman AF (1946) Therapeutic applications of chemical warfare agents. Fed Proc 5:285–292
73. Schomburg L, Hughes and Hepatology DJOJ (2017) The missing link? The potential role of selenium in the development of liver cancer and significance for the general population. 11(8):707–709
74. Schrauzer GN (1976) Selenium and cancer: a review. Bioinorg Chem 5(3):275–281
75. Callejón-Leblic B, Rodríguez-Moro G, Arias-Borrego A, Pereira-Vega A, Gómez-Ariza JL, García-Barrera T (2020) Absolute quantification of selenoproteins and selenometabolites in lung cancer human serum by column switching coupled to triple quadrupole inductively coupled plasma mass spectrometry. J Chromatogr A 1619:460919
76. Puig S, Ramos-Alonso L, Romero AM, Martinez-Pastor MT (2017) The elemental role of iron in DNA synthesis and repair. Metallomics 9(11):1483–1500
77. Laskey J, Webb I, Schulman HM, Ponka P (1988) Evidence that transferrin supports cell proliferation by supplying iron for DNA synthesis. Exp Cell Res 176(1):87–95
78. Brookes MJ, Boult J, Roberts K, Cooper BT, Hotchin NA, Matthews G, Iqbal T, Tselepis C (2008) A role for iron in Wnt signalling. Oncogene 27(7):966–975
79. Perse M (2013) Oxidative stress in the pathogenesis of colorectal cancer: cause or consequence? Biomed Res Int 2013:725710
80. Ji LL, Gomez-Cabrera MC, Vina J (2007) Role of nuclear factor kappaB and mitogen-activated protein kinase signaling in exercise-induced antioxidant enzyme adaptation. Appl Physiol Nutr Metab 32(5):930–935
81. Kramer HF, Goodyear LJ (2007) Exercise, MAPK, and NF-kappaB signaling in skeletal muscle. J Appl Physiol 103(1):388–395
82. Fonseca-Nunes A, Jakszyn P, Agudo A (2014) Iron and cancer risk–a systematic review and meta-analysis of the epidemiological evidence. Cancer Epidemiol Biomarkers Prev 23(1):12–31
83. Paganoni R, Lechel and M. Vujic Spasic (2021). Iron at the Interface of Hepatocellular Carcinoma. Int J Mol Sci 22(8)
84. Broitman SA, Velez H, Vitale JJ (1981) A possible role of iron deficiency in gastric cancer in Colombia. Adv Exp Med Biol 135:155–181
85. Verma S, Cherayil BJ (2017) Iron and inflammation—the gut reaction. Metallomics 9(2):101–111
86. Zacharski LR, Chow BK, Howes PS, Shamayeva G, Baron JA, Dalman RL, Malenka DJ, Ozaki CK, Lavori PW (2008) Decreased cancer risk after iron reduction in patients with peripheral arterial disease: results from a randomized trial. J Natl Cancer Inst 100(14):996–1002
87. Wen CP, Lee JH, Tai YP, Wen C, Wu SB, Tsai MK, Hsieh DP, Chiang HC, Hsiung CA, Hsu CY, Wu X (2014) High serum iron is associated with increased cancer risk. Cancer Res 74(22):6589–6597
88. Mahmood N, Mihalcioiu C, Rabbani SA (2018) Multifaceted role of the urokinase-type plasminogen activator (uPA) and its receptor (uPAR): diagnostic, prognostic, and therapeutic applications. Front Oncol 8:24
89. Roughead ZK, Zito CA, Hunt JR (2005) Inhibitory effects of dietary calcium on the initial uptake and subsequent retention of heme and nonheme iron in humans: comparisons using an intestinal lavage method. Am J Clin Nutr 82(3):589–597
90. Papp B, Launay S, Gelebart P, Arbabian A, Enyedi A, Brouland JP, Carosella ED, Adle-Biassette H (2020) Endoplasmic reticulum calcium pumps and tumor cell differentiation. Int J Mol Sci 21(9)
91. Bong AHL, Monteith GR (2018) Calcium signaling and the therapeutic targeting of cancer cells. Biochim Biophys Acta Mol Cell Res 1865(11 Pt B):1786–1794

92. Prevarskaya N, Skryma R, Shuba Y (2011) Calcium in tumour metastasis: new roles for known actors. Nat Rev Cancer 11(8):609–618
93. Berridge MJ (2009) Inositol trisphosphate and calcium signalling mechanisms. Biochim Biophys Acta 1793(6):933–940
94. Chung FY, Lin SR, Lu CY, Yeh CS, Chen FM, Hsieh JS, Huang TJ, Wang JY (2006) Sarco/endoplasmic reticulum calcium-ATPase 2 expression as a tumor marker in colorectal cancer. Am J Surg Pathol 30(8):969–974
95. Turano C, Gaucci E, Grillo C, Chichiarelli S (2011) ERp57/GRP58: a protein with multiple functions. Cell Mol Biol Lett 16(4):539–563
96. Wulaningsih W, Sagoo HK, Hamza M, Melvin J, Holmberg L, Garmo H, Malmstrom H, Lambe M, Hammar N, Walldius G, Jungner I, Van Hemelrijck M (2016) Serum calcium and the risk of breast cancer: findings from the Swedish AMORIS study and a meta-analysis of prospective studies. Int J Mol Sci 17(9)
97. Pierre F, Tache S, Petit CR, Van der Meer R, Corpet DE (2003) Meat and cancer: haemoglobin and haemin in a low-calcium diet promote colorectal carcinogenesis at the aberrant crypt stage in rats. Carcinogenesis 24(10):1683–1690
98. Huang P, Lan M, Peng AF, Yu QF, Chen WZ, Liu ZL, Liu JM, Huang SH (2017) Serum calcium, alkaline phosphotase and hemoglobin as risk factors for bone metastases in bladder cancer. PLoS ONE 12(9):e0183835
99. Xu QH, Zhu PW, Li B, Shi WQ, Lin Q, Min YL, Ge QM, Yuan Q, Shao Y (2020) Carbohydrate antigen-125, calcium, and hemoglobin as predictive clinical indicator for ocular metastasis in male liver cancer patients. Biosci Rep 40(2)
100. Erem S, Razzaque MS (2018) Dietary phosphate toxicity: an emerging global health concern. Histochem Cell Biol 150(6):711–719
101. Calvo MS, Tucker KL (2013) Is phosphorus intake that exceeds dietary requirements a risk factor in bone health? Ann N Y Acad Sci 1301:29–35
102. Shimada M, Shutto-Uchita Y, Yamabe H (2019) Lack of awareness of dietary sources of phosphorus is a clinical concern. In Vivo 33(1):11–16
103. Anderson JJ (2013) Potential health concerns of dietary phosphorus: cancer, obesity, and hypertension. Ann N Y Acad Sci 1301:1–8
104. Papaloucas CD, Papaloucas MD, Kouloulias V, Neanidis K, Pistevou-Gompaki K, Kouvaris J, Zygogianni A, Mystakidou K, Papaloucas AC (2014) Measurement of blood phosphorus: a quick and inexpensive method for detection of the existence of cancer in the body. Too good to be true, or forgotten knowledge of the past? Med Hypotheses 82(1):24–25
105. Jin H, Xu CX, Lim HT, Park SJ, Shin JY, Chung YS, Park SC, Chang SH, Youn HJ, Lee KH, Lee YS, Ha YC, Chae CH, Beck GR Jr, Cho MH (2009) High dietary inorganic phosphate increases lung tumorigenesis and alters Akt signaling. Am J Respir Crit Care Med 179(1):59–68
106. Chan JM, Pietinen P, Virtanen M, Malila N, Tangrea J, Albanes D, Virtamo J (2000) Diet and prostate cancer risk in a cohort of smokers, with a specific focus on calcium and phosphorus (Finland). Cancer Causes Control 11(9):859–867
107. Kesse E, Boutron-Ruault MC, Norat T, Riboli E, Clavel-Chapelon F, Group EN (2005) Dietary calcium, phosphorus, vitamin D, dairy products and the risk of colorectal adenoma and cancer among French women of the E3N-EPIC prospective study. Int J Cancer 117(1):137–144
108. Brinkman MT, Buntinx F, Kellen E, Dagnelie PC, Van Dongen MC, Muls E, Zeegers MP (2011) Dietary intake of micronutrients and the risk of developing bladder cancer: results from the Belgian case-control study on bladder cancer risk. Cancer Causes Control 22(3):469–478
109. Tavani A, Bertuccio P, Bosetti C, Talamini R, Negri E, Franceschi S, Montella M, La Vecchia C (2005) Dietary intake of calcium, vitamin D, phosphorus and the risk of prostate cancer. Eur Urol 48(1):27–33
110. Berg JW, Burbank F (1972) Correlations between carcinogenic trace metals in water supplies and cancer mortality. Ann N Y Acad Sci 199(1):249–264

111. Luo XM, Wei HJ, Hu GG, Shang AL, Liu YY, Lu SM, Yang SP (1981) Molybdenum and esophageal cancer in china. In: Federation proceedings
112. Stoner GD, Shimkin MB, Troxell MC, Thompson TL, Terry LS (1976) Test for carcinogenicity of metallic compounds by the pulmonary tumor response in strain A mice. Cancer Res 36(5):1744–1747
113. FR: International Agency for Research on Cancer (2006) IWgoteocrthiaolclmoteocrth L
114. Garcia-Leston J, Roma-Torres J, Mayan O, Schroecksnadel S, Fuchs D, Moreira AO, Pasaro E, Mendez J, Teixeira JP, Laffon B (2012) Assessment of immunotoxicity parameters in individuals occupationally exposed to lead. J Toxicol Environ Health A 75(13–15):807–818
115. Liaw FY, Chen WL, Kao TW, Chang YW, Huang CF (2017) Exploring the link between cadmium and psoriasis in a nationally representative sample. Sci Rep 7(1):1723
116. Luevano J, Damodaran C (2014) A review of molecular events of cadmium-induced carcinogenesis. J Environ Pathol Toxicol Oncol 33(3):183–194

Diet, Gut Microbes, and Cancer

7

Asma Saleem Qazi, Ubaid ur Rahman, Bilal Ahmad, Waseem Safdar, Saeed Ahmad, and Sara Mumtaz

Contents

A. S. Qazi (✉) · B. Ahmad · W. Safdar · S. Ahmad · S. Mumtaz
Department of Biological Sciences, National University of Medical Sciences, Islamabad, Pakistan
e-mail: asma.qazi@numspak.edu.pk

B. Ahmad
e-mail: drbilal.uol.edu@gmail.com

W. Safdar
e-mail: waseem.safdar@numspak.edu.pk

S. Ahmad
e-mail: saeed.ahmed@numspak.edu.pk

S. Mumtaz
e-mail: sara.mumtaz@numspak.edu.pk

U. Rahman
Department of Microbiology, Quaid e Azam University, Islamabad, Pakistan
e-mail: ubaid@bs.qau.edu.pk

R. F. Saeed and S. ul. Shaheed (eds.), *Nutrition and Dietary Interventions in Cancer*,
Cancer Treatment and Research 191, https://doi.org/10.1007/978-3-031-55622-7_7

7.1 Overview and Composition of Gut Microbiota

a. **The gut microbiome: Our second genome**

The gut microbiota (GM) comprises of a complex ecosystem mostly present in the colon. The gut microbiota undergoes functional and compositional changes which are reported to take part in both health and disease condition consisting of metabolic, immune, and neuro-behavioral traits [1]. The human microbiome, which includes beneficial and pathogenic bacteria, fungi, viruses, and protozoa, is described as the genetic material of microbes populating the human body [2]. GM is mainly composed of the phyla Firmicutes (64%) which includes the genera Faecalibacterium, Eubacterium, Ruminococcus, Enterococcus, Clostridium, Bacillus, Lactobacillus, Roseburia. Bacteroidetes comprises the second predominant phylum (23%) and includes the genera Prevotella and Bacteroids. It is further followed by the phylum Actinobacteria (3%) and Verrucomicrobia (2%) [3]. The GI system's microbiota is rich in microbial diversity and contributes significantly to the host's physiological activities, such as nutrient absorption and digestion, immunological development, pathogen defense, and other vital physiological functions [4]. The colon is habitat to the majority of gut microorganisms, but they also colonized other parts of the gut, however in lesser quantities in the small intestine, resulting in region-specific distribution [5]. Furthermore, the gut microbiota changes over time, enhancing in variety after birth to around 2 years of age as entire foods are introduced, and decreasing in variety as one aged toward end of life [6].

b. **Factors effecting Gut Microbiota**

The composition of GM is characterized by the variability between individuals, and it might be formed via various factors, such as genetics, age, mode of delivery (either vaginal or cesarean), feeding method of infant (infant formulas or breast milk), drugs such as antibiotics, diet as well as geographical region [7, 8].

7.2 Dietary Patterns Influencing Gut Microbiota

Remarkably, the most significant factor that influences the gut microbiota is "diet", that exhibit a bidirectional and complex relationship between them. Hence, the composition of the GM has a great influence on the absorption and metabolism of nutrients that ultimately effects the physiology of host. In sequence, nutrients, bioactive compounds, specific foods, and dietary patterns also regulate the GM composition and its functionality which effects human health either positively or negatively [7]. Therefore, for reshaping the composition of GM and reducing the imbalance in its activity and composition the adjustment in diet have been recommended (Yang et al. 2012). Thus, a healthy and well-balanced gut microbiota composition is achieved by a diverse and rich microbial community. Current observation studies have been reported, the existence of a close association

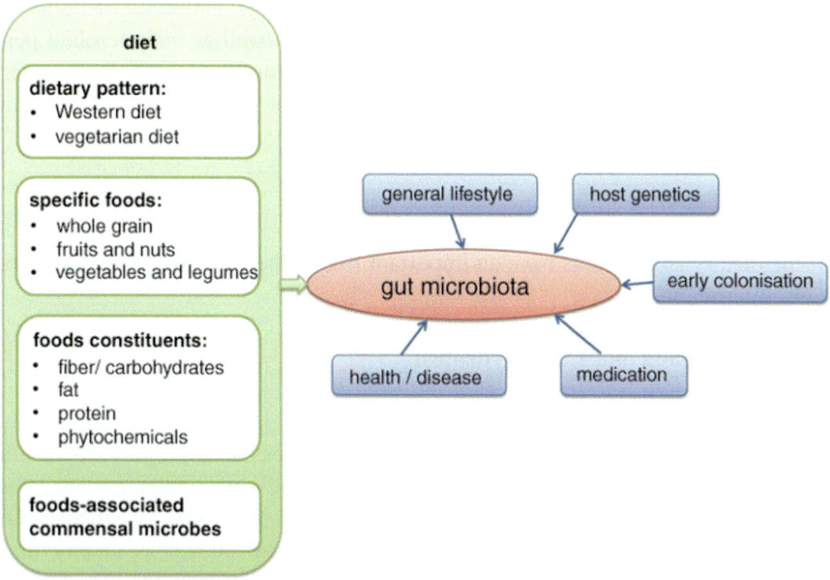

Fig. 7.1 Factor influences human gut microbiota composition based on diet [10]

amongst the intestinal flora dysbiosis and various non-infectious disorders including obesity, diabetes, cardiovascular diseases, cancer, neurological disorders, and GI (gastrointestinal) diseases, e.g., irritable bowel syndrome (IBS) [9] (Fig. 7.1).

a. **Gut Microbiota Function**

Gut microbiota forms a joint advantageous association by the host and performs various vital roles. Certainly gut microbiota shows a main role in intestinal endothelial barrier structure integrity by encouraging intestinal microvasculature, cell regeneration, and wound healing, as well as regulating mucous membranes and changes [11]. Gut bacteria may reactivate mucin glycosylation and contribute to the maintenance of strong connections by activating the signaling of toll-like receptor 2 (TLR2) by peptidoglycan in the cell wall [12]. GM also play an important role in promoting the development of systemic immune system. Gut microbes also contribute in the expansion of T cells and innate lymphoid cells in the lymphoid structures of gut, in raising B cells to produce antibodies IgA, and in pathogens response to regulate the resident macrophages of the lamina propria. Moreover, GM offers protection against microorganisms through its structural elements and metabolites. It stimulates the synthesis of antimicrobial peptides that includes the common immunoglobulins that prevent the growth of pathogenic microbes [13]. To our interest, GM consist of carbohydrate enzymes that have the ability to ferment carbohydrates and produce metabolites (i.e., short chain fatty acids, SCFA), which have important role in the host body. The GM also influence the metabolism of lipids, fats, and proteins by raising hydrolysis of lipids, inhibition of lipogenic enzymes and producing small indicating molecules as well as antimicrobial peptides (bacteriocins). Additionally, GM are also crucial for the production of various vitamins from group B (nicotinic acid, pyridoxine, pantothenic acid, thiamine, and biotin) and vitamin K [14].

b. **Dietary Patterns**

All the dietary components have an important role in the composition and shaping of gut microbiota.

- **Gut Microbiota and Carbohydrates:**

Carbohydrates: Mostly carbohydrates are divided into two categories, i.e., digestible and indigestible carbohydrates. Carbohydrates that are digestible include glucose, galactose, fructose and are degraded in the small intestine enzymatically and quickly released into the bloodstream in the form of glucose. On the other hand, carbohydrates that are indigestible also known as dietary fiber resist digestion in small intestine and pass on to the large intestine. These indigestible dietary fibers consist of lignin, non-starch polysaccharides, non-digestible oligosaccharides, and resistant starches [15].

Resistant starch is mostly discovered in completely or partially crushed seeds or grains. The non-digestible oligosaccharides are composed of oligofructose, raffinose, inulin, and stachyose. Among the dietary fibers some are fermentable and dissolve in water such as pectin, galacto-oligosaccharides (GOSs), beta-glucan, inulin, and fructo-oligosaccharides (FOSs) while other non-fermentable dietary fibers for example resistant starch, cellulose, hemi-cellulose and lignin are considered insoluble in water. In addition, bacteria easily ferment the fermentable fibers in the colon as compared to non-fermentable [16].

Short-Chain Fatty Acids (SCFAs): Saccharolytic fermentation takes place in fermentable dietary fibers by gut bacteria and produce monosaccharides short-chain fatty acids (i.e., acetate (60%), butyrate (15%), propionate (25%), and gases such as carbon dioxide and methane). On the contrary, propionate and acetate are taken up through portal vein by the liver and are used as substrate for the metabolism of glucose, lipid, and cholesterol. While butyrate plats an essential role in the maintenance of tissue barrier functions, immunoregulation and regulation of gene expression. The composition of the gut microbiota and the amount of carbohydrates consumed determines the amount and types of SCFAs. Therefore, the bacterial populations revealed in feces are influenced by the fluctuations in the variety and amount of non-digestible sugars [17].

Prebiotics: We define prebiotics as foods, non-digestible by host which have a vital and positive effect because of their discriminating metabolism in the digestive tract. Microbiota-accessible carbohydrates (MACs) are the carbohydrates which are resistant to host's metabolism for digestion and are presented to the GM in the form of prebiotics to metabolize them into short-chain fatty acids SCFAs [18].

- **Gut Microbiota and Proteins**

Some major microbial phyla, such as Firmicutes, Proteobacteria, and Bacteroidetes, carries out amino acid fermentation in the distal colon. The type of proteins influences its effect on the composition of gut microbiota.

Animal-Based Protein: The intake of animal-based protein diet mostly from dairy products and red meat may result in an increased number of bile-tolerant anaerobic bacteria such as Biolphila, Alistipes, and Bacteroides. These alterations in gut microbiota promotes an increase in trimethylamine N-oxide (TMAO), a compound which is recognized for its proatherogenic ability playing crucial role in cardiovascular disorders [19].

Plant-Based Proteins: The intake of vegetal or plant proteins such as pea proteins results in greater number of gut-commensal Lactobacillus and Bifidobacterium and decreased number of disease-causing Clostridium perfringens and Bacteroides fragilis. The plant-based protein is fermented stimulate SCFA production with an increase of Lactobacillus and Bifidobacterium [20].

- **Gut Microbiota and Fats**

The quality and quantity of dietary fat influence the composition of gut microbiota. According to previous studies the intestinal microbiota is indirectly modulated by dietary fat through its influence on the secretion of bile acid as well as on the composition of bile acid [21]. It is reported that high intake of fat promotes the bile acid secretion and increase the fecal concentration of bile acids, e.g., deoxycholic acid (DCA). Bile acids such as deoxycholic acid DCA have the ability to facilitate fat induced alterations of intestinal microbiota with the help of their selective antimicrobial activity. Wu et al. [22] stated that the Bacteroides enterotype is positively correlated with the consumption of saturated fats, while the Prevotella enterotype is inversely (weakly) related with the total consumption of dietary fat [23].

- **Gut Microbiota and Salts**

The World Health Organization (WHO) suggests a 5 g/day maximum intake of salt. A high-salt diet (HSD) is accompanied with a reduced number of Clostridium XIVa, Pseudoflavonifractor, Oscillibacter, Johnsonella, Lactobacillus spp., and an enhanced number of Christensenellaceae Erwinia genus, Parasutterella spp, and Ruminococcus [24]. HSD may also lead to alterations in composition of gut microbiota, with a potential rise of Bacteroidetes/Firmicutes ratio, which may lead to change in production of SCFAs linked with immune homeostasis and alterations of gut permeability [25].

- **Gut Microbiota and Polyphenols**

More than ten thousand polyphenol compounds have been reported for showing a significant property in the prevention of diabetes, obesity, cardiovascular diseases, and many others. However, the bioavailability and absorption of these polyphenols remains unclear in humans. Nonetheless, researchers strongly agree that the mutual interaction of phenolic compounds and gut microbiota have important effect on the bioavailability of these compounds. For instance, supplementation of quercetin lead to the difference in gut microbiota composition at various taxonomical level that includes comparative Firmicutes and Bacteroidetes ratio and resisting the development of bacteria linked with diet-encouraged obesity such as Eubacterium cylindroides, Bacillus, and Erysipelotrichaceae species. Gut microbiota can control the alteration of phenolic compounds into reduced metabolites, manipulating their bioavailability and altering their properties [26].

c. **Impacts of Dietary Patterns on Gut Microbiota**

Our diet patterns result in the certain combination of a precise mixture of macro and micronutrient, endlessly and indeterminately transported to our gut environment, we thought it beneficial to assess the influence of advanced and present dietary patterns on gut microbiota linked with mucosal barrier of host and immune functions. The Fig. 7.2 demonstrates the effects of various kinds of diet on commensal species of bacteria, lamina propria, and mucus layer hosting the cells of immune system [27].

- **Western Diets**

Nowadays, the common dietary arrangement in high income countries is the western diet. This type of diet is characterized by the increase intake of saturated fat, animal proteins, sugar, and low consumption of plant obtained vegetables and fibers. Several studies have reported the strong impact of western diet pattern on the composition and function of gut microbiota promoting dysbiosis and metabolic diseases [29].

The diet we consume have a strong influence on the gut microbiota, by effecting its composition related to its abundance and diversity. On one side, high consumption of saturated fat, salt, sugar, and animal proteins could promote the development of pathogenic bacteria to the loss of useful bacteria, resulting in possible variations of the intestinal barrier. While on other side, the intake of plant-based protein and complex polysaccharides could be related with a rise of useful and essential bacterial diversity, stimulating the production of SCFA. Additionally, polyphenols, omega-3, and micronutrients seem to have the ability and potential to confer benefits of health through variation of the gut microbiota. The dietary patterns can strongly affect composition of gut microbiota. The Western diet, that includes additives, may decrease gut microbial variety in terms of genus and phyla

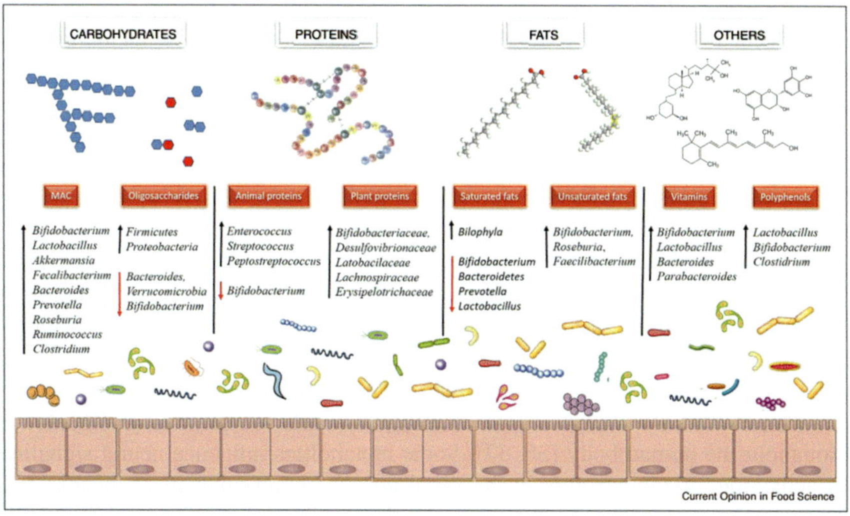

Fig. 7.2 Outline of the major effects of dietary composites on the composition of gut microbiota. Arrows show an induction and reduction of bacterial abundance. *MAC* microbiota-accessible carbohydrates [28]

resulting in dysbiosis, modification of barrier permeability and function, and irregular stimulation of immune cells, resulting in high rates of chronic diseases. Future developments on the data of the interactions between food compounds and specific gut bacteria would result in a better understanding of both positive and negative relations with dietary patterns.

7.3 Epigenetics and Influence of Microbial Metabolites

Host epigenetic mechanisms shows a significant action in gut establishment, comprising the variation of intestinal stem cells into mature, fully functioning cells, which occurs concurrently with the development of gut microbiota [30, 31]. Microbiota significance in the formation and upkeep of proper intestinal growth and physiology, particularly absorption and uptake of nutrient, development of tissue, metabolism, and immunity, has been emphasized in recent decades [32, 33]. Experience to the certain milieu of microbes from birth may influence epigenetic changes. Diet, starting with breast or formula milk, shapes the gut microbiota in early childhood and endures during maturity, depending on someone's dietary and lifestyle preferences. Commonly known phyla of the gastro intestinal tract comprise Bacteriodetes, Actinobacteria, Proteobacteria, and Firmicutes [6]. These are involved in nutrient absorption and digestion, stimulation of the host immune system, deconjugation of bile acid, dietary fiber metabolism, formation of short-chain fatty acids (SCFAs), and epithelial integrity promotion [4]. However, gut dysbiosis, or a harmful reorganization of the gut microbiota, can disturb these mechanisms and lead to the development of a variety of diseases, including obesity, type II diabetes, cardiovascular disease, and nonalcoholic fatty liver disease [34]. The microbiome and microbially derived metabolites have the ability to modulate gene activity epigenetically. While nutrition affects the microbiome, it also affects the epigenetic pathways that involves microbiota. The influence of the gut microbiome's components and metabolites on a variety of processes in the body, including epigenetic processes, contributes to individual variability [35]. Dietary microbial metabolism releases compounds that influence epigenetics by (1) changing the pools of substrates required for modifications like methylation or (2) altering the activity of the enzymes involved in heritable epigenetic alterations. [2].

A wide range of gut microbiota may digest components of our diet, releasing compounds into the gut lumen, many of which are physiologically active throughout the human body [36, 37]. Some metabolites influence neural signaling via activating chemoreceptors in the vagal nerve, among other mechanisms [38]. Enteric neurons can interact directly with the gut microbes. Gut epithelial cells (colonocytes) absorbed metabolites produced by the host and microbiota, which may impact gene expression via epigenetic mechanisms. Many metabolites enter the bloodstream and can circulate across the body, influencing organ systems such as the immune system, where they play an important role in early life programming [39]. Both maternal and neonatal nutrition have a significant impact on epigenome of the offspring, since the food consumed influences the composition of the gut microbiota and hence the metabolites released. Interestingly, host-microbe interactions. Are reciprocal, which means that changes in host epigenetics. Influences the colonization and composition of gut microbiota [40, 41].

Conrad Waddington first coined the term "epigenetics" in 1942 and it is the study of biological processes that alter gene activity without affecting DNA sequence. It include the alteration of genes through (1) covalent modifications to histone proteins like histone acetylation, (2) DNA methylation, such as methylation to cytosine or adenosine residues, (3) expression of enzymes which regulate DNA methylation, like DNA methyl transferase or ten-eleven translocation (TET), or histone acetylation, which include histone deacetylases (HDACs) and histone acyltransferases (HATs), thereby modifying chromatin structure, and (4) post-transcriptional regulation via noncoding RNAs [42, 43].

a. **Histone Modifications**

Histones can be subjected to post-translational modifications (PTMs) such as acetylation, methylation, ubiquitination, SUMOylation, and phosphorylation, all of which influence gene activation and repression. In the existence of microbe-derived SCFAs, histone crotonylation, which modifies chromatin susceptibility to other modifiers, increases [44]. In addition to SCFAs, gut microbes synthesize and release cobalt, selenium, iodine, zinc, and other metabolites as cofactors for histone methylation and acetylation. Histone acetylation causes gene upregulation, whereas histone methylation causes either enhanced or declined expression, grounded on lysine residue. Short-chain fatty acids production by microbes in carbohydrate fermentation have been observed to hinder the deacetylases of histone, indicating that they play a role in epigenetics [45].

b. **DNA Methylation**

In contrast to histone modifications gut microbiome affects DNA's epigenetic state. DNA methylation has different effects dependent on location, with methylation at gene promoters causing methylation and silencing at the gene body that causes activation [46]. The addition of a methyl group to the carbon-5 position of the cytosine pyrimidine ring in DNA is known as methylation, and it happens primarily in cytosine guanine dinucleotide-rich sections known as CpG islands, which are present in the 50 regulatory regions of most genes. By releasing epigenetically active metabolites like folate, acetate, and butyrate to host cells, bacteria can trigger changes in DNA methylation patterns [47]. Despite the fact that endogenous mechanisms predominantly control DNA methylation, the presence of pathogenic microorganisms can significantly alter methylation and cause disease. For example, infection with *H. pylori,* produces abnormal DNA methylation in stomach mucosal cells [48].

- **Effect of Dietary Fiber on GI Immune Barrier**

Fibers have shown indirect positive effect on the gastrointestinal immunological barrier by stimulating the proliferation and metabolic activities of intestinal microbiota communities [49]. Dietary fibers are not digested by human enzymes and are fermented mostly in the colon by the intestinal microbiota [50]. Some dietary fibers facilitate the growth of certain microbial communities and act as substrates for fermentation products including short-chain fatty acids (SCFAs) [49]. Dietary fibers can help you live a healthier life by stimulating the synthesis of SCFAs. These SCFAs have been proven to have a key function in metabolism [31, 51] and immunity [52, 53]. In contrast to the fermentation products of fibers, microbes can produce other metabolites, like secondary bile acids or tryptophan metabolites that have the potential to influence intestinal immunity [54]. Furthermore, dietary fibers may aid in the development of commensal microbiota, which may hinder the growth of pathogens that adhere to the intestinal wall less in the presence of a high population of gut commensals. As a result, dietary fibers have been advocated as a way to protect the gastrointestinal immunological barrier against pathogen harm [55]. Polymorphisms in host genes associated with innate and adaptive immunity have been shown to affect microbial complexity [44].

- **Epigenetics-Based Antimicrobial Therapeutics**

The two-way interaction between microbiota and epigenetics could be exploited to treat and prevent disease. According to new research A number of human clinical trials employing diet probiotics for a wide range of human disorders, from obesity to Alzheimer and disease and cancer, have been conducted based on findings from animal studies [56, 57].

Nutraceuticals, or epigenetically active nutrients, have been shown to protect against a variety of diseases, including cardiovascular disease, gastrointestinal disorders, and cancer [58]. Although research into their mechanisms of action is still in its early stages, epigallocatechin gallate has recently been found to inhibit high-fat diet-induced changes in gut microbiota, DNA methylation, and host gene expression [59].

The gut microbiota, its metabolism, and composition have a bidirectional relationship. Dietary preferences throughout time has a substantial effect on the diversity of microbiota and expression of gene. The gut flora, on the other hand, modulates dietary agent's absorption and produces energy metabolites as cofactors in epigenetic reactions. Dietary substances can influence the epigenome directly or indirectly through microbial metabolites. The microbiome plays a significant role in both health and disease because it affects physiology, endocrinology, and even neurology, influencing the outcome of a variety of diseases and improving drug responses and tolerance.

7.4 Gut Microbiome and Dietary Metabolism

The homeostasis of the gastrointestinal (GI) tract is critically dependent on the diverse ecology of bacteria found in the human gut. Bacteria are the largest of these contributors to ecosystem functioning in terms of the physiology of the human superorganism. In general, a direct advantage is the microbial metabolism of exogenous and endogenous substrates into nutrients usable by the host [60]. Intestinal microflora is formed at an early age, starting from the neonate stage. Neonatal intestinal microflora is influenced by amniotic fluid content, maternal lifestyle, diet, and exposure to antibiotics during pregnancy [61]. The large intestine is the main site because it has favorable conditions for bacterial growth due to its relatively long transit time, high pH, and low cell turnover and redox potential. However, this does not negate the importance of the microbiota in other organs. For example, the microbiota of the small intestine has been shown to control host metabolism and nutrient absorption.

The presence of different metabolic activities may help the microbiota to occupy ecological niches to their full capacity and limit pathogen colonization. The local pH is further lowered by the increasing amount of mostly acidic fermentation byproducts, making the environment less favorable for these incoming invaders [62]. However, toxic chemicals that have the potential to damage the host epithelium and induce inflammation can be produced by certain fermentation processes carried out by intestinal microorganisms. The three macronutrients—carbohydrates, proteins, and fats—from the human diet can either completely resist primary digestion due to the intrinsic structural complexity of some biomolecules, or they can escape primary digestion once the amount consumed exceeds the rate of digestion. The shape and size of food particles (influenced by cooking and processing), food composition (influenced by the relative proportions of macronutrients and the presence of antinutrients such as amylase), and a number of other factors can affect the efficiency of digestion, which in turn modifies the substrates available for gut microflora to consume.

a. **Microbial Metabolism of Dietary Carbohydrates**

Metabolic pathways of gut bacteria can potentially influence the bioavailability of micronutrients to the host. Colonic bacteria have the ability to endogenously produce vitamins and other essential cofactors for host energy/metabolism. Another illustration is the biotransformation of exogenous polyphenols of plant origin by intestinal bacteria, which increases the host's ability to absorb these compounds because they have antioxidant, anticancer, and/or anti-inflammatory effects [62]. Due to the abundance of carbohydrate-activating enzymes, dietary polysaccharides can be linked in complex ways through a wide variety of interactions between monosaccharide units. Bacteroides contains 260 glycoside hydrolases to maximize the consumption of resistant starch and the diversity of fiber present in the human diet. While human cells produce amylase to break down the attached sugar units from starch and can use sugars such as glucose, fructose, sucrose, and lactose in the small intestine, they produce very few of these other enzymes. As a result, human cells must rely on gut microbes to extract energy from the remaining complex carbohydrates.

Monosaccharides can be rapidly consumed by the gut microbiota after undergoing the rate-limiting primary degradation step, and often little interconversion is required for the substrates to enter the Embden-Meyerhof Parnassus pathway, the Entner-Doudoroff pathway, or the Pentose phosphate pathway for pyruvate and subsequent ATP production. Conversely, dietary proteins have conserved peptide bonds that can be cleaved by proteases. Compared to monosaccharides, the 20 proteinogenic amino acid building blocks require more interconversion steps to be included in metabolic pathways, making it unusual for specific species of gut microbes to be able to ferment all amino acids to generate energy. Furthermore, by eliminating the need for amino acid biosynthesis, microbial uptake of amino acids from the environment for anabolic activities would conserve more energy than their catabolic utilization. It follows that the intestinal microflora, depending on the ratio provided to them, preferentially consumes carbohydrates over proteins. Amino acids are not usually considered to be as efficient an energy source as carbohydrates for microorganisms associated with the human gut [62].

The composition and functionality of the intestinal microflora can be attributed mainly to the diet. In fact, a short dietary change from a high-fat/low-fiber diet to a high-fiber/low-fat diet leads to consistent but transient changes in gut flora. High levels of Prevotella have been linked to diets high in fiber and low in animal products. Bacteroides has been shown to be associated with a high-fat/low-fiber diet. On the contrary, our intestinal microflora is mostly shaped by our long-term regular diet. Modern Western diets have seen significant changes in composition in recent decades with increased intake of red meat, high-fat foods, and refined carbohydrates. The "Westernization" of cuisine and lifestyle changes have undoubtedly played a role in the rise of inflammatory diseases such as obesity, diabetes, cardiovascular disease, and cancer.

Comparing the gut microbiomes of rural and western societies can help understand how changes in diet have affected gut symbionts. Studies found that rural populations, who still eat a subsistence, Agrarian diet high in fruits, vegetables, fibrous tubers and roots, and low in animal products [63], are significantly different from urbanized Westerners who consume a high-fat diet and protein (Fig. 7.3). Most of these investigations have highlighted how microbial diversity has decreased in communities that have been exposed to Western culture, and how the traditional community under investigation has similar gut microbiota characteristics [64–68]. Numerous fiber-degrading bacteria, including *Prevotella, Xylanibacter, Treponema, Succinivibrio, Lachnospira*, and others, have been found to be prevalent among traditional cultures that consume agricultural diets. The genetic potential of these strains suggests selective adaptation to the intestinal environment, including the ability to utilize complex polysaccharides that predominate in the diet of non-westernized patients, distinguishing them from known harmful Treponema strains [69].

Numerous variables, including a hypo-perfused gut that enables gut microbial components to be transported into the circulation, might lead to an altered intestinal barrier function. Due to the parallel circulation of the arteries and veins in the villus, which results in a descending tissue gradient in oxygen pressure and tension from the base to the tip of the villus, a decrease in perfusion has a particular impact on the structure of villi in the intestinal mucosa, which are vulnerable to ischemia [70]. As a result, in around 50% of patients, intramucosal acidity might be seen. Additionally, in individuals with chronic heart failure (HF), structural thickening and edema of the intestinal wall can be observed. Notably, intestinal wall thickening was associated with increased indices of intestinal permeability, blood leukocytes, and circulating levels of C-reactive protein (Fig. 7.4). Intestinal ischemia, edema, and inflammation caused by poor cardiac output in heart failure leads to intestinal barrier leakage. Chronic low-grade inflammation is caused by this leak, which facilitates increased entry of inflammatory bacterial products into the circulation. In addition, a leaky gut disrupts the usual microbial population that lives there, which in turn affects the metabolic byproducts produced by those bacteria. Indigestible fiber is converted through metabolic pathways into short-chain

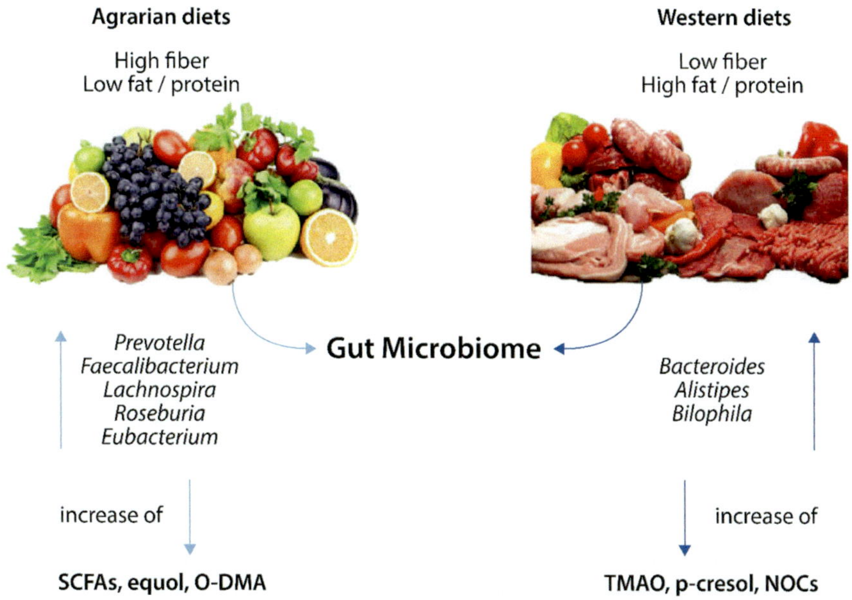

Fig. 7.3 Comparing the gut microbiomes of rural and western societies (adopted with permission from The Gut Microbiome in Health and Disease, edited by Dirk [63])

fatty acids, which have protective properties (reduce inflammation and improve vascular tone) [70].

b. **Microbial Metabolism of High Protein Diet**

Certain metabolites produced by the microbiota from amino acids have been shown to be active on various host activities as described above. These findings suggest that some of the effects of high protein (HP) diets on human metabolism and physiology may be related to some of these metabolites and subsequently to metabolic pathways that are controlled by the microbiota [71]. The effects of increased dietary protein consumption demonstrated in human and animal research are outlined along with potential pathways that may involve compounds derived from gut bacteria (Fig. 7.5). According to two recent meta-analyses of clinical trials, a HP diet marginally reduces body weight, blood pressure, fat mass, and triglyceride levels, while protecting fat-free mass, compared with a normoprotein (NP) diet [69, 72]. These effects are mostly related to the satiety effects of dietary protein. However, the role of gut microflora in these pathways has not yet been studied. The intestinal microflora produces small chain fatty acids (SCFA), indole, tryptamine, and tyramine from precursor amino acids, and these substances are a possibility for mediating the effects of the HP diet on enteroendocrine cell hormone [71].

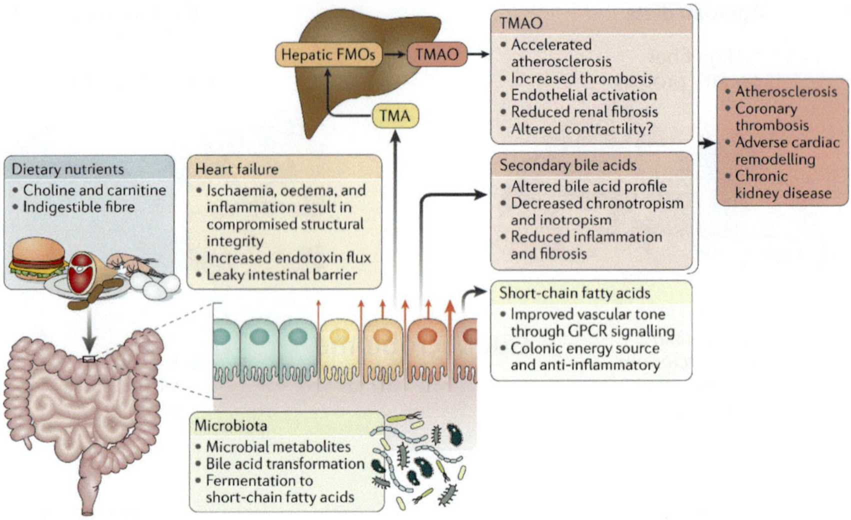

Fig. 7.4 A pathway linking the development of cardiovascular disease, gut bacteria, and food metabolism (Taken with permission from [70])

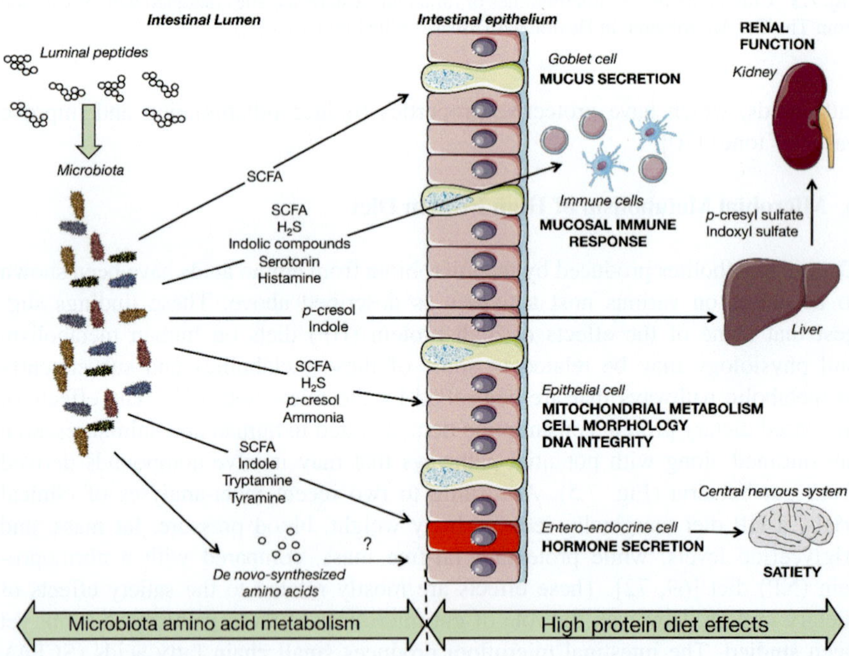

Fig. 7.5 The effect of a diet with a high protein content on the metabolism of intestinal microflora (adopted with permission from [71])

c. Microbial Metabolism of Dietary Lipids

Various bacterial species, including lactobacilli, roseburia, and bifidobacteria, are thought to be able to convert growth-inhibiting polyunsaturated fatty acids (PUFA) into less harmful fatty acids (FA), many of which are beneficial to humans, through microbial metabolism in food. Linoleic acid (LA) is specifically transformed into conjugated linoleic acids (CLAs) during this process (Kochhar and [73]), and these CLAs have been reported to promote gut health, for example by reducing the severity of chemically induced acute colitis in animal models and inhibiting the growth of human colon cancer cells in vitro. Other physiologically active LA metabolites are also formed as intermediates, such as 10-hydroxy-cis-12-octadecenoic acid and 10-oxo-trans-11-octadecenoic acid, which have distinct physiological effects [74].

Although studies have investigated how dietary lipids are delivered to the gut microbiota and how the presence of lipids affects microbial activity, the metabolic pathway by which bacteria consume LA is well established. Dietary lipids are found in dietary components and foods as free oils or emulsions, most of which are triglycerides (95% of total lipids). Gastric and pancreatic lipases hydrolyze most dietary triglycerides and the resulting FA is absorbed in the small intestine [60]. Triglycerides, mono- and diglycerides, and free fatty acids are the most likely form of lipid fraction to enter the colon after escaping small intestinal digestion (5% of total dietary lipids) (FFA). Unlike animal fat, which is readily accessible to digestive fluids, dietary lipids in intact plant tissues have a significant effect on how well the gastrointestinal system absorbs food components. A variable percentage of food components escape digestion in the small intestine and may be digested by the intestinal microflora due to the existence of a cell wall in plant foods that could prevent access to digestive enzymes. The degree of cellular integrity at the time of ingestion largely determines how this fraction fluctuates.

7.5 Functional Contributions Influencing Cancer Susceptibility

The colon contains between 100 billion to one trillion of the bacteria, viruses, archaea, fungi, and protozoa that make up human body. About 90% of the gut microorganisms in healthy people are members of the phyla Bacteroidetes and Firmicutes [65]. Actinobacteria, Fusobacteria, Proteobacteria, and Verrucomicrobia make up the remaining 10% [75]. According to estimates, the oncobiome, a group of carcinogenic microorganisms, is responsible for 2.2 million cancer cases worldwide annually [64]. Escherichia, Citrobacter, Shigella, Flavobacterium, Acinetobacter, and Chryseobacterium species are underrepresented in tumor samples from individuals with colorectal cancer [67].

Lachnospiraceae species, *Bifidobacterium animalis,* and *Streptococcus thermophilus* have low relative abundance, while *Bacteroides clarus, Roseburia intestinalis, Clostridium hathewayi, Fusobacterium nucleatum, Parvimonas micra,* and *Solobacterium moorei* have relatively high relative abundance [63, 65, 76].

These organisms serve as biomarkers of colorectal cancer. A higher risk of colorectal adenocarcinoma is associated with *Helicobacter pylori* infection and CagA protein positivity. *Clostridium septicum* bacterial infection increases the possibility of developing colorectal cancer [65]. Firmicutes and lactococci are more prevalent in the gut microbiota of colorectal cancer tissues compared to nearby non-cancerous colorectal cells. Hepatocellular carcinoma caused by toxins and viruses is promoted by *Helicobacter hepaticus.*

Unlike healthy people, patients with colorectal cancer have relatively higher concentrations of *Clostridium difficile, Enterococcus faecalis, Bacteroides fragilis, Escherichia coli, Streptococcus bovis/gallolyticus, Porphyromonas, Peptostreptococcus, Gemella, Mogibacterium, Klebsiella,* and *Prevotella* [63, 65, 68, 76, 77]. Human cancer has been linked to certain diets. A lower incidence of cancer is associated with diets high in fiber, fruit, yogurt, whole grains, extra virgin olive oil, vegetables, and low in animal products. On the other hand, an increased risk of cancer is associated with a diet rich in processed foods, animal fats, red meat, and a lack of fiber. Human colon cancer cells are inhibited from proliferation by Bacteroides species and Bacillus polyfermenticus [78], while Lactobacillus and Bifidobacterium inhibit colorectal cancer growth by reducing intestinal inflammation and angiogenesis [65].

A number of bacteria have been associated with tumorigenesis, including *F. nucleatum, enterotoxic Bacteroides fragilis, E. faecalis, Peptostreptococcus anaerobius, Helicobacter pylori.* However, for the vast majority of microbial-cancer correlations, it is unclear whether the relationship is causal, unidirectional or bidirectional, or merely correlational [68]. To better understand the relationships between these factors, it is important to investigate the processes underlying the interactions between nutrition, microorganisms, and cancer. Examples of plausible processes that could explain these associations include resource availability in the gut, resource limitation, inflammation, production of growth factors, and even cell signaling between bacteria and malignant or pre-cancerous cells.

The fact that the vast majority of microbiome species are still unknown is another limitation to consider. Despite the fact that advances in metagenomics have sequenced 806 microbial genomes from 124 individuals and 5000 from approximately 180 wild and domesticated species, there is still insufficient genome coverage for many microbial genomes that are underrepresented in the gut microbiome [68, 79]. Furthermore, for many years, interventions involving dietary therapies, food-induced microbial treatments, probiotics and prebiotics, microbial biomarkers, and personalized medicine have been shown to be successful. To reduce the burden of cancer in non-human animals and to find new treatments that might be more effective, future research should examine dietary and microbial therapies across species.

a. **Diet-Microbiome Interactions in Cancer Treatment**

Studies suggest that the microbiome may play a role in some adverse outcomes of cancer therapy. Numerous studies in animal models show that altering the gut microbiome by fecal microbiome transplantation (FMT), antibiotics or probiotics can alleviate the effects of inflammatory and neuropathic pain caused by cancer therapy [64, 67, 68, 72, 78, 79]. A small number of studies show benefits for side effects of cancer treatment with the use of dietary prebiotics and/or probiotics (such as pectin and inulin). However, a more recent study suggests that probiotics may counteract the effectiveness of immunotherapy [61, 64, 65].

Nevertheless, a number of clinical trials are being conducted to address the knowledge gap regarding nutritional interventions in cancer patients. Overall, addressing malnutrition and developing tailored nutritional therapy will involve a thorough understanding of genetics, food and drug metabolism at diagnosis and during cancer treatment, as well as the role of gut microbiota in malnutrition. The lack of standardized dietary capture techniques is, among others, one of the main obstacles to offering customized nutritional therapy for cancer patients. These methods would significantly improve the early detection of at-risk individuals after diagnosis in order to manage and treat malnutrition and improve treatment response.

Despite the availability of various screening techniques for malnutrition, Multidimensional Screening Tool (MST), NUTRISCORE, and Patient-Generated Subjective Global Assessment (PG-SGA). In addition, dietary screening methods including food frequency questionnaires (FFQ), healthy eating index (HEI), food diaries, 24-h recall, and brief dietary screeners are designed for healthy populations and do not include questions specifically for cancer patients. In nutritional studies involving cancer patients, the most commonly used techniques are the 24-h recall and/or food FFQ (unpublished data). The advantage of the 24-h recall is the ability to record specific short-term nutritional consumption, such as dietary supplements or medical nutrition formulas often used by cancer patients similar to FFQs, which are limited to a small number of items, they record long-term eating habits (from the previous month or year) based on the likelihood that a food was consumed and in what quantity on a given day. This estimate of typical consumption is based on the assumption that a person's diet does not change much over the course of a month or year—an assumption that could be violated during cancer treatment. These limitations are well discussed and point to the requirement to create more suitable dietary methods of cancer detection [64].

More than 90% of the diet in healthy people is absorbed in the small intestine and nutrients are dispersed to maintain physical health. Dietary residues that pass into the large intestine are mostly composed of complex carbohydrates (fiber), followed by protein residues and primary bile acids that the liver secretes in response to dietary fat. These are key players in maintaining the health of the large intestine based on fermentation, as they control the composition and function of the intestinal microflora. In a healthy diet, short-chain fatty acids are mostly produced by saccharolytic fermentation of complex carbohydrates (fiber) (SCFA). Butyrate, the most prominent member of the SCFA family, with its mucosal anti-inflammatory and anticancer properties, functions as a beneficial resource for colonocytes through cellular metabolism, microbiota homeostasis, antiproliferative, immunomodulatory, and genetic/epigenetic control. Conversely, with an

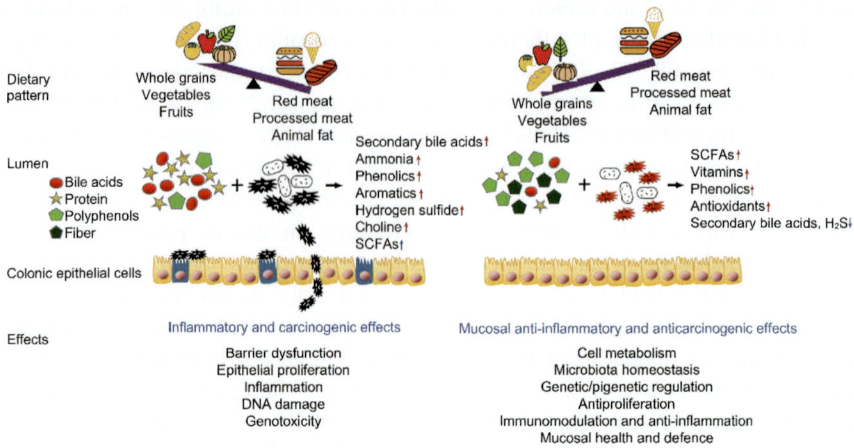

Fig. 7.6 Dietary factors influence CRC risk through gut microbiota and related metabolites (adopted with permission [72])

unbalanced Western diet, protein fermentation and bile acid deconjugation are the most common processes in the colonic lumen, which damage colonic cells in a proneoplastic and pro-inflammatory manner and increase the risk of CRC [72] (Fig. 7.6).

b. **The Microbiome and the Immune System**

The gut microbiota and the growth and control of the innate and adaptive immune systems are interdependent. The immune system is essential for maintaining a healthy balance between oral food antigen tolerance, microbiota, and prevention of pathogenic causes. The composition and shape of the intestinal microflora are influenced by the host's immune system. The development of distal lymphoid tissues, such as the spleen or peripheral lymph nodes, is influenced by the intestinal microflora. It directs lymphocyte subpopulations in secondary immune organs and helps direct the immune system for local mucosal immunity. Gut microflora supports the host's immune system, which is anticancer, maintains bacterial diversity and protects against pathogens colonizing the gastrointestinal tract.

Lymphoid structures, epithelial cells, and the host's intestinal microflora work together to maintain this balance. Consequently, there is a two-way interaction between gut bacteria and the host's immune system. The microbiome uses a number of pathways to communicate with the host. Immune cell recognition receptors (PRRs), such as toll-like receptors (TLRs), on leukocytes and epithelial cells recognize pathogen-associated molecular patterns (PAMPs), such as flagellin, lipopolysaccharide, and peptidoglycan. These PAMPs control how the host's immune system responds to bacteria. Immune cells that contain a significant number of PRRs are present on the surface of the microbiota cluster.

Immune system cells that are activated by PRRs identify pathogens and amplify B- and T-cell-related responses by activating a number of intracellular signaling pathways. Differentiation of naive T cells in mesenteric lymph nodes is influenced by gut microbes. PAMPs could encourage dendritic cells and other antigen-presenting cells (DCs) to mature. Interactions between dendritic cells encourage naïve T cells to differentiate into T helper (Th) and Treg cells. CD8-positive T lymphocytes can be directly stimulated by DCs and Th cells. Through the activation of immune cells, the microbiome can modify systemic immunological responses in addition to influencing local immunity. Toll-like receptors activate dendritic cells and other innate immune effectors, which can then release cytokines and interferons that function in both a paracrine and endocrine manner at distant sites.

An important role is also played by Treg lymphocytes, which suppress the pro-inflammatory response and promote immunological tolerance and immunosuppression. This can be achieved by producing substances such as IL-10, TGF-, IL-35, IL-2, and others. TGF-, IL-10, IL-25, and IL-33 are examples of anti-inflammatory mediators secreted by certain gut bacteria. It is thought that some bacterial species can activate alternative pathways that depend on polysaccharide A (PSA) binding to TLR2 on dendritic cells to promote Treg maturation and TGF production. According to research, the gut, which contains the commensal microbiome, is where T cells differentiate into Treg cells and mature functionally, unlike the thymus.

Lactobacillus acidophilus and Bacteroides some strains of Clostridia, Faecalibacterium, *Helicobacter hepaticus*, *Lactobacillus murinus*, and *Lactobacillus reuteri* may promote the proliferation of Treg cells or promote the production of anti-inflammatory cytokines, which inhibits the host's immune response. Short-chain fatty acids are produced by the bacteria *Faecalibacterium prausnitzii, Eubacterium, Roseburia, Bifidobacterium longum, Ruminococcus, Alistipes,* and *Lactobacillus* (SCFAs). SCFAs boost Treg cells while impairing T cells. The production of myeloid dendritic cells in the bone marrow may be stimulated by microbial SCFAs and dietary fiber fermentation products. The ability of mucosal B lymphocytes to generate IgM and IgA antibodies is enhanced by intestinal flora. SCFAs may affect a local immune system by inducing plasmocytes to produce more IgA. Putrescine, spermine, and spermidine are examples of polyamines (byproducts of gut microbiota metabolism) that can increase IgA production in the intestine [76].

7.6 Mechanism of Carcinogenesis

Colorectal carcinoma is a complex process, driven by genetic and environmental variables and there are various causal processes many of these systems including inflammation immune modulation metabolism of food items and generation of genotoxins is closely related to the gut microbiome. Some microbiome related components in the carcinogenicity of CRC which can be adapted and interpreted to the clinical setting [80]. Many different bacteria have been drawn to their link and contribution to colon cancer or colorectal carcinogenesis in the previous 10 years. Some species, such as *Fusobacterium nucleatum* (*F. nucleatum*), were the first to emerge from ongoing studies of human colorectal cancer (CRC) models, and mechanistic data from the clinical models of the time played a significant role in *F. nucleatum* in many areas of in vitro biology; in mice, the presence of *F. nucleatum* increased tumor growth in patients derived from CRC xenografts (mimicking CRC samples in patients with mice), *F. nucleoatum* binds to an Ecadherin on FadA on the surface of CRC cells and induces cancer-causing Wnt/-catenin signaling. This may explain these findings that TIGIT (T-cell immune receptor) in the ITIM and Ig domains was used to bind binders and assemble tumor-infiltrating phospholipids and natural killer (NK) cells with Fap2 as the underlying disaccharide to [galactose N-acetyl] binds-d-galactosamine (GalGalNAc)], which is abundant in tumor cells and other cells. Which promotes *F. nucleatum* CRC cell growth and enrichment of CRC [81].

The process by which *F. nucleatum* is associated with carcinogenesis also includes suggesting resistance to treatment. Tumors resistant to treatment with oxaliplatin CRC were widely used in a preclinical CRC model with a large number of *F. nucleatum.* Through toll-like receptor 4 (TLR4) expressed on CRC cells, *F. nucleatum* activates autophagy (cell processing process that regulates cell survival), which makes tumors resistant to oxalipla-induced apoptosis [80, 81].

For example, Enterotoxigenic *Bacteroides fragilis* (ETBF) is a well-studied human digestive disorder. It causes diarrhea and gastrointestinal inflammation. ETBF is also found in human CRC biofilms and pre-cancerous intestinal lesions called adenomas, and promotes the development of colon cancer in animals (Fig. 7.7). Similarly, *Escherichia coli* strains with genome-island polyketide synthase (pks +) promote carcinogenicity in preclinical CRC models and are found in many human CRC tissues. In colon epithelial cells, pks + *E. coli* produces genotoxin colibactin, which alkylates DNA and forms DNA adducts (a type of DNA damage that can cause mutations). How host versus microbes can lead to cancer [81, 82] (Fig. 7.8).

7.7 Cancer Prevention and Treatment Strategies

a. **Probiotics Administration**

Probiotics are living microorganisms that, when eaten in sufficient proportions, are good for health. The concept of probiotics has been around for over a century. And these microbes are considered to have cancer-fighting properties through many hypothesized immune pathways. In preclinical studies for CRC, several bacterial species, such as *Bifidobacterium* and *Lactobacillus* spp., have shown antitumor properties by various mechanisms including inhibiting cell proliferation inducing cancer cell death host immune modulation inhibition of carcinogenic toxin and production of anticancer agents [83]. The effectiveness of human probiotics for

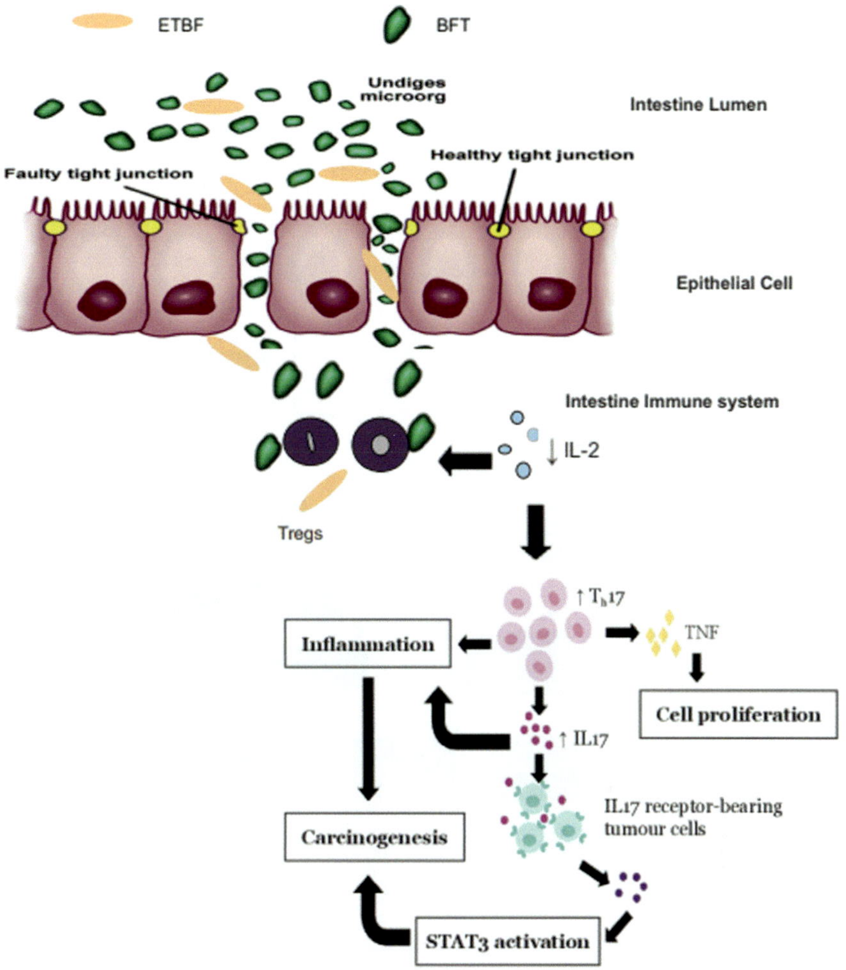

Fig. 7.7 Example of Enterotoxigenic *Bacteroids fragilis* (ETBF) which influence the colorectal cancer (Wong 2019, #3)

CRC has been studied in only a few clinical studies. In patients who had undergone resection, oral treatment of *Lactobacillus casei* reduced the incidence rate of moderate- or high-grade dysplastic tumors, but not the overall number of tumors. Furthermore, in patients with a history of colonic polyps, a synbiotic intervention containing the prebiotic inulin and the probiotics *Lactobacillus rhamnosus* GG and *Bifidobacterium lactis* Bb12 induced changes in the faecal microbiota (decreased *Clostridium perfringens*, increased Lactobacillus and Bifidobacterium), as well as reduced cell proliferation and improved epitheli (Konishi et al. 2016). However, despite changes in the intestinal microflora with a proportion of infected patients. Lachnospiraceae spp was elevated with a combination intervention followed by

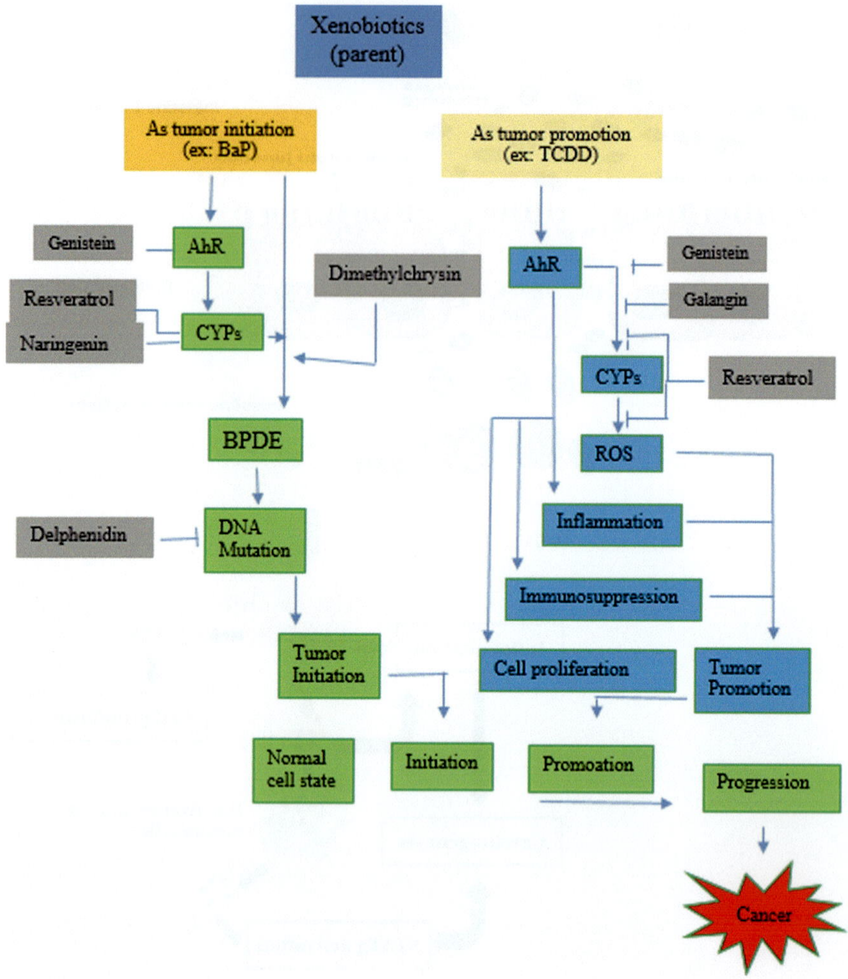

Fig. 7.8 Schematic mechanism of xenobiotics-induced carcinogenesis (Wu 2017, #6)

resistant starch and *B. lactis* in 20 human volunteers failed to induce changes in cell proliferation or other physiological markers. Despite in vitro and in vivo experimental data but there is only preliminary evidence supporting the use of probiotics in preventing CRC. More clinical trials are needed to determine the therapeutic value of probiotics in preventing CRC (Wong et al. 2019).

b. **Gut Microbiota to Treat CRC**

In addition to its role in carcinogenesis and tumor development, there is still growing evidence. How intestinal microflora influences the efficacy and toxicity of chemotherapy and immunotherapy the gut microbiome can therefore be used as

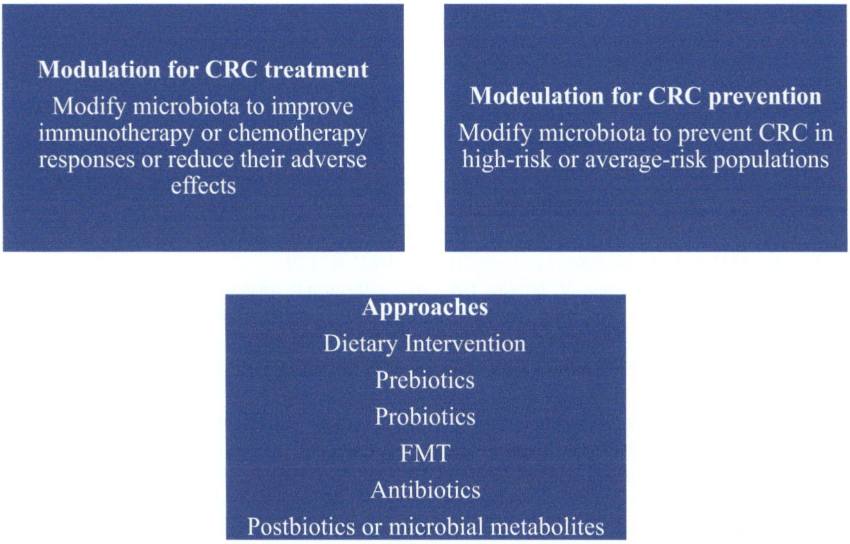

Fig. 7.9 Different approaches and treatment pattern for CRC

a biomarker to predict treatment response or poor response and can also be modified to improve cancer treatment and patient outcomes. Some research has offered insights into managing these patients using innovative and customized strategies, however, they are still in the early stages of development (Wong et al. 2019) (Fig. 7.9).

7.8 Conclusion

Human health is affected by interaction of gut microbiome, diet, immune strength, and physiological state of the host. In this chapter the emphasis was on highlighting importance of dietary pattern in influencing gut microbiota. Epigenetics also plays crucial role in influencing microbial metabolites. Yet there are microbially mediated pathways that are associated with cancers and influence the mechanism of carcinogenesis. Microbial metabolism may alter inflammation, influence the epigenetics and gene silencing or modify the DNA leading to mutations. Dietary patterns influence the composition of microbial community associated with tumor and non-tumor regions especially in the colon. So, the variation in cancer risk and disease severity may be dependent on the microbial biomass, composition, dietary pattern, host interactions, and immune status of the body. Some detail studies are required to consider gut microbiome, body physiology, and host exposures to better understand the impact of cancer risk. Not only in diagnosis but it will also help in designing appropriate therapeutic and preventive strategies.

References

1. Jackson MA, Verdi S, Maxan ME, Shin CM, Zierer J, Bowyer RCE, Martin T, Williams FMK, Menni C, Bell JT, Spector TD, Steves CJ (2018) Gut microbiota associations with common diseases and prescription medications in a population-based cohort. Nat Commun 9. https://doi.org/10.1038/S41467-018-05184-7
2. Hullar MAJ, Fu BC (2014) Diet, the gut microbiome, and epigenetics. Cancer J 20:170–175. https://doi.org/10.1097/PPO.0000000000000053
3. Valdes AM, Walter J, Segal E, Spector TD (2018) Role of the gut microbiota in nutrition and health. BMJ 361:36–44. https://doi.org/10.1136/BMJ.K2179
4. Martinez-Guryn K, Leone V, Chang EB (2019) Regional diversity of the gastrointestinal microbiome. Cell Host Microbe 26:314–324. https://doi.org/10.1016/J.CHOM.2019.08.011
5. Tropini C, Earle KA, Huang KC, Sonnenburg JL (2017) The gut microbiome: connecting spatial organization to function. Cell Host Microbe 21:433–442. https://doi.org/10.1016/J.CHOM.2017.03.010
6. Laursen MF, Andersen LBB, Michaelsen KF, Mølgaard C, Trolle E, Bahl MI, Licht TR (2016) Infant gut microbiota development is driven by transition to family foods independent of maternal obesity. mSphere 1. https://doi.org/10.1128/MSPHERE.00069-15
7. Rinninella E, Cintoni M, Raoul P, Lopetuso LR, Scaldaferri F, Pulcini G, Miggiano GAD, Gasbarrini A, Mele MC (2019) Food components and dietary habits: keys for a healthy gut microbiota composition. Nutrients 11. https://doi.org/10.3390/NU11102393
8. Rinninella E, Raoul P, Cintoni M, Franceschi F, Miggiano GAD, Gasbarrini A, Mele MC (2019) What is the healthy gut microbiota composition? A changing ecosystem across age, environment, diet, and diseases. Microorganisms 7. https://doi.org/10.3390/MICROORGANISMS7010014
9. Collins SM, Surette M, Bercik P (2012) The interplay between the intestinal microbiota and the brain. Nat Rev Microbiol 10:735–742. https://doi.org/10.1038/NRMICRO2876
10. Graf D, Di Cagno R, Fåk F, Flint HJ, Nyman M, Saarela M, Watzl B (2015) Contribution of diet to the composition of the human gut microbiota. Microbiol Ecol Health Dis 26. https://doi.org/10.3402/MEHD.V26.26164
11. Allam-Ndoul B, Castonguay-Paradis S, Veilleux A (2020) Gut microbiota and intestinal trans-epithelial permeability. Int J Mol Sci 21:1–14. https://doi.org/10.3390/IJMS21176402
12. Soderholm AT, Pedicord VA (2019) Intestinal epithelial cells: at the interface of the microbiota and mucosal immunity. Immunology 158:267–280. https://doi.org/10.1111/IMM.13117
13. Sánchez-Tapia M, Tovar AR, Torres N (2019) Diet as regulator of gut microbiota and its role in health and disease. Arch Med Res 50:259–268. https://doi.org/10.1016/J.ARCMED.2019.09.004
14. Rowland I, Gibson G, Heinken A, Scott K, Swann J, Thiele I, Tuohy K (2018) Gut microbiota functions: metabolism of nutrients and other food components. Eur J Nutr 57. https://doi.org/10.1007/S00394-017-1445-8
15. Mudgil D, Barak S (2013) Composition, properties and health benefits of indigestible carbohydrate polymers as dietary fiber: a review. Int J Biol Macromol 61:1–6. https://doi.org/10.1016/J.IJBIOMAC.2013.06.044
16. Galanakis CM (n.d.) Dietary fiber: properties, recovery, and applications
17. Klampfer L, Huang J, Sasazuki T, Shirasawa S, Augenlicht L (2003) Inhibition of interferon γ signaling by the short chain fatty acid butyrate. Mol Cancer Res 1:855–862
18. Sonnenburg ED, Smits SA, Tikhonov M, Higginbottom SK, Wingreen NS, Sonnenburg JL (2016) Diet-induced extinction in the gut microbiota compounds over generations. Nature 529:212. https://doi.org/10.1038/NATURE16504
19. David LA, Maurice CF, Carmody RN, Gootenberg DB, Button JE, Wolfe BE, Ling AV, Devlin AS, Varma Y, Fischbach MA, Biddinger SB, Dutton RJ, Turnbaugh PJ (2014) Diet rapidly and reproducibly alters the human gut microbiome. Nature 505:559–563. https://doi.org/10.1038/NATURE12820

20. Dominika Ś, Arjan N, Karyn RP, Henryk K (2011) The study on the impact of glycated pea proteins on human intestinal bacteria. Int J Food Microbiol 145:267–272. https://doi.org/10.1016/J.IJFOODMICRO.2011.01.002
21. Rafter JJ, Child P, Anderson AM, Alder R, Eng V, Bruce WR (1987) Cellular toxicity of fecal water depends on diet. Am J Clin Nutr 45:559–563. https://doi.org/10.1093/AJCN/45.3.559
22. Wu GD, Chen J, Hoffmann C, Bittinger K, Chen YY, Keilbaugh SA, Bewtra M, Knights D, Walters WA, Knight R, Sinha R, Gilroy E, Gupta K, Baldassano R, Nessel L, Li H, Bushman FD, Lewis JD (2011) Linking long-term dietary patterns with gut microbial enterotypes. Science 334:105–108. https://doi.org/10.1126/SCIENCE.1208344
23. Islam KBMS, Fukiya S, Hagio M, Fujii N, Ishizuka S, Ooka T, Ogura Y, Hayashi T, Yokota A (2011) Bile acid is a host factor that regulates the composition of the cecal microbiota in rats. Gastroenterology 141:1773–1781. https://doi.org/10.1053/J.GASTRO.2011.07.046
24. Li J, Sun F, Guo Y, Fan H (2019) High-salt diet gets involved in gastrointestinal diseases through the reshaping of gastroenterological milieu. Digestion 99:267–274. https://doi.org/10.1159/000493096
25. Miranda PM, De Palma G, Serkis V, Lu J, Louis-Auguste MP, McCarville JL, Verdu EF, Collins SM, Bercik P (2018) High salt diet exacerbates colitis in mice by decreasing Lactobacillus levels and butyrate production. Microbiome 6:57. https://doi.org/10.1186/S40168-018-0433-4
26. Ozdal T, Sela DA, Xiao J, Boyacioglu D, Chen F, Capanoglu E (2016) The reciprocal interactions between polyphenols and gut microbiota and effects on bioaccessibility. Nutrients 8. https://doi.org/10.3390/NU8020078
27. Moszak M, Szulińska M, Bogdański P (2020) You are what you eat—the relationship between diet, microbiota, and metabolic disorders—a review. Nutrients 12. https://doi.org/10.3390/NU12041096
28. Ramos S, Martín MÁ (2021) Impact of diet on gut microbiota. Curr Opin Food Sci 37:83–90. https://doi.org/10.1016/J.COFS.2020.09.006
29. Wan Y, Yuan J, Li J, Li H, Zhang J, Tang J, Ni Y, Huang T, Wang F, Zhao F, Li D (2020) Unconjugated and secondary bile acid profiles in response to higher-fat, lower-carbohydrate diet and associated with related gut microbiota: a 6-month randomized controlled-feeding trial. Clin Nutr 39:395–404. https://doi.org/10.1016/J.CLNU.2019.02.037
30. Kazakevych J, Sayols S, Messner B, Krienke C, Soshnikova N (2017) Dynamic changes in chromatin states during specification and differentiation of adult intestinal stem cells. Nucleic Acids Res 45:5770–5784. https://doi.org/10.1093/NAR/GKX167
31. Kim TH, Li F, Ferreiro-Neira I, Ho LL, Luyten A, Nalapareddy K, Long H, Verzi M, Shivdasani RA (2014) Broadly permissive intestinal chromatin underlies lateral inhibition and cell plasticity. Nature 506:511–515. https://doi.org/10.1038/NATURE12903
32. Fan Y, Pedersen O (2020) Gut microbiota in human metabolic health and disease. Nat Rev Microbiol 191(19):55–71. https://doi.org/10.1038/s41579-020-0433-9
33. Hooper LV, Littman DR, Macpherson AJ (2012) Interactions between the microbiota and the immune system. Science 336:1268–1273. https://doi.org/10.1126/SCIENCE.1223490
34. Newsholme P, De Bittencourt PIH (2016) Gut associated bacteria are critical to metabolism, inflammation and health. Curr Opin Clin Nutr Metab Care 19:245–249. https://doi.org/10.1097/MCO.0000000000000293
35. Riscuta G, Xi D, Pierre-Victor D, Starke-Reed P, Khalsa J, Duffy L (2018) Diet, microbiome, and epigenetics in the era of precision medicine. Methods Mol Biol 1856:141–156. https://doi.org/10.1007/978-1-4939-8751-1_8
36. Levy M, Thaiss CA, Elinav E (2016) Metabolites: messengers between the microbiota and the immune system. Genes Dev 30:1589. https://doi.org/10.1101/GAD.284091.116
37. Mischke M, Plösch T (2016) The gut microbiota and their metabolites: potential implications for the host epigenome. Adv Exp Med Biol 902:33–44. https://doi.org/10.1007/978-3-319-31248-4_3

38. Berding K, Donovan SM (2016) Microbiome and nutrition in autism spectrum disorder: current knowledge and research needs. Nutr Rev 74:723–736. https://doi.org/10.1093/NUTRIT/NUW048
39. Shapiro H, Thaiss CA, Levy M, Elinav E (2014) The cross talk between microbiota and the immune system: metabolites take center stage. Curr Opin Immunol 30:54–62. https://doi.org/10.1016/J.COI.2014.07.003
40. Alenghat T (2015) Epigenomics and the microbiota. Toxicol Pathol 43:101–106. https://doi.org/10.1177/0192623314553805/ASSET/IMAGES/LARGE/10.1177_0192623314553805-FIG1.JPEG
41. Cortese R, Lu L, Yu Y, Ruden D, Claud EC (2016) Epigenome-microbiome crosstalk: a potential new paradigm influencing neonatal susceptibility to disease. Epigenetics 11:205–215. https://doi.org/10.1080/15592294.2016.1155011
42. Ling C, Rönn T (2019) Epigenetics in human obesity and type 2 diabetes. Cell Metab 29:1028–1044. https://doi.org/10.1016/J.CMET.2019.03.009
43. Rosen ED, Kaestner KH, Natarajan R, Patti ME, Sallari R, Sander M, Susztak K (2018) Epigenetics and epigenomics: implications for diabetes and obesity. Diabetes 67:1923–1931. https://doi.org/10.2337/DB18-0537
44. Bonder MJ, Kurilshikov A, Tigchelaar EF, Mujagic Z, Imhann F, Vila AV, Deelen P, Vatanen T, Schirmer M, Smeekens SP, Zhernakova DV, Jankipersadsing SA, Jaeger M, Oosting M, Cenit MC, Masclee AAM, Swertz MA, Li Y, Kumar V, Joosten L, Harmsen H, Weersma RK, Franke L, Hofker MH, Xavier RJ, Jonkers D, Netea MG, Wijmenga C, Fu J, Zhernakova A (2016) The effect of host genetics on the gut microbiome. Nat Genet 48:1407–1412. https://doi.org/10.1038/NG.3663
45. Ye J, Wu W, Li Y, Li L (2017) Influences of the gut microbiota on DNA methylation and histone modification. Dig Dis Sci 62:1155–1164. https://doi.org/10.1007/S10620-017-4538-6
46. Shock T, Badang L, Ferguson B, Martinez-Guryn K (2021) The interplay between diet, gut microbes, and host epigenetics in health and disease. J Nutr Biochem 95. https://doi.org/10.1016/J.JNUTBIO.2021.108631
47. Paul B, Barnes S, Demark-Wahnefried W, Morrow C, Salvador C, Skibola C, Tollefsbol TO (2015) Influences of diet and the gut microbiome on epigenetic modulation in cancer and other diseases. Clin Epigenetics 7:1–11. https://doi.org/10.1186/S13148-015-0144-7/TABLES/2
48. Yamashita S, Nanjo S, Rehnberg E, Iida N, Takeshima H, Ando T, Maekita T, Sugiyama T, Ushijima T (2019) Distinct DNA methylation targets by aging and chronic inflammation: a pilot study using gastric mucosa infected with Helicobacter pylori. Clin Epigen 11:1–14. https://doi.org/10.1186/S13148-019-0789-8/FIGURES/5
49. Holscher HD (2017) Dietary fiber and prebiotics and the gastrointestinal microbiota. Gut Microbes 8:172–184. https://doi.org/10.1080/19490976.2017.1290756
50. Nicholson JK, Holmes E, Kinross J, Burcelin R, Gibson G, Jia W, Pettersson S (2012) Host-gut microbiota metabolic interactions. Science 336:1262–1267. https://doi.org/10.1126/SCIENCE.1223813
51. Bellahcene M, O'Dowd JF, Wargent ET, Zaibi MS, Hislop DC, Ngala RA, Smith DM, Cawthorne MA, Stocker CJ, Arch JRS (2013) Male mice that lack the G-protein-coupled receptor GPR41 have low energy expenditure and increased body fat content. Br J Nutr 109:1755–1764. https://doi.org/10.1017/S0007114512003923
52. Li M, van Esch BCAM, Wagenaar GTM, Garssen J, Folkerts G, Henricks PAJ (2018) Pro- and anti-inflammatory effects of short chain fatty acids on immune and endothelial cells. Eur J Pharmacol 831:52–59. https://doi.org/10.1016/J.EJPHAR.2018.05.003
53. Smith PM, Howitt MR, Panikov N, Michaud M, Gallini CA, Bohlooly-Y M, Glickman JN, Garrett WS (2013) The microbial metabolites, short-chain fatty acids, regulate colonic Treg cell homeostasis. Science 341:569–573. https://doi.org/10.1126/SCIENCE.1241165
54. Roager HM, Dragsted LO (2019) Diet-derived microbial metabolites in health and disease. Nutr Bull 44:216–227. https://doi.org/10.1111/NBU.12396

55. Desai MS, Seekatz AM, Koropatkin NM, Stappenbeck TS, Núñez G, Martens EC (2016) A dietary fiber-deprived gut microbiota degrades the colonic mucus barrier and enhances pathogen susceptibility. Cell 167:1339–1353.e21. https://doi.org/10.1016/j.cell.2016.10.043
56. Lynch SV, Pedersen O (2016) The human intestinal microbiome in health and disease. N Engl J Med 375:2369–2379. https://doi.org/10.1056/NEJMRA1600266
57. Zmora N, Zeevi D, Korem T, Segal E, Elinav E (2016) Taking it personally: personalized utilization of the human microbiome in health and disease. Cell Host Microbe 19:12–20. https://doi.org/10.1016/J.CHOM.2015.12.016
58. Ahmad I, Nasiruddin M, Khan MA, Zafaryab M, Mehdi SH, Rizvi MMA (2016) Nutraceuticals as chemopreventive and therapeutic agents in gut associated pathogenesis. Biochem Anal Biochem 5. https://doi.org/10.4172/2161-1009.1000298
59. Remely M, Ferk F, Sterneder S, Setayesh T, Roth S, Kepcija T, Noorizadeh R, Rebhan I, Greunz M, Beckmann J, Wagner KH, Knasmüller S, Haslberger AG (2017) EGCG prevents high fat diet-induced changes in gut microbiota, decreases of DNA strand breaks, and changes in expression and DNA methylation of Dnmt1 and MLH1 in C57BL/6J male mice. Oxid Med Cell Longev. https://doi.org/10.1155/2017/3079148
60. Huyan Z, Pellegrini N, Steegenga W, Capuano E (2022) Insights into gut microbiota metabolism of dietary lipids: the case of linoleic acid. Food Funct 4513–4526. https://doi.org/10.1039/d1fo04254h
61. Fujita K, Matsushita M, Banno E, De Velasco MA, Hatano K, Nonomura N, Uemura H (2022) Gut microbiome and prostate cancer. Int J Urol 29(8):793–798. https://doi.org/10.1111/iju.14894
62. Oliphant K, Allen-Vercoe E (2019) Macronutrient metabolism by the human gut microbiome: major fermentation by-products and their impact on host health. Microbiome 7(1):1–15. https://doi.org/10.1186/s40168-019-0704-8
63. Haller D (2018) In: Haller D (ed) The gut microbiome in health and illness, 1st edn. Springer Nature. Springer Berlin Heidelberg. https://doi.org/10.1007/978-3-319-90545-7
64. Greathouse KL, Wyatt M, Johnson AJ, Toy EP, Khan JM, Dunn K, Clegg DJ, Reddy S (2022) Diet-microbiome interactions in cancer treatment: opportunities and challenges for precision nutrition in cancer. Neoplasia 29(C):100800. https://doi.org/10.1016/j.neo.2022.100800
65. Kapsetaki SE, Alcaraz GM, Maley CC, Whisner CM, Aktipis A (2022) Diet, microbes, and cancer across the tree of life: a systematic review. Curr Nutr Rep 508–525. https://doi.org/10.1007/s13668-022-00420-5
66. Murga-Garrido SM, Hong Q, Tzu WL, Cross ER, Hutchison JH, Thomas SP, Vivas EI et al (2021) Gut microbiome variation modulates the effects of dietary fiber on host metabolism. Microbiome 9(1):1–26. https://doi.org/10.1186/s40168-021-01061-6
67. Todd E, Elnour R, Simpson R, Castaneda M, Shanahan ER (2021) Munching microbes: diet-microbiome interactions shape gut health and cancer outcomes. Microbiol Aust 42(2):60–64. https://doi.org/10.1071/MA21026
68. Tong Y, Gao H, Qi Q, Liu X, Li J, Gao J, Li P, Wang Y, Du L, Wang C (2021) High fat diet, gut microbiome and gastrointestinal cancer. Theranostics 11(12):5889–5910. https://doi.org/10.7150/thno.56157
69. Vernocchi P, Chierico FD, Putignani L (2020) Gut microbiota metabolism and interaction with food components. Int J Mol Sci 21(10). https://doi.org/10.3390/ijms21103688
70. Tang WHW, Li DY, Hazen SL (2019) Dietary metabolism, the gut microbiome, and heart failure. Nat Rev Cardiol 16(3):137–154. https://doi.org/10.1038/s41569-018-0108-7
71. Portune KJ, Beaumont M, Davila AM, Tomé D, Blachier F, Sanz Y (2016) Gut microbiota role in dietary protein metabolism and health-related outcomes: the two sides of the coin. Trends Food Sci Technol 57:213–232. https://doi.org/10.1016/j.tifs.2016.08.011
72. Yang J, Yu J (2018) The association of diet, gut microbiota and colorectal cancer: what we eat may imply what we get. Protein Cell 9(5):474–487. https://doi.org/10.1007/s13238-018-0543-6
73. Kochhar S, François-Pierre M (2015) Metabonomics and gut microbiota in nutrition and disease. Transactions of the Royal Academy of Medicine in Ireland

74. Pray L, Pillsbury L, Tomayko E (2013) The human microbiome, diet, and health. In: The human microbiome, diet, and health. https://doi.org/10.17226/13522.
75. Jardon KM, Canfora EE, Goossens GH, Blaak EE (2022) Dietary macronutrients and the gut microbiome: a precision nutrition approach to improve cardiometabolic health. Gut 71(6):1214–1226. https://doi.org/10.1136/gutjnl-2020-323715
76. Szczyrek M, Bitkowska P, Chunowski P, Czuchryta P, Krawczyk P, Milanowski J (2021) Diet, microbiome, and cancer immunotherapy—a comprehensive review. Nutrients 13(2217):1–23. https://doi.org/10.1190/1.9781560802662.ch1
77. Rinninella E, Raoul P, Cintoni M, Palombaro M, Pulcini G, Gasbarrini A, Mele MC (2021) Nutritional interventions targeting gut microbiota during cancer therapies. Microorganisms 9(7):1–16. https://doi.org/10.3390/microorganisms9071469
78. Lampe JW (2016) Dietary modulation of the microbiome and cancer risk diet, the gut microbiome and cancer dietary exposures and cellular processes linked to cancer involvement of microbial metabolism
79. Appunni S, Rubens M, Ramamoorthy V, Tonse R, Saxena A, McGranaghan P, Kaiser A, Kotecha R (2021) Emerging evidence on the effects of dietary factors on the gut microbiome in colorectal cancer. Front Nutr 8(October):1–20. https://doi.org/10.3389/fnut.2021.718389
80. Wong SH, Yu J (2019) Gut microbiota in colorectal cancer: mechanisms of action and clinical applications. Nat Rev Gastroenterol Hepatol 16(11):690–704
81. Garrett WS (2019) The gut microbiota and colon cancer. Sci 364(6446):1133–1135. viewed 19 December 2022, https://www.science.org/doi/10.1126/science.aaw2367
82. Wu JC, Lai CS, Tsai ML, Ho CT, Wang YJ, Pan MH (2017) Chemopreventive effect of natural dietary compounds on xenobiotic-induced toxicity. J Food Drug Anal 25(1):176–186
83. Thirabunyanon M, Boonprasom P, Niamsup P (2009) Probiotic potential of lactic acid bacteria isolated from fermented dairy milks on antiproliferation of colon cancer cells. Biotech Lett 31(4):571–576

Dietary Pattern and Cancer

8

Sara Mumtaz, Nosheen Akhtar, Awais Ahmed,
and Asma Saleem Qazi

Contents

8.1 What Are Dietary Pattern

Traditionally, a dietary pattern can be defined as "the amounts, proportions, variety, or combination of different foods, liquids, and nutrients in diet, as well as the frequency with which they are consumed on a daily basis." However, there are two important aspects of dietary consumption, the first one is dynamic and the second one is multidimensional [114]. Diet is frequently based on a single evaluation and

S. Mumtaz (✉) · N. Akhtar · A. S. Qazi
National University of Medical Sciences (NUMS), Rawalpindi, Pakistan
e-mail: sara.mumtaz@numspak.edu.pk

A. Ahmed
University of Concepcion, Concepcion, Chile

R. F. Saeed and S. ul. Shaheed (eds.), *Nutrition and Dietary Interventions in Cancer*,
Cancer Treatment and Research 191, https://doi.org/10.1007/978-3-031-55622-7_8

implies that it is either a constant or a one-time exposure of interest. The majority of people's diets, on the other hand, change throughout the course of a week, year, and lifetime as well as at various stages of cancer, including prevention, treatment, and survivorship. Researchers have typically used a summary index to assess the comprehensiveness of diets, ranking each component on the same scale. It has recently become understood that the many features or dimensions of food have various effects and ought to be researched individually yet in combination. Some aspects will be improved, while others will be restricted. Some features of food have strong connections to other aspects, but others have links that are opposite, inverse, or completely absent. Some aspects of diet can have both positive and negative effects. It depends on the outcome that is under observation. The several attributes of food intake, as well as the underlying dynamics of interconnectedness and harmony, are referred to as multidimensionality [114].

8.2 Analysis of Dietary Pattern

To assess dietary patterns, usually interviewer-administered or self-reported questionnaires are used based on dietary recalls. A questionnaire was employed to measure ordinary or habitual previous diet in the majority of epidemiological investigations on dietary patterns and cancer. The questionnaire typically contains various food or drink items, and questions related to portion sizes. Using a questionnaire to rate people based on their relative consumption of dietary components is generally accepted as suitable, despite the fact that measurement error in nutritional assessment methodologies has been highly disputed [39, 52, 126, 131, 132]. Depending on whether dietary patterns are identified directly or through the use of parameters set by the investigator, dietary pattern examination is typically divided into two groups. The first category includes posteriori diet patterns. These patterns are established using data-driven methods from the studied population such as principle components analysis (PCA), factor analysis, or cluster analysis [92, 146]. Diet patterns such as "Western" and "Prudent" are commonly labeled. Western diet is considered as unhealthy and Prudent is considered as healthy. Higher intake of red and processed meat, fried meals, solid fats, sweets, and refined grains characterizes the "Western" pattern, while greater intake of a range of fruits and vegetables, as well as whole grains, characterizes the "Prudent" pattern. Numerous dietary patterns exist, and essentially countless combinations of foods and beverages are regularly consumed [92, 146]. The second category includes priori dietary patterns that is also known as investigator-defined or score-based patterns. These patterns are established by criteria set in advance, frequently based on external evidence such as dietary recommendations or assumptions concerning diet–disease processes [156]. The posteriori method has the advantage of considering numerous components of the diet rather than concentrating on a few suggested key food groups. Furthermore, the most priori scores employ broad definitions of food groupings that may not account for small changes in nutrients and phytochemicals in particular food items. Focusing on broad categories may cause critical differences to be ignored. A posteriori dietary patterns, on the other hand, do not rely on existing research and so do not evaluate present diet–disease patterns [91].

8.3 Dietary Pattern and Cancer

There is an established link between diet and cancer. Numerous studies have been conducted on specific nutrients or phytochemicals in relation to cancer. And researches have come out that a few nutrients are related to an increased cancer risk. Individual dietary components are interconnected and interrelate with one another to determine risk of disease. As a result, investigating dietary patterns in connection to disease development, progression, and prevention has a greater impact on the development of disease prevention strategies in the form of dietary guidelines [114]. If we look into epidemiological data, we can see that in early years of research on dietary pattern, only a few studies reported association of dietary pattern with cancer. These investigations are based on a posteriori classification of dietary patterns into healthy and unhealthy categories. A healthy diet is also linked with a decreased lung and colorectal cancer risk, while an unhealthy diet is linked with an increased colorectal cancer risk [31, 126]. Basically, posteriori diet pattern is a data-driven method. In this approach, diet patterns are shaped by using statistical methods such as factor analysis, principal components analysis (PCA), or cluster analysis [127]. However, this trend changed with passage of time and various dietary patterns and indexes, such as the Dietary Guidelines of America (DGAs), the new Nordic diet, the Chinese food pagoda, and the World Health Organization's (WHO) healthy diet indicator, have been established to represent the dietary requirements of various organizations or countries. In order to assess compliance with the DGAs, an eating index called the Healthy Eating Index (HEI) was developed. It has changed throughout time to reflect the revisions to the DGAs, which happens every five years. Other indexes were developed to prevent chronic diseases like alternate HEI (aHEI) and the Dietary Approaches to Stop Hypertension (DASH) [26, 86]. According to DGAs 2020–2025, people's health is greatly influenced by the foods and beverages they consume. Scientists have known for decades that leading a healthy lifestyle, which normally includes a balanced diet, can help people attain and maintain good health and prevent chronic diseases at all stages of life. The essential components of a healthy eating habit are strikingly stable throughout life and across health outcomes. According to a growing body of evidence, a healthy eating pattern is linked to better results for a variety of diseases, including certain types of cancer. In the same way, the World Cancer Research Fund/American Institute for Cancer Research (WCRF/ AICR) 2018 Third Expert Report has recommended healthy dietary pattern, rich in wholegrains, fruits, vegetables, and beans, which is good to reduce cancer risk as well as other weight-related health conditions. Other recommendations were related to reduce intake of fast food and other kinds of processed food [25]. Many less studies on diet indexes that are used in specific countries also show some association with risk of cancer. The healthy Nordic Food Index (HNFI), well known as the Baltic Sea Diet, is used for Nordic populations to check recommended dietary guidelines. This dietary index includes items that are considered beneficial with high consumption. One of its versions consist of six items including fish, rye bread, cabbage, apples or pears, root vegetables, and oatmeal. It is another version known as the New Nordic Diet combines dietary items with physical activity. It gives equal weight to all components including proteins, carbohydrates, fats, fiber alcohol, vitamins, minerals, salt, and physical activity. Various researches have been carried out on communities whose diet is based on HNFI. A Danish study showed that in women, the HNFI was linked to a lower risk of colorectal cancer, but not in men. However, a Swedish study found no link for HNFI with breast cancer. Likewise, a case control Swedish study on the New Nordic Diet could not find it association with the risk of prostate cancer.

The Healthy Diet Indicator (HDI) is a global metric that measures adherence to dietary guidelines of the World Health Organization (WHO). In 1990, the WHO has presented dietary recommendation for the chronic diseases prevention, and the original HDI was created based on these recommendations. Then, in 2003, an upgraded version based on the WHO dietary recommendations was released. It includes eight dietary components: protein, polyunsaturated fatty acid, cholesterol, saturated fat, dietary fiber, free sugar, vegetables, fruits, and sodium [62]. In British population, no association was found for HDI and risk of breast cancer. In the European study, it was not found related with cancer risk.

In 2007, the Chinese Food Pagoda (CHFP) or the dietary Guidelines for Chinese were presented by the Chinese Nutrition Society and Ministry of Health. It is recommended to eat plenty of vegetables, whole grains, fruits, and beans plus it is encouraged to consume suitable quantities of poultry, fish, lean meats, and egg and limited amount of fats and salt. It was reported that great adherence to CHFP is linked with reduced mortality due to chronic diseases including cancer in adult population of China. Studies based on Shanghai population reported that CHPF is associated with reduced colorectal cancer risk. This will provide help in prevention of colorectal cancer in China where its prevalence is high. Such information will assist in reducing colorectal cancer in China, where it is one of the major causes of cancer-related death [95]. However, in the same studies, no link was found for aHEI and DASH with colorectal cancer. This indicated that country-specific guidelines are important to influence the health of people within country.

The DASH diet is recommended for people to reduce hypertension. It emphasizes on the consumption of vegetables and fruits while appropriate amount of lean protein from fish and chicken is also recommended. But this diet is low in fat, red meat, and added sugars and salts. This diet is considered healthy and many studies were conducted to find association of DASH diet and cancer. In 2018, an observational study reported that the DASH diet is inversely related to risk of colorectal cancer in men. But this inverse relation was not found in women [105]. In another study, a modest inverse link between DASH diet and risk of aggressive prostate cancer was reported. Furthermore, additional dietary patterns are linked to cultural eating habits or biological processes that have been linked to carcinogenesis [126].

In this chapter, we will look at the association of some of famous dietary pattern with cancer risk.

8.4 Cancer Association with Some Major Dietary Patterns

8.4.1 Mediterranean Diet (MD)

The United Nations Educational, Scientific, and Cultural Organization (UNESCO) in 2010 stated that the Mediterranean diet is a unique cultural heritage of Italy, France, Spain, Greece, and Morocco. It is also a major dietary pattern in many other Mediterranean countries and considered beneficial for human health. Ancel Keys and his colleagues considered it for the first time as a low saturated lipids diet and capable of protecting the cardiovascular system because of a lower level of blood cholesterol [69]. In thereafter years, it has been discovered as a dietary pattern consisting of food items high in preventive nutrients capable of preventing a variety of ailments. Furthermore, because of MD's protective effect against DNA damage, it has been studied extensively in the assessment of general mortality as a possible and advantageous lifestyle that is associated with an increase in longevity in healthy persons [69, 83]. So, the Mediterranean diet is a cuisine paradigm that encompasses not only a way of life, but it is a culture too, and it has been identified as a key to enhancing quality of life, health, and lifespan [31]. However, the Mediterranean diet according to each country has some different characteristics that are based on specificities of that country and it even varies within different locations of a country [123, 142]. As a result, in order to consistently apply various models of Mediterranean diet with relation to foods and their recommended consumption amounts, it was essential to establish common features in various Mediterranean diet models. An alimentary pyramid was made by doing this (Fig. 8.1). In this pyramid, the primary foods of each distinct type of Mediterranean diet and frequency of their consumption were described [31]. On the whole, the Mediterranean diet comprises a high consumption of whole grains (around 50–60% of calories) and a great intake of legumes, fruits, and vegetables; utilization of extra virgin olive oil to encompass approximately 70% needs of lipid; but use of red wine on regular basis during major meals; consistent intake of fresh fish and an optimum quantity of omega-3 both from vegetable and animal sources [31, 50, 74].

8.4.1.1 Mechanism of Mediterranean Diet for the Cancer Prevention

The high content of anti-inflammatory and antioxidants' nutrients is found in many Mediterranean diet foods (fruits, vegetables, legumes, olive oil, nuts, and fish), which have a protecting influence in proliferation of cancer cells and fighting cell

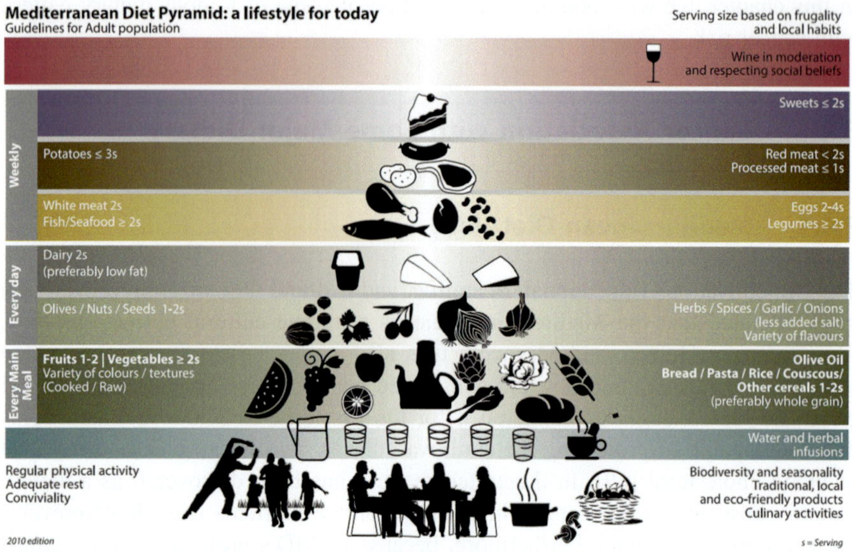

Fig. 8.1 Mediterranean diet pyramid (https://dietamediterranea.com/nutricion-saludable-ejercicio-fisico/)

degeneration and are a major reason of positive effects of Mediterranean diet on prevention of cancer [24].

Olive oil and vegetables are high in polyphenols, which are rich in nutrients that might slow down growth of cancer cell and shield cell membranes from metastasis, which may be responsible for the Mediterranean diet's cancer-preventive effects [24, 38, 110, 119].

Additionally, a large number of vitamins, including vitamins E and C, flavonoids and folates, compounds with antioxidant properties that aid in preventing DNA damage, are present in fruit and vegetables [104, 108]. Lastly, omega-3 fatty acids, which are abundant in fish, notably mackerel and sardines, and nuts (walnuts, almonds, and pumpkin seeds), help to prevent cancer by regulating cell survival, proliferation, angiogenesis, inflammation, and metastasis [22]. Modest levels of animal fat intake and low levels of meat consumption serve to mitigate the unfavorable effects of high-temperature meat cooking [77].

According to numerous studies, a constant intake of Mediterranean diet is frequently associated with a lower risk of cancer [88, 122]. However, due to an unclear description of the Mediterranean diet score or confounding variables, several researchers have found it challenging to draw a strong connection between the cancer and Mediterranean diet. The reason for these issues is that it is difficult to prove a link between the beginning of cancer and adherence to Mediterranean diet. This impossibility results from the absence of a linear link between the two variables; instead, the cancer onset is governed by cell degeneration brought on by a number of circumstances [13, 72, 88].

Cancer incidence can be influenced by lifestyle factors like diet and nutrition, but given the relevance of few investigations and the absence of a straight connection between cancer and nutrition, other lifestyle features (like a sedentary lifestyle and physical inactivity) may also participate to the global rise in cancer incidence. More than half of malignancies today may be avoided if food, nutrition, and physical activity were properly managed, as well as sedentary lifestyles were reduced [88]. This factor contributes to decrease obesity that contributes in the incidence of many types of cancer. Furthermore, it is important to emphasize that the Mediterranean diet is a way of life, where eating right and participating in normal activities help maintain the original Mediterranean diet. As a result, it can be concluded that the current technique, which distinguishes between the physical activity and Mediterranean diet, is not totally accurate. Indeed, this strategy can be an exact cause for the dearth of evidence supporting the relation between cancer risk, Mediterranean diet, and physical activity. Indeed, because it was often difficult to assess the risk of cancer connected straight with Mediterranean diet due to the variety of neoplasia and the varying influences of risk factors, there was a lack of uniformity across studies. It is indeed critical to stress that the Mediterranean diet is a way of life, where healthy eating and engaging in everyday activities support the preservation of the original Mediterranean diet [44]. However, there are a slew of biological concerns that could be at the root of this link. Some of these questions can be answered by considering the mechanism of relationship between food items of Mediterranean diet and types of cancer. A detailed analysis of the micro- and macro-elements found in each Mediterranean diet item or produced by each in response to a particular cooking style is necessary to comprehend interaction mechanism between the Mediterranean diet and cancer. Phytochemicals and polyphenols included in many Mediterranean food items have an antioxidant protective impact, even helping to balance the fatty acids found in some Mediterranean foods, such as olive oil. In addition, vegetables, whole grains, fruit, and legumes all contain fiber that help in inhibiting cholesterol synthesis in liver and its absorption in the intestine and reduction of insulin resistance [57, 74]. A series of mechanism were proposed to explain the role of Mediterranean diet in reducing risk of cancer such as fish intake which help in reduction of tumor cell growth, vegetables, fruits, and olive oils which have anti-inflammatory and antioxidative effect, and olive oil which increases chemoprotective effects and prevents tumor development [48, 80]. It also has beneficial effects on gut microbiota. However, there are controversial results about the intake of red wine in Mediterranean diet. On the whole, Mediterranean diet produces many beneficial effects [88, 141].

8.4.1.2 Types of Cancer and Mediterranean Diet Components

Breast Cancer

Breast cancer affects mainly women, and less than 1%, it occurs in men. In women about 25% new cases were diagnosed with breast cancer in 2018. Both lifestyle and environmental factors have a significant impact on breast cancer development. There has been a concerning rise in the frequency of this breast cancer among women in developing nations, who had previously been less susceptible to it due to a lack of exposure to hormonal and environmental factors. This increase appears to be attributable to the adaptation of Western lifestyle, which has changed their habits as well as their traditional diets to a non-healthy food patterns with high contents of saturated fats [136]. Mediterranean diets can help in reduction of breast cancer occurrence because it contains vitamins, antioxidants, carotenoids, and fiber, which can increase sex-hormone levels and reduce estrogens. Hence, it can neutralize free radicals, reduce oxidative stress, and protect DNA [143]. Numerous studies established an opposite link between with constant eating of Mediterranean diet and the incidence of breast cancer. Overall, it was discovered that when strong MD adherence, the incidence dropped by 6%. For postmenopausal women, the drop was slightly higher (7%) than for pre-menopausal women and it was much greater in case of ER-(ER negative)/PR-(PR negative) breast cancer [15]. Additionally, a current study found that completely eliminating alcohol use could boost the benefits of following a moderate Mediterranean diet. However, in the case of firm adherence to Mediterranean diet, no affects were noted on its associated benefits. A direct relation was observed for the intake of unhealthy diet and incidence of breast cancer. The unhealthy diet rises breast cancer risk by many times and it increases to seven times in case of intake of fried meat [73, 137].

Colorectal Cancer

Diet has a significant impact on the development of colorectal cancer. As health and unhealthy eating habit eating habits are important risk factor for this cancer. In fact, good eating habits and a good quality diet reduce the risk of colorectal cancer independently from genetic, environmental, and traditional factors [7, 113, 128]. A 70% reduction in the incidence of colorectal cancer can be attributed to healthy diet, physically activity, and the exclusion of smoking [128]. It has been discovered that calcium, fiber, a regular consumption of garlic may be protective factors in dropping colorectal cancer incidence [9, 124]. While unhealthy eating habits, such as eating a lot of meat or drinking a lot of alcohol, are unfavorable factors that rise colorectal cancer risk [5, 19, 59, 82]. As far as Mediterranean diet and colorectal cancer are concerned, a high adherence to this diet is linked with 30% and 45% reduction of colorectal cancer risk in men and women respectively [21]. The significant protective power of Mediterranean diet was also validated in a current which found that high MD adherence can lower mortality rates in colorectal cancer patients [112].

Prostate Cancer

Wilson and Giovannucci's 2012 study provides conclusive evidence that food and lifestyle are important variables in the preventing the most fatal kinds of prostate cancer [148]. An increase in the prostate cancer incidence with the use of fats, especially animal-derived fat, dairy, and calcium, has been noted [6, 33, 40]. Alternatively, diet rich in vegetables, fiber, legumes, tomatoes, and soya is beneficial for the reduction of cancer risk. Studies of Richard and Kenfield also confirm a firm connection between prostate cancer and dietary intake. A high level of Mediterranean diet adherence is connected to a less prostate cancer risk and lower death rate in subjects that are without metastasis due to this neoplasia [65, 120].

Gastric Cancer

Though the main factor of stomach cancer is the presence of *Helicobacter pylori*, however, epidemiological investigations provide a connection between dietary factors and stomach cancer [134]. When we look more thoroughly at Mediterranean diet items and their links to gastric cancer, we can see that a greater consumption of fresh vegetables and fruits in Mediterranean diet can help to minimize gastric cancer risk. Antioxidants are high in fruits and vegetables are high, which help to prevent oxidative DNA damage by removing free radicals and participating in a variety of biological changes connected to cancer (e.g., angiogenesis and inflammation, cell signaling, cell regulation circle, and bioactivation of carcinogens). However, in case of gastric cancer, a high consumption of fruits and vegetables may specifically link to decrease the adverse effect of *H. pylori* [22]. Overall, an inverse relation is present between Mediterranean diet consumption and gastric cancer [88, 110].

Bladder Cancer

The global incidence of bladder cancer is 3.2% with men being more affected than women. Because numerous metabolites and contaminants from consumed meals are eliminated from body through the urinary system and so directly make a connection with the bladder mucosa, diet plays a major role in this type of cancer [103, 109]. Olive oil, a typical Mediterranean product, has a prevent role in reducing risk of bladder cancer of 38% and 50% with a moderate and high consumptions, respectively [13, 14]. The global impact of Mediterranean diet on bladder cancer incidence while taking into account some confounding variable like obesity, age, sex, and smoking demonstrates that inverse relation exists between bladder cancer risk and Mediterranean diet [13]. Among confounding factors, smoking exerts an influence on the effect of Mediterranean diet, especially heavy smoking [13]. This indicates that the advantages of MD and its protecting role are more apparent when they are viewed in the context of a healthy lifestyle aimed at avoiding all risk factors that not only contribute to the onset of bladder cancer, but also may reduce the beneficial effects of a healthy diet [88].

Female Reproductive System Cancer

Endometrial cancer and cervical cancer are two separate kinds of female reproductive cancer that may have a relation to nutrition intake. More precisely, consumption of vegetables and fruits is substantially linked with lower cervical cancer risk. As a result, frequent intake of vitamins A, C, and E, carotenoids, folates, and minerals may help lower the risk of cervical cancer [8]. Since the there is substantial link between high-risk human papillomavirus and cervical cancer [18], it was noted that Mediterranean diet strongly affects the development of this neoplasia. Since Mediterranean diet slows down the progression of high-risk human papilloma virus thus reduce the likelihood that bladder cancer will occur [8]. As far as endometrial cancer is concerned, it is mainly linked with an unbalanced estrogen level in body. Such hormonal problems are directly related to being obese or overweight [100]. So, it is reasonable to believe that nutrition plays a role in preventing the onset of endometrial cancer through modulating estrogen production [154]. Thus, a regular consumption of Mediterranean diet that includes high amount of fruits and vegetables could reduce endometrial cancer risk particularly in women who are not taking hormonal therapies or contraceptives and in elderly women [37, 88].

Head-Neck Cancer

Excessive alcohol use, smoking, and in rare circumstances infections such the human papillomavirus are the main risk factors for head and neck cancer. But diet also plays important role and many epidemiological studies showed that dietary items like fruits and vegetables have a protective effect in cancer particularly in cases where tumors are in oral cavity [41, 78]. As a result, it is found that a constant intake of Mediterranean is inversely linked with head and neck cancer risk and a significant reduction in the development of this cancer has been noticed both in women and men when the strictly consume Mediterranean diet [78, 88].

Lung Cancer

One of the main causes of death in West is lung cancer and it is strong associated with air pollution and smoking. However, the identification of lung cancer association with diet is complicated. In a study, positive effects of Mediterranean diet adherence are noted in case of heavy smokers. So, an inverse relation between lung cancer and adherence to Mediterranean diet in smokers is noted. It could be concluded that lung cancer risk can be reduced with a greater intake of Mediterranean diet [3].

8.4.2 Vegetarian Diet

Vegetarianism is becoming more popular than other dietary patterns and some data recommend that vegetarian diet may be linked to a lower overall cancer risk. The term "vegetarian" refers to a diet that is free of any meats (pork, beef, fish, poultry, lamb, etc.) and is also known as plant-based diet. These diets cover a wide range of dietary patterns, all of which are defined by a high adherence to whole grains, vegetables, fruits, and legumes, as well as a limited intake of animal foods [140]. For cultural or socioeconomic reasons, many people around the world eat diets that contain only a limited amount of meat from any source. Specific people avoid red meat and/or some types of meat. Although results for individual malignancies are less clear, the majority of large epidemiological studies demonstrate that plant-based diets are modestly cancer preventive. Various plant-based diets, including vegetables and fruits, plant-based nutrients like antioxidants, fiber, and other phytochemicals help to maintain healthy weight, which is linked to a lower cancer risk and recurrence. Studies that identify the health benefits of particular foods or nutrients from plant sources as well as communities that eat plant-based diets provide the majority of the evidence used to justify the use of vegetarian diets for cancer risk reduction. Different studies indicated the association of different cancer and vegetarian diet. A diet high in whole plant foods is essential for cancer prevention, according to the Cornell-Oxford China Study, and found strong connections between cancer risk and dietary patterns [20]. According to WCRF/AICR, plant-based diets are good in the cancer prevention because intake of fruits, vegetables, legumes, and whole grains decrease risk of cancer. According to the study of the large British cohorts that compared meat eaters and vegetarians documented that overall risk of cancer is approximately 12% lower among Britons vegetarians. This is probably due to lower relative risk of bladder, stomach, lymphatic, and ovarian cancers [67, 68].

Regarding the connections between diet and disease in clinical context, different types of vegetarian diets produced different results [121]. This emphasized the requirement for creating a continual scoring system as a strict method for assessing adherence to such dietary patterns [84]. An overall plant-based diet index (PDI), indicating intake of all plant foods, was created using this scoring system. A healthy PDI (hPDI), which shows consumption of good quality plant foods with known benefits on health, and an unhealthy PDI (uPDI), which shows intake of less nutrient-dense plant foods with a negative influence on the risk of adverse situations, were also proposed [121].

8.4.2.1 Mechanism of Vegetarian Diet in Cancer Prevention

Physiological factors like obesity are frequently linked to lower risk of cancer across food groups. There is evidence that vegetarian diets in western nations result in lower body mass indices than meat-eating ones [4, 118, 138], and it is significant because obesity is a known risk factor for a number of cancer types [25]. When BMI was taken into account as a potential mediator and confounder, it did not significantly affect the estimations, excluding postmenopausal breast cancer. It is challenging to determine whether BMI mediates or confounds the correlations between cancer risk and diet group, since it is unclear if differences in BMI by diet group are entirely caused by differences in food or other factors of lifestyle. Another likely explanation for the lower cancer risk reported in vegetarians is possible variations at the levels of hormones [25], such as testosterone and insulin-like growth factor-I (IGF-I). Different studies reported that the variations in these hormones may be linked to the dietary intakes [25]. The occurrence of prostate, breast, and colorectal cancer has been described to be linked with levels of IGF-I. Similarly, prostate cancer and postmenopausal breast cancer have both been linked to increased levels of free testosterone [147].

8.4.2.2 Types of Cancer and Vegetarian Diet Components

Breast Cancer

A plant-based diet may have a vital role in breast cancer. In reality, epidemiologic research suggests that a prudent or healthy eating pattern can reduce breast cancer incidence, particularly ER- and PR-positive tumors, along with ER-and PR-negative tumors [150]. According to the study that included the nurses, eating more vegetables overall was linked to a lower risk of breast cancer, especially for more aggressive tumors. The study pooled the repeated measures and followed up for over 30 years [34]. This links with the previous research that found both dietary and circulatory carotenoids to be inversely related to ER-breast cancer. These chemicals may have the ability to bind and remove toxic free radicals, repair DNA damage, suppress cell growth, induce cell death, and block angiogenesis, among other things [17]. Similarly, researchers from two large p cohort studies in US discovered that a higher hPDI score—a metric for eating a high-quality plant-based diet—was linked to a lower risk of developing all types of breast cancer, regardless of changes in weight, fiber, or total carotenoid consumption. The connection was strongest in regard to ER-negative cancers, which may be most affected by non-hormonal exposures. Studies providing the link between plant-based diet and breast cancer are not steady [63, 116]. When comparing healthy and unhealthy provegetarian dietary patterns independently, the SUN research found that modest, but not greater, adherence to a provegetarian diet was related with a lower risk of breast cancer. Moreover, enriched proplant diet score was connected with a lower overall risk of developing cancer, but no association with breast cancer was found, which may partly be explained by the small number of cases [117]. A higher hPDI score, which assesses adherence to a high-quality plant-based diet, was linked to a decreased risk of all breast cancer in two large prospective cohort studies conducted in the USA. This association was observed regardless of changes in weight, total carotenoid intake, or dietary fiber. The connection was strongest in respect to ER-negative cancers, which may be most affected by non-hormonal exposures. Less weight gain might statistically account for 7.3% of the negative relationship with hPDI [117].

Lung Cancer

Lung cancer is one of the many cancers that can be affected by diet. Carotene supplements have been found to raise the lung cancer incidence, but eating fruits and other foods rich in carotenoids may have protective effects, according to the World Cancer Research/American Institute for Cancer Research. The study showed that higher consumption of fruits decreased the risk of lung cancer by 8–18%. When the study was stratified based on smoking status, the risk reduction associated with vegetable consumption was reduced. Numerous nutrients included in fruits and vegetables have protective effects, primarily by lowering DNA oxidative damage, stimulating the immune system, boosting the activity of enzymes that can detoxify carcinogens, and engaging in antiproliferative activities regulating hormone levels [11, 66]. The true link between vegetarian diet and lung cancer may be better understood by studying a never-smokers' population due to the significant confounding effect of smoking, but since lung cancer is a rare disease in never-smokers, the information currently available is insufficient to make a reliable conclusion. A meta-analysis proposed the protecting role of vegetarian diet in lung cancer etiology. A diet with significant amount of pulses, whole grains, vegetables, fruits, which are enriched with a high content in antioxidants and phytonutrients in balanced doses, might reduce the lung cancer risk [145]. The study suggested that increasing the daily intake of vegetables and fruits by 100 g would result in substantial inverse dose–response correlations [145]. Additionally, smoking cigarettes is linked to a decline in the levels of provitamin A carotenoid in the blood [2]. Additionally, smokers are known to consume less fruit than non-smokers, and smoking is strongly linked to lung cancer. Overall, a normal weight, eating a balanced, diverse diet, and getting regular exercise can lower your risk of developing lung cancer.

Colorectal Cancer

Few studies show that the vegetarian diets are linked with risk of colorectal cancers. Olrich and his coworkers showed that the Pescovegetarians in particular have a much lower incidence in comparison to non-vegetarians [101]. Vegetarians and non-vegetarians consume different types of food, according to [157]. In addition to consuming fewer animal products than non-vegetarians, vegetarians consume more of a wide range of plant foods and consumed fewer added fats, refined grains, sweets, snack foods, and caloric beverages. As a result, such pattern would decrease in hyperinsulinemia, which has been suggested as a potential mechanism by which food may raise the risk of colon cancer. The vegetarian diets are higher in fiber content; these are associated with the lower BMI [93]. The amount of fecal bile acids in vegetarians was found to be lower than in non-vegetarians. Vegetarians had a 22% lower overall risk of colorectal cancer than non-vegetarians, according to a study. When compared to meat eaters, vegetarians had a risk of colon cancer that was 19% lower and a risk of rectal cancer that was 29% lower [149]. However, vegetarian diets in Britain have not been linked to a decline in the incidence of colorectal cancer [67, 68]. According to the EPIC-Oxford study's preliminary findings, vegetarians have a roughly 50% higher chance of developing colorectal cancer [67, 68].

Gastric Cancer

The vegetarian diet has his impact on the occurrence of gastric cancer. Dietary factors play a significant role in gastric cancer development, especially when it comes to the intestinal subtype of gastric adenocarcinoma. A lower risk of gastric cancer is linked to having a healthy diet and keeping a healthy weight. Consistent evidence suggests that gastric *H. pylori* infection plays a significant role in the development and spread of gastric cancers of the body. By supplying noxious chemicals that increase the pathogenicity of *H. pylori*, dietary variables are thought to play a role in the development of the infection. Numerous fruits have bacteriostatic properties against *H. pylori*. Fruit extracts are thought to have antibacterial properties due to phenolic compounds [97]. High bush blueberry extract has been shown to be effective in vitro at reducing the adherence of *H. pylori* to mucus, erythrocytes in gastric epithelial cell culture. Raspberries, strawberries, blackberries, and bilberries exhibit powerful bacteriostatic activity against strains of *H. pylori* that are resistant to clarithromycin, according to a study [23]. In a prospective, randomized, double-blinded study, 189 adults with *H. pylori* infections drank 250 ml of blueberry juice daily for 90 days. On the 35th day, the urea breath test was negative in 14.46% of patients. On the 90th day, this result persisted [155]. Meat eaters and vegetarians were examined in a study using large British populations, and the findings showed significant heterogeneity and a decreased overall relative risk (RR) for stomach cancer [67, 68]. In a different study, carried out in Tokyo, 5765 middle-aged men workers were studied prospectively. Using a food consumption questionnaire, four dietary patterns including vegetable and fruit were discovered. Following up for ten years, between 1988 and 1998, 84 incident cases of stomach cancer were recorded. In their estimation of risk ratios using proportional hazards regression, the scientists discovered no conclusive link between any food pattern and the incidence of stomach cancer [85].

Prostate Cancer

It is shown by a study that plant-based diets may confer a lower risk of prostate cancer. Over a mean follow-up of 7.8 years, 1079 incident cases of prostate cancer were identified in the study. And about 237 advanced/high-grade cases were found among them. A study was conducted on a large British cohort with the title of EPIC-Oxford and the Oxford Vegetarian Study. In this study, it was found that a significant lower prostate cancer risk was found in fish eater than meat eaters and no risk was found among vegetarian [133].

8.4.3 Western-Style Diet or High-Fat Diet

The western style diet is also known as high-fat diet. Such diet consists of great intake red and processed meat, dairy products rich in fats, sweets, refined grains, potatoes, butter and high-fat gravy, and less consumption of vegetables and fruits [36]. It is substantially causative for the onset of metabolic diseases and the global obesity epidemic. Metabolic pathologies brought on by excessive body fat include cancer, insulin resistance, type 2 diabetes, non-alcoholic fatty liver disease, dyslipidemia, cardiovascular disease, and dyslipidemia. Among adults, 500 million are obese and 1.5 billion are overweight in accordance with the World Health Organization report [99]. It is assessed that overweight and obesity are linked to 5.5% cases of cancer in the UK. According to several research, the relative risk of cancer mortality related to obesity was approximately 14.2% for men and 19.8% for women [102, 129].

So in human populations, the link between fat and cancer is very strong [107]. Studies have focused on postmenopausal women's breast cancer, endometrial cancer, colon cancer, gall bladder cancer, esophageal adenocarcinoma, and kidney cancer in an effort to pinpoint the cancers most closely associated with obesity [10, 111, 115, 129].

8.4.3.1 Mechanism of Western Diet in Cancer Development and Progression

Western diet encourages a number of changes that could make someone more likely to get cancer or could make the microenvironment of tissue more favorable for the growth of cancerous cells, which would favor the spread of the disease and its metastasis. In general, hypercaloric diets cause oxidative stress, which produces reactive oxygen species and endoplasmic reticulum stress [55]. Many molecular mechanisms underpinning the association between high-fat induced obesity and cancer development have been presented such as dysregulated hormonal signaling, fatty acid metabolism, an aberrant insulin/IGF-1 axis, and chronic inflammation [129]. Numerous studies have been conducted to find role of chronic inflammation in development of cancer. It is concluded that inflammation triggers the kynurenine pathway. It also affects the aryl hydrocarbon receptor (AHR) and modulates synaptic transmission in the brain and in this way plays an important role in feeding and metabolism. The evidence for the kynurenine pathway's involvement in carcinogenesis then establishes a potentially significant connection between cancer and obesity. The second new theory is supported by data showing that the tumor suppressor genes deleted in colorectal cancer and neogenin can be removed from cells by serine proteases. Mammalian chymotryptic proteases, such as those produced by macrophages and proinflammatory neutrophils, are among these enzymes. Chymotrypsin levels in the blood rise concurrently with dietary consumption. The bacterial enzyme subtilisin, which functions similarly, is found in abundance in the environment, cleaning products, meat processing, and animal probiotics. Simple public health initiatives in these places with AHR antagonists and selective serine protease inhibitors could prevent a variety of malignancies, including those of the intestine [129].

8.4.3.2 Types of Cancer and High-Fat Diet Components

Breast Cancer

Breast cancer development is strongly affected by the obesity caused by western diet. Adipose tissue is thought to be involved in breast cancer development as there is a strong correlation between the amount of adipose tissue in breast, breast cell density, and collagen (which often correlates with overall breast size) [12, 30]. The CD36 is a common membrane protein reversed expression of this protein is involved in cell growth and intercellular communication and it is thought that this may be the cause of breast cancer. Breast tissue with lower levels of CD36 deposits more collagen at the expense of less adipose tissue. Increase in the collagen to adipose ratio leads to denser tissue in the breasts and a higher risk of cancer [12, 30]. The potential impact of estrogens produced in adipose tissue has been mentioned as a further factor impacting the development of breast cancer through obesity and breast adiposity. These steroids are likely to contribute to estrogen stimulation through pregnancy, hormone replacement therapy, oral contraceptives, as well as the occurrence of cancer [43, 129].

Gastrointestinal Cancer

Due to the change of various carcinogenic compounds and metabolic reprogramming, a high-fat diet can significantly raise the risk of gastrointestinal malignancies [43]. Here we will discuss link of high-fat diet with different types of gastrointestinal cancer. Clinical epidemiological investigations revealed a connection between meat consumption and esophageal cancer, gastric esophageal cancer, and squamous cell carcinoma. Additionally, according to research, a higher fat intake increased the risk of esophageal carcinoma and esophageal gastric adenocarcinoma, whereas a higher carbohydrate intake decreased those risks. A meta-analysis on observational studies in 2017 reported association of esophageal carcinoma with high-fat intake, but no association was found for esophageal squamous cell carcinoma [51]. However, large-scale epidemiological studies are warranted to confirm association of high-fat diet with esophagus cancer.

Gastric Cancer

According to numerous epidemiological studies, high-fat diet is a risk factor for gastric cancer [51]. Leptin plays an important role in apoptosis, angiogenesis, and cell proliferation, and due to this, it is thought that it is crucial in the development of gastrointestinal cancers associated with obesity. It has been demonstrated to influence STAT3, mTOR, and ERK-dependent pathways, promoting mucin synthesis and the growth of gastrointestinal tumors [61]. Gastric cancers are known to be brought on by high levels of leptin and leptin signaling activation. Increased expression of ectopic molecules associated with the intestinal epithelium is one of the identified mechanisms for it [76, 144]. According to Arita and coworkers, tissue integrity, the disturbance of gastric epithelial organelle homeostasis, and stemness gene expression caused by lipotoxicity linked with high-fat diet led to precancerous lesions that leads to gastric adenocarcinoma [29, 135].

Liver Cancer

Liver cancer is also known as hepatocellular carcinoma (HCC). Among HCCs, the most prevalent form is primary liver cancer that is an obesity-related cancer. Its development is linked with non-alcoholic fatty liver disease (NAFLD). About 20% of these people develop non-alcoholic steatohepatitis (NASH) from simple liver steatosis (hepatosteatosis). The NASH is marked by chronic liver damage, inflammation, and fibrosis and significantly raises the risk of HCC in addition to liver failure. With the rising prevalence of insulin resistance and obesity in the next years, NASH and NASH-associated HCC will become an even bigger global health issue. NAFLD and HCC are highly connected with insulin resistance, obesity, and the metabolic syndrome and can be controlled through changes in lifestyle, particularly food patterns and inactive habits. High-fat diet or western diet is one of the main cause of the development of these conditions. Such kind of diet worsens the accumulation of free Chol in liver that affects negatively [71]. For HCC prevention, a focus on lifestyle changes is required that includes healthy diet and physical activity.

Pancreatic Cancer

By 2030, colorectal cancer will lose ground to pancreatic cancer, which is presently the third highest cause of cancer-related death in the USA. The development of pancreatic cancer is linked with high-fat diet, obesity, excess body weight, and excessive caloric consumption [42]. As far as diet is concerned, saturated fatty acids (FAs) present in high-fat diet are the kind of fat related to a higher pancreatic cancer risk [47, 152, 153]. In contrast, low-fat diets are linked to a reduced risk of pancreatic cancer [58] and research has revealed that diets rich in omega-3 FAs can reduce pancreatic cancer risk [130]. In fact, high-fat diet causes obesity that is a risk factor for pancreatic cancer. High-fat diets have been linked to an increase in obesity via modifying the intestinal flora, which can increase energy absorption, intestinal permeability, and systemic inflammation [89]. Obesity itself can exacerbate inflammation, as adipokines and cytokines interact intricately to cause the growth of fat tissue [45]. A favorable environment for carcinogenesis is created in obesity by cytokines and leptin, which encourage monocyte conversion to macrophages [46]. The current theories on how fat encourages cancer include increased insulin and IGF-1 levels [75, 106], increased sex hormones like estrogen [56], altered levels of adipocytokines like leptin, adiponectin, and visfatin [32], low-grade inflammation influencing cytokines and immune modulation [27], and altered intestinal gut bacteria are just a few of the changes that have been observed [90]. Most research on the impact of inflammation on pancreatic carcinogenesis has used obese animal models and studies on human are needed to understand this mechanism.

Colorectal Cancer

A link between colorectal cancer and Western dietary pattern has been demonstrated by epidemiological studies [81]. High content of fat in such kind of diet raises the risk of colorectal cancer and its metastases [16]. It has been predicted that Western dietary pattern scores are more significantly related with distal colon and rectal malignancies in two American prospective cohort studies [87]. High intake of processed and red meat was found to raise colorectal cancer risk in a statement by the World Cancer Research Fund and the American Institute for Cancer Research [36]. In addition, worldwide and particularly in high-income nations, the occurrence of early-onset colorectal cancer (CRC), which affects people under 50, has been rising due to Western life style [1].

Numerous molecular pathways that are essential in a high-fat diet's promotion of colon cancer have been found. The JNK pathway encourages cell growth and malignant transformation and is crucial for insulin resistance and obesity [53]. Niku et al. discovered a heterozygous APC gene deletion and downregulation of the mTOR, ERK1/2 and AKT signaling pathways, and they linked these findings to colorectal cancer that developed by consuming a western diet [96]. The STRA6 pathway establishes a link between colorectal cancer and a high-fat diet which is crucial for maintaining colorectal cancer stem cells [64, 139]. A strong link of high-fat diet with colorectal cancer has been identified and its prevention depends on the change of life style including adaptation of a health dietary pattern [36].

8.5 Animal Models' Based Research on Dietary Pattern and Cancer Risk

The epidemiological literature on cancer risk and dietary patterns has received some support from animal models, which have also provided insights into the probable molecular mechanisms at play. However, up to now, the major animal studies investigating the relationship between cancer and nutrition have concentrated on the use of a single macronutrient and research on actual dietary patterns is still scarce [126]. Regarding the Mediterranean diet, there has only been one study that has been reported on its impact on tumors in mice. In mice, colon tumorigenesis was found to be decreased by a Mediterranean diet mix, which was related with gut dysbiosis and regulation of apoptosis. This Mediterranean diet mix contained eicosapentaenoic acid. It is an omega-3 polyunsaturated fatty acid that can be found in the Mediterranean diet in the form of free fatty acids together with a number of bioactive phytochemical extracts. Further studies on animals that closely mimic the dietary patterns reported in the epidemiological investigations are required in order to elucidate the effects of the Mediterranean diet on cancer risk and to explain the underlying processes [126]. According to a plant-based diet study in mice, the prenatal/maternal broccoli sprouts' treatment is more effective in preventing development of breast cancer when compared to postnatal early-life and adult broccoli sprouts treatment. This was true for two mouse models that were transgenic in nature and could develop breast cancer. The prenatal/maternal broccoli sprout treatment was more successful in preventing breast cancer than the postnatal early-life broccoli sprout treatment, which began before the onset of puberty. However, the consumption of broccoli sprouts during maturity had no impact on the development of breast tumors. These results suggest that embryonic development may be effected by prenatal/maternal broccoli sprouts treatment by regulating global differential gene expression that in later life leads to differential susceptibility to breast cancer. And it is bioactive natural compounds in plants that regulate this activity. Furthermore, these findings imply that cruciferous vegetables, which have an epigenetic-modulating influence on diet, may be a crucial element in increasing chemopreventive effects on human breast cancer. By properly administering important dietary components, this study may have the potential to translate into early breast cancer prevention in humans [79]. However further studies on plant-based dietary pattern that include all components of such diet are warranted to get a clear picture of molecular mechanism that how such diet is protective in cancer prevention and treatment. Undoubtedly, the most thoroughly researched dietary treatments in mice are those that examine the relationship between cancer development, progression, and mortality and Western-style diets or high-fat diets.

These widely accessible commercial diets trigger the phenotypic development of obesity because they frequently include up to 60% fat [125].

Most mice studies show a favorable correlation between colon and breast cancer and diets high in fat [28, 49, 151]. Consideration of the link between maternal intake of high-fat food and transgenerational occurrence of cancer and its progression is also noteworthy. Many studies have shown that when mice are prenatally expose to high-fat diet, it increases rises the risk of prostate and breast cancer in offspring [94, 98]. The gut microbiota, inflammatory processes, metabolic variables, adipokines, and estrogen metabolism and signaling are a few of the mechanisms influencing the association between high-fat diets and cancer occurrence and progression in these animal models [35, 60, 70]. Despite evidence from animal studies linking a high dietary fat intake to cancer incidence and development, the current work has some limitations that raise questions about its translatable usefulness. Many mouse research employ diets with excessively high dietary fat content about 40–60% of energy from fat, which are not normal diets consumed by human [125]. Lack of consideration for other dietary components while consuming a single source of fat, such as beef tallow, coconut oil, or milk fat, may have an impact on health consequences. To completely assess the processes relating high-fat dietary practices to incidence of cancer and development in mice, more research using realistic high-fat diets is required [126].

8.6 Conclusion

The scientific data are oversaturated with studies finding a relationship between dietary patterns and cancer. Herein, we review few main dietary patterns prevalent in the world and their link with different types of cancer. Overall, western dietary pattern is linked with cancer development and progression in human and animal bodies. The prevailing consensus is that plant-based foods are cancer-preventative. Even early research found that the risk of cancer was roughly twice as high for those who consumed fewer fruits and vegetables than for those who consumed more of these foods. More recent work confirms these finding. Plants are known to contain diverse secondary metabolites that are used in the disease prevention and treatment or in the promotion of well-being. These metabolites have antioxidant characteristics and can interact with free radicals like hydroxyl, peroxyl, and superoxide groups to prevent them from attaching to biological macromolecules (proteins, lipids, and DNA). As a result, the interaction's potential for lipid peroxidation, oxidative DNA damage, and protein degradation will be greatly diminished, which will significantly lessen the likelihood of genetic events that encourage the development of cancer. The design of such research will be made easier by a greater understanding of polyphenol bioavailability characteristics, such as the kinetics of accumulation, absorption, and elimination.

References

1. Akimoto N, Ugai T et al (2021) Rising incidence of early-onset colorectal cancer—a call to action. Nat Rev Clin Oncol 18(4):230–243
2. Alberg AJ, Chen JC et al (2000) Household exposure to passive cigarette smoking and serum micronutrient concentrations. Am J Clin Nutr 72(6):1576–1582
3. Anic G, Park Y et al (2016) Index-based dietary patterns and risk of lung cancer in the NIH–AARP diet and health study. Eur J Clin Nutr 70(1):123–129
4. Appleby PN, Key TJ (2016) The long-term health of vegetarians and vegans. Proc Nutr Soc 75(3):287–293
5. Aune D, Chan DS et al (2013) Red and processed meat intake and risk of colorectal adenomas: a systematic review and meta-analysis of epidemiological studies. Cancer Causes Control 24(4):611–627
6. Aune D, Navarro Rosenblatt DA et al (2015) Dairy products, calcium, and prostate cancer risk: a systematic review and meta-analysis of cohort studies. Am J Clin Nutr 101(1):87–117
7. Bamia C, Lagiou P et al (2013) Mediterranean diet and colorectal cancer risk: results from a European cohort. Eur J Epidemiol 28(4):317–328
8. Barchitta M, Maugeri A et al (2018) The association of dietary patterns with high-risk human papillomavirus infection and cervical cancer: a cross-sectional study in Italy. Nutrients 10(4):469
9. Barrubés L, Babio N et al (2018) Dairy product consumption and risk of colorectal cancer in an older mediterranean population at high cardiovascular risk. Int J Cancer 143(6):1356–1366
10. Bhaskaran K, Douglas I et al (2014) Body-mass index and risk of 22 specific cancers: a population-based cohort study of 5·24 million UK adults. Lancet 384(9945):755–765
11. Boffetta P, Couto E et al (2010) Fruit and vegetable intake and overall cancer risk in the European prospective investigation into cancer and nutrition (EPIC). J Natl Cancer Inst 102(8):529–537
12. Boyd NF, Guo H et al (2007) Mammographic density and the risk and detection of breast cancer. N Engl J Med 356(3):227–236
13. Bravi F, Spei M-E et al (2018) Mediterranean diet and bladder cancer risk in Italy. Nutrients 10(8):1061
14. Brinkman MT, Buntinx F et al (2011) Consumption of animal products, olive oil and dietary fat and results from the Belgian case–control study on bladder cancer risk. Eur J Cancer 47(3):436–442
15. Buckland G, Travier N et al (2013) Adherence to the mediterranean diet and risk of breast cancer in the European prospective investigation into cancer and nutrition cohort study. Int J Cancer 132(12):2918–2927
16. Bufill JA (1990) Colorectal cancer: evidence for distinct genetic categories based on proximal or distal tumor location. Ann Intern Med 113(10):779–788
17. Buja A, Pierbon M et al (2020) Breast cancer primary prevention and diet: an umbrella review. Int J Environ Res Public Health 17(13)
18. Cai Q, Yuan Z et al (2017) Infectious agents associated cancers: epidemiology and molecular biology. Springer
19. Cai S, Li Y et al (2014) Alcohol drinking and the risk of colorectal cancer death. Eur J Cancer Prev 23(6):532–539
20. Campbell TC, Parpia B et al (1998) Diet, lifestyle, and the etiology of coronary artery disease: the Cornell China study. Am J Cardiol 82(10):18–21
21. Castelló A, Amiano P et al (2019) Low adherence to the western and high adherence to the mediterranean dietary patterns could prevent colorectal cancer. Eur J Nutr 58(4):1495–1505
22. Castello A, Boldo E et al (2017) Adherence to the Western, Prudent and Mediterranean dietary patterns and breast cancer risk: MCC-Spain study. Maturitas 103:8–15
23. Chatterjee A, Yasmin T et al (2004) Inhibition of *Helicobacter pylori* in vitro by various berry extracts, with enhanced susceptibility to clarithromycin. Mol Cell Biochem 265(1–2):19–26

24. Ciancarelli MGT, Di Massimo C et al (2017) Mediterranean diet and health promotion: evidence and current concerns. Med Res Arch 5(7)
25. Clinton SK, Giovannucci EL et al (2020) The world cancer research fund/American institute for cancer research third expert report on diet, nutrition, physical activity, and cancer: impact and future directions. J Nutr 150(4):663–671
26. Conlin PR, Chow D et al (2000) The effect of dietary patterns on blood pressure control in hypertensive patients: results from the dietary approaches to stop hypertension (DASH) trial. Am J Hypertens 13(9):949–955
27. Coussens LM, Werb Z (2002) Inflammation and cancer. Nature 420(6917):860–867
28. Cranford TL, Velázquez KT et al (2019) Effects of high fat diet-induced obesity on mammary tumorigenesis in the PyMT/MMTV murine model. Cancer Biol Ther 20(4):487–496
29. De Stefani E, Deneo-Pellegrini H et al (1999) Meat intake and risk of squamous cell esophageal cancer: a case-control study in Uruguay. Int J Cancer 82(1):33–37
30. DeFilippis RA, Chang H et al (2012) CD36 repression activates a multicellular stromal program shared by high mammographic density and tumor tissues. Cancer Discov 2(9):826–839
31. Divella R, Daniele A et al (2020) Anticancer effects of nutraceuticals in the Mediterranean diet: an epigenetic diet model. Cancer Genomics Proteomics 17(4):335–350
32. Dutta D, Ghosh S et al (2012) Leptin and cancer: pathogenesis and modulation. Indian J Endocrinol Metab 16(Suppl 3):S596-600
33. Erdrich S, Bishop KS et al (2015) A pilot study to investigate if New Zealand men with prostate cancer benefit from a Mediterranean-style diet. PeerJ 3:e1080
34. Farvid MS, Chen WY et al (2019) Fruit and vegetable consumption and breast cancer incidence: repeated measures over 30 years of follow-up. Int J Cancer 144(7):1496–1510
35. Feakins RM (2016) Obesity and metabolic syndrome: pathological effects on the gastrointestinal tract. Histopathology 68(5):630–640
36. Feng Y-L, Shu L et al (2017) Dietary patterns and colorectal cancer risk: a meta-analysis. Eur J Cancer Prev 26(3):201–211
37. Filomeno M, Bosetti C et al (2015) Mediterranean diet and risk of endometrial cancer: a pooled analysis of three Italian case-control studies. Br J Cancer 112(11):1816–1821
38. Fitó M, Cladellas M et al (2008) Anti-inflammatory effect of virgin olive oil in stable coronary disease patients: a randomized, crossover, controlled trial. Eur J Clin Nutr 62(4):570–574
39. Freedman LS, Midthune D et al (2018) Combining a food frequency questionnaire with 24-hour recalls to increase the precision of estimation of usual dietary intakes—evidence from the validation studies pooling project. Am J Epidemiol 187(10):2227–2232
40. Gann PH (2002) Risk factors for prostate cancer. Rev Urol 4(Suppl 5):S3
41. Garavello W, Lucenteforte E et al (2009) Diet diversity and the risk of laryngeal cancer: a case–control study from Italy and Switzerland. Oral Oncol 45(1):85–89
42. Garcia DI, Hurst KE et al (2021) High-fat diet drives an aggressive pancreatic cancer phenotype. J Surg Res 264:163–172
43. Gérard C, Brown KA (2018) Obesity and breast cancer—role of estrogens and the molecular underpinnings of aromatase regulation in breast adipose tissue. Mol Cell Endocrinol 466:15–30
44. Gerber M, Hoffman R (2015) The Mediterranean diet: health, science and society. Br J Nutr 113(S2):S4–S10
45. Gilbert CA, Slingerland JM (2013) Cytokines, obesity, and cancer: new insights on mechanisms linking obesity to cancer risk and progression. Annu Rev Med 64:45–57
46. Goodwin PJ, Stambolic V (2015) Impact of the obesity epidemic on cancer. Annu Rev Med 66:281–296
47. Gordon-Dseagu VLZ, Thompson FE et al (2017) A cohort study of adolescent and midlife diet and pancreatic cancer risk in the NIH-AARP diet and health study. Am J Epidemiol 186(3):305–317
48. Grosso G, Buscemi S et al (2013) Mediterranean diet and cancer: epidemiological evidence and mechanism of selected aspects. BMC Surg 13 (Suppl 2):S14

49. Guffey CR (2013) Linking obesity to colorectal cancer: recent insights into plausible biological mechanisms
50. Hardin J, Cheng I et al (2011) Impact of consumption of vegetable, fruit, grain, and high glycemic index foods on aggressive prostate cancer risk. Nutr Cancer 63(6):860–872
51. He D, Huang X et al (2017) Dietary fat intake and risk of esophageal carcinoma: a meta-analysis of observational studies. Oncotarget 8(58):99049–99056
52. Hébert JR, Hurley TG et al (2014) Considering the value of dietary assessment data in informing nutrition-related health policy. Adv Nutr 5(4):447–455
53. Hirosumi J, Tuncman G et al (2002) A central role for JNK in obesity and insulin resistance. Nature 420(6913):333–336
54. https://dietamediterranea.com/nutricion-saludable-ejercicio-fisico/
55. Imbroisi Filho R, Ochioni AC et al (2021) Western diet leads to aging-related tumorigenesis via activation of the inflammatory, UPR, and EMT pathways. Cell Death Dis 12(7):643
56. Iyengar NM, Hudis CA et al (2015) Obesity and cancer: local and systemic mechanisms. Annu Rev Med 66:297–309
57. Jacobs DR Jr, Gross MD et al (2009) Food synergy: an operational concept for understanding nutrition. Am J Clin Nutr 89(5):1543S-1548S
58. Jiao L, Chen L et al (2018) Low-fat dietary pattern and pancreatic cancer risk in the women's health initiative dietary modification randomized controlled trial. J Natl Cancer Inst 110(1):49–56
59. Johnson IT (2017) The cancer risk related to meat and meat products. Br Med Bull 121(1)
60. Jordan BF, Gourgue F et al (2017) Adipose tissue metabolism and cancer progression: novel insights from gut microbiota? Curr Pathobiol Rep 5(4):315–322
61. Kabat GC, Ng SK et al (1993) Tobacco, alcohol intake, and diet in relation to adenocarcinoma of the esophagus and gastric cardia. Cancer Causes Control 4(2):123–132
62. Kanauchi M, Kanauchi K (2018) The World Health Organization's healthy diet indicator and its associated factors: a cross-sectional study in central Kinki, Japan. Prev Med Rep 12:198–202
63. Kane-Diallo A, Srour B et al (2018) Association between a pro plant-based dietary score and cancer risk in the prospective NutriNet-santé cohort. Int J Cancer 143(9):2168–2176
64. Karunanithi S, Levi L et al (2017) RBP4-stra6 pathway drives cancer stem cell maintenance and mediates high-fat diet-induced colon carcinogenesis. Stem Cell Rep 9(2):438–450
65. Kenfield SA, DuPre N et al (2014) Mediterranean diet and prostate cancer risk and mortality in the health professionals follow-up study. Eur Urol 65(5):887–894
66. Key TJ (2011) Fruit and vegetables and cancer risk. Br J Cancer 104(1):6–11
67. Key TJ, Appleby P et al (2009) Cancer incidence in British vegetarians. Br J Cancer 101(1):192–197
68. Key TJ, Appleby PN et al (2009) Cancer incidence in vegetarians: results from the European prospective investigation into cancer and nutrition (EPIC-Oxford). Am J Clin Nutr 89(5):1620s–1626s
69. Keys A, Mienotti A et al (1986) The diet and 15-year death rate in the seven countries study. Am J Epidemiol 124(6):903–915
70. Khadge S, Sharp JG et al (2018) Immune regulation and anti-cancer activity by lipid inflammatory mediators. Int Immunopharmacol 65:580–592
71. Kim JY, He F (2021) From liver fat to cancer: perils of the western diet. Cancers (Basel) 13(5)
72. Kontou N, Psaltopoulou T et al (2013) The mediating effect of Mediterranean diet on the relation between smoking and colorectal cancer: a case-control study. Eur J Public Health 23(5):742–746
73. Krusinska B, Hawrysz I et al (2018) Associations of Mediterranean diet and a posteriori derived dietary patterns with breast and lung cancer risk: a case-control study. Nutrients 10(4):470
74. Lăcătușu C-M, Grigorescu E-D et al (2019) The mediterranean diet: From an environment-driven food culture to an emerging medical prescription. Int J Environ Res Public Health 16(6):942

75. Lashinger LM, Harrison LM et al (2013) Dietary energy balance modulation of Kras- and Ink4a/Arf$^{+/-}$-driven pancreatic cancer: the role of insulin-like growth factor-I. Cancer Prev Res (Philadelphia) 6(10):1046–1055
76. Launoy G, Milan C et al (1998) Diet and squamous-cell cancer of the oesophagus: a French multicentre case-control study. Int J Cancer 76(1):7–12
77. Li F, An S et al (2014) Red and processed meat intake and risk of bladder cancer: a meta-analysis. Int J Clin Exp Med 7(8):2100
78. Li W-Q, Park Y et al (2014) Index-based dietary patterns and risk of head and neck cancer in a large prospective study. Am J Clin Nutr 99(3):559–566
79. Li Y, Buckhaults P et al (2018) Temporal efficacy of a sulforaphane-based broccoli sprout diet in prevention of breast cancer through modulation of epigenetic mechanisms. Cancer Prev Res (Philadelphia) 11(8):451–464
80. Li Y, Li S et al (2017) Dietary natural products for prevention and treatment of breast cancer. Nutrients 9(7)
81. Louis P, Hold GL et al (2014) The gut microbiota, bacterial metabolites and colorectal cancer. Nat Rev Microbiol 12(10):661–672
82. Magalhães B, Bastos J et al (2011) Dietary patterns and colorectal cancer. Eur J Cancer Prev 20(5):389–395
83. Martinez-Gonzalez MA, Bes-Rastrollo M et al (2009) Mediterranean food pattern and the primary prevention of chronic disease: recent developments. Nutr Rev 67(suppl_1):S111–S116
84. Martínez-González MA, Sanchez-Tainta A et al (2014) A provegetarian food pattern and reduction in total mortality in the Prevención con Dieta Mediterránea (PREDIMED) study. Am J Clin Nutr 100(suppl_1):320S–328S
85. Masaki M, Sugimori H et al (2003) Dietary patterns and stomach cancer among middle-aged male workers in Tokyo. Asian Pac J Cancer Prev 4(1):61–66
86. McCullough ML, Feskanich D et al (2002) Diet quality and major chronic disease risk in men and women: moving toward improved dietary guidance. Am J Clin Nutr 76(6):1261–1271
87. Mehta RS, Song M et al (2017) Dietary patterns and risk of colorectal cancer: analysis by tumor location and molecular subtypes. Gastroenterology 152(8):1944-1953.e1941
88. Mentella MC, Scaldaferri F et al (2019) Cancer and Mediterranean diet: a review. Nutrients 11(9):2059
89. Mulders RJ, de Git KCG et al (2018) Microbiota in obesity: interactions with enteroendocrine, immune and central nervous systems. Obes Rev 19(4):435–451
90. Nadella S, Burks J et al (2018) Dietary fat stimulates pancreatic cancer growth and promotes fibrosis of the tumor microenvironment through the cholecystokinin receptor. Am J Physiol Gastrointest Liver Physiol 315(5):G699–g712
91. Nettleton JA, Schulze MB et al (2008) A priori-defined dietary patterns and markers of cardiovascular disease risk in the multi-ethnic study of atherosclerosis (MESA). Am J Clin Nutr 88(1):185–194
92. Newby P, Tucker KL (2004) Empirically derived eating patterns using factor or cluster analysis: a review. Nutr Rev 62(5):177–203
93. Newby PK, Tucker KL et al (2005) Risk of overweight and obesity among semivegetarian, lactovegetarian, and vegan women. Am J Clin Nutr 81(6):1267–1274
94. Nguyen NM, de Oliveira Andrade F et al (2017) Maternal intake of high n-6 polyunsaturated fatty acid diet during pregnancy causes transgenerational increase in mammary cancer risk in mice. Breast Cancer Res 19(1):1–13
95. Nguyen S, Li H et al (2020) Adherence to dietary recommendations and colorectal cancer risk: results from two prospective cohort studies. Int J Epidemiol 49(1):270–280
96. Niku M, Pajari AM et al (2017) Western diet enhances intestinal tumorigenesis in Min/+ mice, associating with mucosal metabolic and inflammatory stress and loss of Apc heterozygosity. J Nutr Biochem 39:126–133
97. Nohynek LJ, Alakomi HL et al (2006) Berry phenolics: antimicrobial properties and mechanisms of action against severe human pathogens. Nutr Cancer 54(1):18–32

98. Okeyo-Owuor T, Benesh E et al (2017) Exposure to maternal obesogenic diet worsens some but not all pre-cancer phenotypes in a murine genetic model of prostate cancer. PLoS ONE 12(5):e0175764
99. Okreglicka K (2015) Health effects of changes in the structure of dietary macronutrients intake in western societies. Rocz Państw Zakładu Hig 66(2)
100. Onstad MA, Schmandt RE et al (2016) Addressing the role of obesity in endometrial cancer risk, prevention, and treatment. J Clin Oncol 34(35):4225
101. Orlich MJ, Singh PN et al (2015) Vegetarian dietary patterns and the risk of colorectal cancers. JAMA Intern Med 175(5):767–776
102. Parkin D, Boyd L (2011) 8. Cancers attributable to overweight and obesity in the UK in 2010. Br J Cancer 105(2):S34–S37
103. Pelucchi C, Bosetti C et al (2006) Mechanisms of disease: the epidemiology of bladder cancer. Nat Clin Pract Urol 3(6):327–340
104. Pérez-Jiménez J, Elena Díaz-Rubio M et al (2015) Contribution of macromolecular antioxidants to dietary antioxidant capacity: a study in the Spanish Mediterranean diet. Plant Foods Hum Nutr 70(4):365–370
105. Petimar J, Smith-Warner SA et al (2018) Recommendation-based dietary indexes and risk of colorectal cancer in the nurses' health study and health professionals follow-up study. Am J Clin Nutr 108(5):1092–1103
106. Pisani P (2008) Hyper-insulinaemia and cancer, meta-analyses of epidemiological studies. Arch Physiol Biochem 114(1):63–70
107. Pischon T, Lahmann PH et al (2006) Body size and risk of renal cell carcinoma in the European prospective investigation into cancer and nutrition (EPIC). Int J Cancer 118(3):728–738
108. Pitsavos C, Panagiotakos DB et al (2005) Adherence to the Mediterranean diet is associated with total antioxidant capacity in healthy adults: the ATTICA study. Am J Clin Nutr 82(3):694–699
109. Piyathilake C (2016) Dietary factors associated with bladder cancer. Invest Clin Urol 57(Suppl 1):S14–S25
110. Praud D, Bertuccio P et al (2014) Adherence to the Mediterranean diet and gastric cancer risk in Italy. Int J Cancer 134(12):2935–2941
111. Price AJ, Allen NE et al (2012) Insulin-like growth factor-I concentration and risk of prostate cancer: results from the European prospective investigation into cancer and nutrition. Cancer Epidemiol Biomarkers Prev 21(9):1531–1541
112. Ratjen I, Schafmayer C et al (2017) Postdiagnostic Mediterranean and healthy Nordic dietary patterns are inversely associated with all-cause mortality in long-term colorectal cancer survivors. J Nutr 147(4):636–644
113. Reedy J, Mitrou P et al (2008) Index-based dietary patterns and risk of colorectal cancer: the NIH-AARP diet and health study. Am J Epidemiol 168(1):38–48
114. Reedy J, Subar AF et al (2018) Extending methods in dietary patterns research. Nutrients 10(5):571
115. Renehan AG, Tyson M et al (2008) Body-mass index and incidence of cancer: a systematic review and meta-analysis of prospective observational studies. Lancet 371(9612):569–578
116. Romanos-Nanclares A, Toledo E et al (2020) Healthful and unhealthful provegetarian food patterns and the incidence of breast cancer: results from a Mediterranean cohort. Nutrition 79–80:110884
117. Romanos-Nanclares A, Willett WC (2021) Healthful and unhealthful plant-based diets and risk of breast cancer in U.S. women: results from the nurses' health studies. Cancer Epidemiol Biomarkers Prev 30(10):1921–1931
118. Rosell M, Appleby P et al (2006) Weight gain over 5 years in 21966 meat-eating, fish-eating, vegetarian, and vegan men and women in EPIC-Oxford. Int J Obes 30(9):1389–1396
119. Rossi M, Turati F et al (2013) Mediterranean diet and glycaemic load in relation to incidence of type 2 diabetes: results from the Greek cohort of the population-based European prospective investigation into cancer and nutrition (EPIC). Diabetologia 56(11):2405–2413

120. Russo GI, Solinas T et al (2019) Adherence to Mediterranean diet and prostate cancer risk in Sicily: population-based case-control study. Int J Impot Res 31(4):269–275
121. Satija A, Bhupathiraju SN et al (2016) Plant-based dietary patterns and incidence of type 2 diabetes in US men and women: results from three prospective cohort studies. PLoS Med 13(6):e1002039
122. Schwingshackl L, Hoffmann G (2016) Does a Mediterranean-type diet reduce cancer risk? Curr Nutr Rep 5(1):9–17
123. Sofi F (2009) The Mediterranean diet revisited: evidence of its effectiveness grows. Curr Opin Cardiol 24(5):442–446
124. Song M, Garrett WS et al (2015) Nutrients, foods, and colorectal cancer prevention. Gastroenterology 148(6):1244–1260. e1216
125. Speakman JR (2019) Use of high-fat diets to study rodent obesity as a model of human obesity. Nat Publ Group 43:1491–1492
126. Steck SE, Murphy EA (2020) Dietary patterns and cancer risk. Nat Rev Cancer 20(2):125–138
127. Steffen LM, Hootman KC (2016) A posteriori data-derived dietary patterns and incident coronary heart disease: making sense of inconsistent findings. Curr Nutr Rep 5(3):168–179
128. Stone RAT, Waring ME et al (2017) The association of dietary quality with colorectal cancer among normal weight, overweight and obese men and women: a prospective longitudinal study in the USA. BMJ Open 7(6):e015619
129. Stone TW, McPherson M et al (2018) Obesity and cancer: existing and new hypotheses for a causal connection. EBioMedicine 30:14–28
130. Strouch MJ, Ding Y et al (2011) A high omega-3 fatty acid diet mitigates murine pancreatic precancer development. J Surg Res 165(1):75–81
131. Subar AF, Freedman LS et al (2015) Addressing current criticism regarding the value of self-report dietary data. J Nutr 145(12):2639–2645
132. Subar AF, Kushi LH et al (2017) Invited commentary: the contribution to the field of nutritional epidemiology of the landmark 1985 publication by Willett et al. Am J Epidemiol 185(11):1124–1129
133. Tantamango-Bartley Y, Knutsen SF et al (2016) Are strict vegetarians protected against prostate cancer? Am J Clin Nutr 103(1):153–160
134. Tay SW, Li JW et al (2021) Diet and cancer of the esophagus and stomach. Curr Opin Gastroenterol 37(2):158–163
135. Terry P, Lagergren J et al (2000) Reflux-inducing dietary factors and risk of adenocarcinoma of the esophagus and gastric cardia. Nutr Cancer 38(2):186–191
136. Tfayli A, Temraz S et al (2010) Breast cancer in low-and middle-income countries: an emerging and challenging epidemic. J Oncol 2010
137. Toklu H, Nogay N (2018) Effects of dietary habits and sedentary lifestyle on breast cancer among women attending the oncology day treatment center at a state university in Turkey. Niger J Clin Pract 21(12):1576–1584
138. Tong TY, Key TJ et al (2018) Anthropometric and physiologic characteristics in white and British Indian vegetarians and nonvegetarians in the UK Biobank. Am J Clin Nutr 107(6):909–920
139. Tong Y, Gao H et al (2021) High fat diet, gut microbiome and gastrointestinal cancer. Theranostics 11(12):5889–5910
140. Tonstad S, Stewart K et al (2013) Vegetarian diets and incidence of diabetes in the Adventist Health Study-2. Nutr Metab Cardiovasc Dis 23(4):292–299
141. Tosti V, Bertozzi B et al (2018) Health benefits of the Mediterranean diet: metabolic and molecular mechanisms. J Gerontol Ser A 73(3):318–326
142. Trichopoulou A, Lagiou P (1997) Healthy traditional Mediterranean diet: an expression of culture, history, and lifestyle. Nutr Rev 55(11):383–389
143. Turati F, Carioli G et al (2018) Mediterranean diet and breast cancer risk. Nutrients 10(3):326
144. Tzonou A, Lipworth L et al (1996) Diet and risk of esophageal cancer by histologic type in a low-risk population. Int J Cancer 68(3):300–304

145. Vieira AR, Abar L et al (2016) Fruits, vegetables and lung cancer risk: a systematic review and meta-analysis. Ann Oncol 27(1):81–96
146. Waijers PM, Feskens EJ et al (2007) A critical review of predefined diet quality scores. Br J Nutr 97(2):219–231
147. Watts EL, Fensom GK et al (2021) Circulating insulin-like growth factor-I, total and free testosterone concentrations and prostate cancer risk in 200 000 men in UK Biobank. Int J Cancer 148(9):2274–2288
148. Wilson KM, Giovannucci EL et al (2012) Lifestyle and dietary factors in the prevention of lethal prostate cancer. Asian J Androl 14(3):365
149. Wise J (2015) Vegetarians have lower risk of colorectal cancers, study finds. BMJ 350
150. Xiao Y, Xia J et al (2019) Associations between dietary patterns and the risk of breast cancer: a systematic review and meta-analysis of observational studies. Breast Cancer Res 21(1):16
151. Xiu L, Yang Z et al (2019) High-fat diets promote colon orthotopic transplantation tumor metastasis in BALB/c mice. Oncol Lett 17(2):1914–1920
152. Yao X, Tian Z (2015) Saturated, monounsaturated and polyunsaturated fatty acids intake and risk of pancreatic cancer: evidence from observational studies. PLoS ONE 10(6):e0130870
153. Yu M, Liu H et al (2015) Four types of fatty acids exert differential impact on pancreatic cancer growth. Cancer Lett 360(2):187–194
154. Zhang C, Mumford S et al (2009) Effect of daily fiber intake on reproductive function: the BioCycle study
155. Zhang L, Ma J et al (2005) Efficacy of cranberry juice on *Helicobacter pylori* infection: a double-blind, randomized placebo-controlled trial. Helicobacter 10(2):139–145
156. Zheng J, Guinter MA et al (2017) Dietary patterns and risk of pancreatic cancer: a systematic review. Nutr Rev 75(11):883–908
157. Orlich MJ, Jaceldo-Siegl K, Sabaté J, Fan J, Singh PN, Fraser GE (2014) Patterns of food consumption among vegetarians and non-vegetarians. Br J Nutr. 2014 Nov 28 112(10):1644–53. https://doi.org/10.1017/S000711451400261X. Epub 2014 Sep 23. PMID: 25247790; PMCID: PMC4232985

Nutritional Genomics and Cancer Prevention

9

Shaista Aslam, Riffat Iqbal, Rida Fatima Saeed, Nuzhat Akram, Farhat Ijaz, Irfana Liaqat, and Ahmed Sohaib Aslam

Contents

S. Aslam (✉) · R. F. Saeed
Department of Biological Sciences, National University of Medical Sciences (NUMS), Rawalpindi, Pakistan
e-mail: shaista.aslam@numspak.edu.pk

R. F. Saeed
e-mail: rida.saeed@numspak.edu.pk

R. Iqbal · I. Liaqat
Department of Zoology, Government College University, Lahore, Pakistan
e-mail: riffatiqbal@gcu.edu.pk

I. Liaqat
e-mail: irfana.liaqat@gcu.edu.pk

N. Akram
Hamdard College of Medicine, Hamdard University, Karachi, Pakistan
e-mail: Nuzhat.akram@hamdard.edu.pk

F. Ijaz
CMH Lahore Medical College & IOD (NUMS), Lahore, Pakistan
e-mail: farhat_khurram_rana@cmhlahore.edu.pk

A. S. Aslam
Leiden University Medical Centre, Leiden, The Netherlands

R. F. Saeed and S. ul. Shaheed (eds.), *Nutrition and Dietary Interventions in Cancer*, Cancer Treatment and Research 191, https://doi.org/10.1007/978-3-031-55622-7_9

Abbreviations

AGEs	Advanced glycation end products
ADR	Adverse drug reaction
ACE	Angiotensic converting enzyme
CR	Calorie restriction
CA	Cancer
COMT	Catechol-*O*-amyltransferase
INK4b(p15)	Cyclin-dependent kinase 4 inhibitor B/
CpG	Cytosine and guanine separated by phosphate
DNA	Deoxyribonucleic acid
DDRs	DNA damage responses
DNMT	DNA methyltransferase
p300	E1A binding protein P300
EGCG	Epigallocatechin-3-gallate
HAT	Histone acetyl transferases
HDAC	Histone deacetylase
HDAC	Histone deacetylases
HDA	Histone deacetylases
HT-29	Human colorectal adenocarcinoma cell line
KYSE 150 cells	Human esophageal squamous cell carcinoma
PC3 cells	Human prostate cancer cell line
HIC1	Hypermethylated in cancer 1 protein
kb	Kilobase
LoVo and LoVo	Metastatic cell lines
CH3	Methyl group
MTHFR	Methylenetetrahydrofolate reductase
miRNA	MicroRNA
PUFA	Poly unsaturated fatty acids

ROS	Reactive oxygen species
RDAs	Recommended daily allowances
SAH	*S*-Adenosyl L-homocysteine
SAM	*S*-Adenosyl-L-methionine
SAM	*S*-Adenosylmethionine
SNPs	Single-nucleotide polymorphisms
SIRT-1	Sirtuin 1
TYMS	Thymidylate synthase
TP3	Tilapia piscidin 3
TIMP3	TIMP metallopeptidase inhibitor 3
WHO	World Health Organization

9.1 Basic Concept of the Nutrigenomics

Nutrigenomics is an interdisciplinary field that examines the relationship between nutrients, diet, and gene expression as well as how different people react to different dietary components [1]. It explains how genes and nutrients interact. It further explains how DNA and genetic makeup influence an individual's demand for particular nutrients in certain amounts and how this affects overall health. It establishes the relationship between nutrition and genes and determines if diet has a positive or negative impact on health [2]. The potential impact of nutrigenomics on healthcare include therapy, lifestyle guidance, and monitoring focused on disease prevention and diet may be personalized appropriately to fit individual need [3]. Nutrigenomics is still a young and rapidly developing area, having the potential to provide the groundwork for "personalized nutrition" strategies [4]. It may aid in the development of more enduring strategies for promoting dietary change at the community level [5] and may help to reduce the rising worldwide burden of nutrition-related non-communicable diseases [6].

The basic principles of nutrigenomics include:

1. Micro- and macronutrients in food can directly or indirectly modify the gene's structure and expression in the human genome.
2. The food can have a significant role in the development of a number of diseases under specific conditions and in some people.
3. The development, progression, incidence, and severity of the disease are significantly influenced by several genes that are controlled by nutrients in the diet.
4. A person's genetic makeup may influence the effects of nutrition on the harmony between sickness and health.
5. Nutritional intervention is based on understanding a person's nutritional status, needs, and genotype (specific dietary requirements) and can be utilized for chronic illness prevention/treatment and mitigation. [2, 7].

The nutrigenomics studies have revealed that common food substances (nutrients) have an impact on gene expression, which affects the balance between health and sickness. Different pathways have the potential to modify nutritional needs and metabolism. Additionally, dietary substances may have a direct or indirect impact on gene expression. By functioning as ligands for transcription factor receptors, being processed by primary or secondary metabolic pathways, or negatively or positively impacting signal pathways, nutrients may have an impact on the amounts of substrates or intermediates at the cellular level [7]. Nutrients can influence genes in a variety of ways like serve as an enzyme building block, a cofactor in metabolism, a regulator of hormones, and a transcription factor. In order to prevent, delay, and treat diseases like obesity, cardiovascular disease, asthma, type 2 diabetes, and cancer, dietary therapies aim to affect a person's genetic makeup. Raising public knowledge about health, receiving tailored meals, and leveraging genetic predispositions as a powerful driver of dietary and lifestyle modifications [8].

The nutrient-gene interactions are conceptually divided into three main groups:

1. **Direct interactions**: Nutrients act as binding transcription factors for DNA and abruptly increase gene expression after engaging with a receptor.
2. **Epigenetic interactions**: Nutrients may change the shape of DNA or the histone proteins in chromatin, which may result in a long-term change in gene expression.
3. **Genetic variations**: Single-nucleotide polymorphisms (SNPs) might change how genes express themselves or function [8].

9.2 Influence of Bioactive Food Components on Expression of Genes and Gene Products

Bioactive dietary components are biomolecules that can influence a broad spectrum of metabolic processes in the body. They alter the expression of specific genes in human genome to promote health or minimize the chance of sickness. Overconsumption of bioactive nutrients, on the other hand, could contribute to the disease progression or alter the course of the disease's natural history. Genes and nutrition have a two-way relationship: nutrients influence gene expression (nutrigenomics) and genes influence food (nutrigenetics) [9]. Therefore, a deeper comprehension of these basic characteristics can aid in the treatment and avoidance of human disorders. Progress in biological sciences has allowed for a better understanding of the disease's physiopathology, as well as the recognition of the role of numerous bioactive constituents in food in metabolic mechanism. Individualized dietary advice is now achievable because of advances in nutrigenetics and nutrigenomics. Gene expression is influenced by diet, exercise, and medications, which increases the chance of pathological changes in an organism's biological system [10]. According to the study, eating habits are a critical environmental factor in cancer. Managing the consumption of dietary factors and/or their bioactive constituents may appear to be a smart, non-invasive, and cost-effective way to reduce cancer burden, but it is far from simple. Differences in gene sequences that are exclusive to individuals, especially SNPs, have been emphasized since the completion of the Human Genome Project. With 500–2000 bp every 500–2000 bp in the human genome, SNPs are the most common type of genetic variation [11]. These mutations resulted in the production of novel RNA molecules as well as alterations in protein structure/function encoded by mutant genes, both of which can disrupt an organism's system and lead to sickness [12].

There are various contradictions in the literature, despite the fact that observational and experimental evidence continues to point to dietary factors ranging from macro- to micro-constituents as potential cancer modifiers [13]. These differences could be owing to the combined effects of a number of factors that alter the bioactive component's potential to cause biochemical or morphological changes. Dietary elements that are bioactive can alter phenotypes through a variety of interactions with genes and their expression. Unquestionably, genes can influence the site of action, metabolism, or transport of a bioactive dietary component, and thus, the overall response to the diet. Similar to this, bioactive food ingredients can affect cancer outcomes by changing how certain cellular processes are expressed genetically. It has long been understood that several mechanisms, such as phosphorylation, methylation, and other genetic pathways, can cause nutrients to modify proteins after they have been produced [14] explain in detail in Sect. 9.5. As a result, nutritional proteomics is expected to play a role in changes in tumour incidence or aspect in model systems following dietary modifications, as demonstrated by epidemiology research and limited clinical trials. The variety of dietary elements that have been suggested to modify one or more steps in the cancer process serves as an example of how complex the diet is [13, 15]. There is evidence that some dietary components can influence cancer progression. Table 9.1 listed major food components that play a significant role in cancer risk and tumour activity.

9.3 Dietary Components Effect on Gene Expression Interaction Mechanisms

The effect of dietary elements on epigenetic modifications in the genome is an important and exciting topic in nutrigenetics and nutrigenomics. The most frequent epigenetic modifications are DNA methylation and histone modifications, which are heritable changes in gene expression and chromatin. Food components are one of the factors that can cause epigenetic changes, and aberrant epigenetic change profiles can lead to disorders like cancer [1, 16].

One of the most well-known epigenetic modifications is DNA methylation. It entails the methyl groups of nucleotides being attached to their nitrogen bases. Gene expression regulation and chromatin structure modification, are both tied to DNA methylation. DNA methylation profiles can be influenced by SNPs, environmental factors, and dietary components, and many ailments have been

Table 9.1 A comprehensive list of bioactive food components and its dietary sources

Class	Bioactive component	Dietary source
Vitamins	Folic acid	Vegetables
	Vitamin C (ascorbic acid)	Vegetables, fruits
	Vitamin A	Vegetables
	Vitamin D	Dairy products
	Vitamin E (tocopherol)	Vegetable oils
Minerals	Selenium	Cereal grains, fish, meat,
	Zinc	Vegetables, meat,
Carotenoids	β-carotene	Orange-yellow vegetables
Flavonoids	Quercetin	Vegetables, fruits
	(−)-Epigallocatechin-3-gallate	Green tea
Indoles	Indole-3-carbinol	Cruciferous vegetables
Phenolic acids	Curcumin	Turmeric, curry, mustard
	Caffeic acid	Coffee beans, fruits, soybeans
Chlorophyll	Chlorophyll	Green vegetables

Modified and adapted from [29]

linked to variations in this mechanism. The tumour suppressors cyclin dependent kinases, phosphatase, insulin-like growth factor-II, E-cadherin, and Glutathione-*S*-transferase are all affected by DNA hypermethylation. Vitamin A and zinc, for example, have shown to change the patterns of DNA methylation in a variety of foods and/or combinations of foods; even non-essential dietary components may be involved [17]. Researchers were able to discover correlations between diets and telomere length (TL) because to nutrigenomics and nutrigenetics. Rich diet in fruits, vegetables, good fats, and fibre leads to telomere fragments that are longer [18]. Dietary components may influence microRNA (miRNA), which has epigenetic regulatory functions, causing miRNA expression to change, affecting gene expression and phenotype. Fat soluble vitamins (vitamins A, D, and E), polyphenols (catechins, resveratrol, quercetin), fatty acids (omegas-3 and -6), and minerals (selenium, zinc) are some of the nutrients found in food [19].

In 2016, the existence of plant microRNA named as miR159 in human sera was detected, and its level was found to be negatively linked with the onset and progression of breast cancer [20]. Despite an increasing body of evidence suggesting miRNA can be absorbed through the food, the topic remains unanswered and requires more research. *S*-adenosylmethionine (SAM) is a methyl donor made from a number of dietary precursors, including methionine, folate, and vitamins B1 and B2 [21]. Folate and folic acid are the forms of a water-soluble vitamin B, most commonly found in dark leafy green vegetables.

Researchers exploring the impact of dietary components on DNA methylation have become interested in folic acid. Because it transforms into N-5-methyltetrahydrofolate, which is then changed into SAM, the CH3 donor in

DNA methylation, folate is essential for C1 metabolism. Folate is also necessary for DNA synthesis, repair, and methylation. Following dietary consumption, this molecule goes through a series of chemical processes [22]. During the metabolism of folate, the folic acid contained in food is absorbed by the intestine and converted into 5-methyltetrahydrofolate by a series of chemical catabolism and synthesis processes. This chemical component is required for the production of methionine, which is employed in the DNA mutilation process. As a result, a low-folic acid diet can disrupt this process and interfere with DNA replication, increasing the risk of cancer formation [21]. It is advised to take folic acid supplements since folic acid obtained through food may not always be properly utilized by the body due to storage and preparation conditions, as well as specific problems with absorption and metabolism [23]. Zinc serves as a cofactor for several enzymes involved in the creation of methyl group donors. Zinc deficiency can lead to a lack of methyl groups, which can affect gene expression and increase the likelihood of issues with cell development [24]. Histone modification, which largely affects the N-terminus of histones, is another epigenetic mechanism linked to chromatin structure. This includes acetylation, methylation, phosphorylation, biotinylation, and ubiquitination. Nutrients can also alter histone modification. Inhibitors include butyrate, sulforaphane, polyphenols (green tea, garlic, or cinnamon), and diallyl sulphide [25].

Numerous chronic diseases (linked to oxidative damage), such as cancer, diabetes, cardiovascular disease, metabolic disease, and obesity, can be prevented by phytochemicals and phytonutrients, which are produced by plants [26]. Polyphenols (resveratrol, curcumin, quercetin), isoprenoid derivatives (carotenoids and tocopherols), and organo-sulphur compounds are all part of this group. Flavonoids are phenolic compounds found in fruits and vegetables that reduce the risk of cardiovascular disease, metabolic disorders, and certain types of cancer when consumed. Flavonoids' physiological activity in reducing oxidative stress, lowering platelet aggregation and low-density lipoprotein oxidation, as well as functioning as vasodilators in blood vessels is responsible for these benefits [27]. Quercetin, a plant pigment that can inhibit DNA methylases and is found in a variety of vegetables, fruits, nuts, tea, red wine, and propolis, is a powerful antioxidant flavonoid [28].

Because a range of environmental factors, such as climate, soil conditions, season, horticulture practises, and the age and type of the plant, can affect the concentration of food components in plants, a single database may be insufficient. Large fluctuations in exposures at putative cancer prevention target areas can be caused by changes in dietary content. Polyphenols like (−)-epigallocatechin-3-gallate (EGCG) inhibit DNA methyltransferase and reawaken methylation-silenced genes in cancer cell lines (human colon cancer HT-29 cells, esophageal cancer KYSE 150 cells, and prostate cancer PC3 cells) [29]. Gene expression is regulated by bioactive dietary components in a variety of ways. It would be possible to make more effective food recommendations for groups or individuals if their mechanisms of action could be identified and elucidated. Bioactive diet components are used to prevent and treat a variety of food-related illnesses, including cancer. To develop more successful dietary recommendations, it appears that more research into nutrigenetics and nutrigenomics is required.

9.4 Modulation of Multiple Cellular Processes Through Dietary Patterns and Dietary Components

The study of nutritional modification of gene expression at the cellular and subcellular levels has generated a significant amount of data as a result of the area of nutrigenomics' rapid advancement. Research is increasingly concentrating on how diet and nutrition can reduce oxidative damage in the onset of disease. Dietary habits control the mechanisms that have a beneficial impact on a number of diseases, including cancer. Positive effects of the dietary pattern include lowering of lipid and modulating of their effects, impacts on cancer-prone mediators (hormones or growth factors), reduction in the activation of hormones or other extracellular or intracellular transmission pathways involved in cancer through changes in amino acid content, and changes in gut microbiota [30]. Gene expression is regulated by epigenetic mechanisms throughout normal development, and their abnormal regulation may result in human disorders like cancer. Natural phytochemicals have potential to be beneficial due to their reverse effects in the epigenetic alterations in tumour suppressor genes and oncogenes, as well as its ability to modulate and restore protein expression levels. The high levels of antioxidants and anti-inflammatory nutrients present in many foods like fresh fruit, nuts, vegetables, legumes, fish, and olive oil have a protective effect to combat against cell ageing and cancer cell growth (Table 9.2) [31]. It has been noted that curcumin has a significant impact on cancer cells and functions as an antioxidant and an anti-inflammatory [32]. High polyphenol concentrations in foods like olive oil, wine, and vegetables have been shown to have preventive benefits against cancer by slowing down the growth of cancer cells, arresting the cell cycle, causing apoptosis in tumour cells, and preventing metastasis of cell membranes [33–37]. Through a plethora of epigenetic targets, including oncogenes, tumour suppressor genes, inhibitors of DNA methyltransferase (DNMT) and histone deacetylase (HDAC), polyphenol sensitize tumour cells. Additionally, a lot of carotenoids and vitamins, like C and E, folates, and flavonoids, are present in fruit and vegetables. These nutrients are recognized for their antioxidant capabilities, which help prevent DNA damage [38, 39]. Blueberries, plums, kiwis, cherries, and coffee, which contains significant amounts of chlorogenic acid, are just a few examples of the numerous types of fruit that contain this combination of caffeic and quinic acids [40]. Fish and nuts (walnuts, almonds, and pumpkin seeds) are rich sources of omega-3, which slows the growth of cancer through altering angiogenesis, metastasis, cell survival, and inflammation [41].

Table 9.2 Major food categories, their bioactive compounds and their effect on cancer

Food type	Elements	Function
Fruits and vegetables	Antioxidants and micronutrients (carotenoids, protease inhibitors, selenium, vitamins C and E, dithiolthiones, dietary fibre, glucosinates, polyphenols, plant sterols, allium compounds, and limonene)	Tumour-preventing impact
Fish	Omega-3 long-chain fatty acids Eicosapentaenoic and docosahexaenoic acids When cooking fish on a grill or barbecue, heterocyclic amines, and polycyclic aromatic hydrocarbons may be produced	Limiting the development of cancerous cells Modulation of signal transduction and transcription factor activity Alteration in the metabolism of oestrogen Creation of mutagenic substances
Olive oil	Polyphenols including hydroxytyrosol and oleuropein Poly unsaturated fatty acids (PUFA), Oleic acid, low n-6 PUFA/n-3 PUFA ratio	Anti-inflammatory, antioxidant, and anti-mutagenic properties Chemoprotective
Meat	In meat cooked at high temperatures, heterocyclic amines and polycyclic aromatic hydrocarbons are produced High levels of hemeo iron are found Advanced glycation end products (AGEs may be produced more easily when red and processed meats are cooked at a high temperature) Meat consumption may result in insulin resistance and hyperinsulinemia, which encourage the development of cancer cells	Carcinogens Stimulation of endogenous production of cancer-causing N-nitroso compounds to promote carcinogenesis Produce various effects that are cancer-promoting Fostering the expansion of malignant cells
Whole grains	Offer a variety of nutrients, including dietary fibre, selenium, vitamin E, zinc, copper, and bioactive non-nutrients (phytoestrogens, lignans, and phenolic compounds) Aflatoxin (mycotoxin produced by moulds of the Aspergillus species)	Anti-oxidative activity and anti-carcinogenic qualities Lowering insulin resistance TP3 has a high mutation burden
Dairy products	Calcium, vitamin D, linoleic acids, lactic acid-producing bacteria, lactoferrin, High calcium content	Inhibit the growth of tumours Downregulating the production of the physiologically active vitamin D form that promotes cellular growth

Modified and adapted from [42]

9.5 Individual's Genetic Background, Dietary Components, and Health Consequences

The majority of infections and acute diseases have been successfully treated by healthcare, but the majority of non-communicable diseases, or illnesses that are typically not contagious between people, have not been successfully treated or even well managed [43]. In actuality, these diseases related death rates are rising [44]. The World Health Organization (WHO) [45] reports that these diseases currently cause the deaths of nearly 40 million people annually. Non-communicable illnesses frequently have a long lifespan and are a result of lifestyle factors like smoking and drinking [46]. They include, among others, cardiovascular and pulmonary illnesses, malignancies, diabetes mellitus, and obesity. In terms of both health and quality of life, these diseases pose a significant worldwide burden on humanity, particularly for the poorest countries [47]. This section reviews how nutrigenetics and nutrigenomics can be used to prevent and possibly treat conditions like type 2 diabetes, obesity, cardiovascular disease, and cancer.

WHO states that cancer is the second biggest cause of mortality worldwide, accounting for about 1 in 6 fatalities [48]. According to this, a number of factors, including low fruits and vegetable intake, drinking and using cigarettes, having a high body mass index, and not exercising, approximately one-third of all cancer-related deaths. The risk of carcinogenesis has also been linked to a person's diet [49, 50].

Breast cancer is among most frequent malignancies with predominantly female patients worldwide. In 2020, there were 2.26 million new cases of breast cancer, making it the primary reason for cancer-related deaths in women globally [51]. It is a heterogenous disease involving both genetic and environmental factors. The aetiology of breast cancer is connected to a number of dietary components, including calorie consumption, different carbohydrates, proteins, and fats, as well as numerous vitamins, trace elements, and minerals [52]. Additionally, it is also believed that the lack or reduction of some nutrients in the diet can cause carcinogenesis. For instance, a diet low in folate may contribute in cancer development, particularly pancreatic and colorectal tumours [53, 54]. Reduced dietary levels lead to genomic instability through epigenetic pathways since folate is an active agent in preserving DNA integrity through DNA repair [55]. Exogenous carcinogens, which can turn off tumour suppressor genes or turn up oncogenes make up a large portion of the factors that are hypothesized to contribute to tumorigenesis [56]. While food and nutrition are known to be risk factors in the development of cancer, they may also help prevent and even treat the disease [57].

An important objective of nutrigenomics/nutrigenetics research is to examine this involvement. For instance, it has been proposed that dietary polyphenols may have a role in epigenetic pathways that protect or reverse a number of malignancies, including breast cancer and prostate cancer [1, 58]. Because epigenetic modifications like methylation may be reversible, diet is thought to be helpful [59]. Additionally, studies based on nutrigenomics reveal that macronutrients like dietary fibre and micronutrients like certain trace minerals and vitamins are useful both in preventing and treating cancer. This is particularly true in regards to a half-dozen characteristics of tumour cells, such as their endless capacity for replication and capacity to metastasize, which are the hallmarks of cancer [60]. For instance, it has been shown that including flaxseeds in diet can help treat breast cancer [61]. The method involves the conversion of a lignan found in flaxseed into a compound that binds to estrogen receptors and inhibits cell development [62]. It's interesting to note that a recent meta-analysis that combines data mining from nutrigenomics-based research identified a characteristic group of 18 genes that are engaged in controlling the cell cycle [63]. This group of genes reacts to specific bioactive substances, including sulforaphane and withaferin A, which can be found in a variety of diets and dietary supplements [64]. Finally, diets that reduce the negative effects of conventional cancer chemotherapy and radiation therapy can be created using nutrigenomics [65, 66].

9.6 Prevention of Cancer Through Nutrigenomics Approach

Research on nutritional genomics focuses on how chemicals in food and drink affect the integrity of DNA and gene expression. The approaches used for studying the effects of nutrients on DNA synthesis, damage/repair, and expression encompass a wide range of topics including nutrition, food science, biochemistry, molecular biology, genetics, and genomics. Hence nutrigenomic studies investigate the interaction between nutrients and DNA/gene with a multidimensional approach where integration of disciplines can explain the heterogeneity of the individual or specific population response to different nutrients in the diet. Thus, epidemiological variation on the phenomenon of diet-DNA interaction is also observed. Moreover, the interaction between nutrient and DNA/gene expression is not a straightforward mechanism instead many factors can influence this interaction directly or remotely.

Bioactive nutrients can affect the DNA and gene expression through both genetic and epigenetic mechanisms. DNA repair, DNA damage prevention, and nucleotide synthesis are all components of the genetic system. Without altering the coding DNA sequences, epigenetic mechanisms can modify how genes are expressed. Conrad Hal Waddington, a British developmental biologist, created the phrase "epigenetics" in 1942. It includes RNA, histone covalent modifications, and DNA methylation. These epigenetic processes control gene expression and maintain stability of chromatin structure.

The importance of epigenetic mechanisms can explicitly be described by the fact that critical changes in cancer cell genomes like silencing of tumour suppressor genes, defects in DNA repair mechanism, and activation of oncogenes are largely affected if not initiated by epigenetic events.

Nutritional factors can alter the expression of genes that play an important role for both physiological growth and pathological changes. For example, embryonic

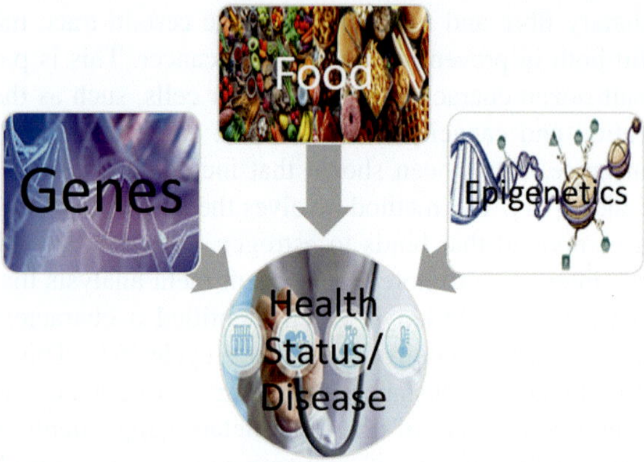

Fig. 9.1 The inter-relationship of individual genes, epigenetics, diet, and health status/disease

growth, foetal development, and the ageing process are few of the physiological processes affected by nutrition. On the other hand, role of nutrients has also been observed in etiological aspects of diseases like cardiovascular diseases, diabetes, breast, colon, and lung cancers. Epigenetic processes involved in cancer development are shown in Fig. 9.1.

Some of the nutrients show the predominant effect just like cancer therapeutic agents and some as cancer preventive agents. Cancer therapeutic nutrients usually initiate oxidative stress through Reactive Oxygen Species (ROS) in mutant cancer cell lines while cancer preventive agents halt cellular processes that can initiate mutation and cell uncontrolled propagation and supports cellular processes that are helpful in stabilizing DNA.

In order to understand the epigenetic mechanism, cell differentiation and lineage specific expression, which are also time bound processes present an exemplary phenomenon. It is quite obvious that the somatic cells in the body have identical genomes, i.e. 22 autosomes and a pair of sex chromosomes. However, each cell has a lineage specific expression profiles created and maintained by specific sets of epigenetic instructions. Each cell genome has built in programme to express specific sets of genes, even the genes are scheduled to express at specific time points during the lifetime. Epigenetic instruction also carries a memory of cell identity once it is differentiated. Surprisingly epigenetic mechanisms also show the capability of causing changes in chromosomal structure hence modulating gene expression.

In the presence of modifiers (factors, elements, or processes in the body that can affect epigenetic mechanisms) such as polymorphic forms of different enzymes, life style factors, intake of other nutrients effect of nutrients on epigenetic modulation cannot be precisely described. Similarly, association of nutrients or bioactive food with physiological, biochemical, or pathological events in the human body cannot be predicted with accuracy and specificity. For example, deficiencies of vitamin B6 and B12, folic acid, and niacin, may raise the risk of neurological dysfunction, heart disease, and colon cancer through neurological dysfunctions and defects in DNA repair mechanisms. A wide range of investigation and exhaustive research need to be conducted to establish a link between a nutrient and physiological or pathological process including cancer.

Some epigenetic mechanisms are explained here that play a vital role in tumorigenesis and if they are blocked or stimulated by suitable therapies growth of cancer cells can be arrested.

9.6.1 DNA Methylation

The differentiation of cells during embryonic development depends on DNA methylation. With the exception of CpG islands, or specific DNA sections (about 1 kilobase (kb) in length), where significant CpG contents are present, methylation is found sparingly but generally across the whole genome of mammals. CpG is abbreviated for Cytosine base (C) linked to Guanine base (G) by a phosphate group in such a manner that Cytosine being 5-prime to Guanine, i.e. 5′-C-phophate-G-3′. CpG islands are mostly associated with promoter regions of genes. Around 50% of promoter regions of genes are having these CpG clusters. CpG clusters in CpG islands are mostly unmethylated as compared to those heavily methylated CpG dinucleotides that are not associated with islands. In mammals approximately 60–90% of CpG dinucleotides are methylated. Rest of CpGs are unmethylated found in clusters in CpG islands. DNA methyltransferases (DNMTs), are principally responsible for maintaining DNA methylation. They catalyse the transfer of a methyl group (CH3) from the methyl precursor SAM to the cytosine of the CpG cytosine. Humans and other species both contain a number of DNMTs.

Low frequency of CpG content is due to the spontaneously occurring deamination of a methylated cytosine resulting in a thymine and transformation of CpG to ApT. If cytosine is unmethylated its deamination results in an Uracil which is quickly replaced by the base excision repair mechanism. Cytosine methylation disturbs the binding of proteins and transcription factors due to changes in structure of major grooves. If cytosine methylation involves a specific site such as upstream of a promoter region genes transcription is disturbed, and it may not get translated into specific proteins. That's how epigenetic phenomenon of DNA methylation disrupts genes transcription and protein translation.

Studies have shown that hypermethylation in the tumour suppressor genes' heritable promoter region results in the transcriptional silence of those genes in cancer cells (Fig. 9.2). It's interesting to note that hypermethylation events at genes play a role in DNA repair, tumour cell invasion, cell cycle regulation, and other processes that silence promote metastasis. In fact, hypermethylation can act as a diagnostic for the disease and is evident early in some cancers, such as CA colon. DNA methylation silences transcription of a number of putative tumour suppressor genes, such as INK4b(p15), HIC1, and TIMP3. DNA methylation is a reversible process and plays a vital role in suppression of specific genes that lead to progression of cancer. Numerous bioactive dietary ingredients have demonstrated promising benefits in DNMTs inhibition.

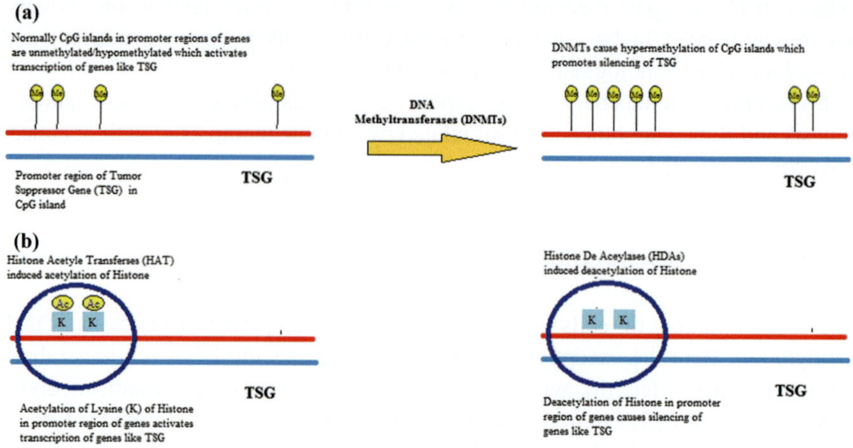

Fig. 9.2 Epigenetic landscape of cancer. **a** DNA methylation and **b** histone acetylation

9.6.2 Histone Chemical Modifications

In eukaryotic nuclei genetic material forms a complex with a globular protein named histones. This complex is called nucleosome. The key histone proteins H2A, H2B, H3, and H4 are wrapped around 147 base pairs of DNA to form a nucleosome. Acetylation and methylation are the two important chemical modifications in histone which can bring about a change in chromatin state, i.e. relaxed/ open or closed. Open state activates transcription and closed state suppresses transcription. Interaction between histone modifications and histone modifiers complexes is referred as "histone code" which ensures that transcription remains inactive unless needed. Therefore, specific genes are switched off/on in a timely manner. Deregulation of the histone code increases the risk of oncogenic transformation, genomic instability, and the emergence of cancer by causing mutations in three important genes, i.e. oncogenes, tumour suppressor genes, and DNA repair genes.

Histone Acetyle Transferases (HAT) and Histone DeAcetylases (HDA) are the two major modifiers of chromatin state. The tumour suppressor gene is silenced as a result of histone hypoacetylation at a promoter region, which is brought on by either a deficiency in HAT function or an increase in HDA activity (Fig. 9.2). There are more than 18 classes of HDAs. Class I HDAs are more linked to malignant tumours when compared with other classes. Various bioactive nutrients like EGCG, suforaphane, curcumin showed to induce alterations in both HATs and HDAs.

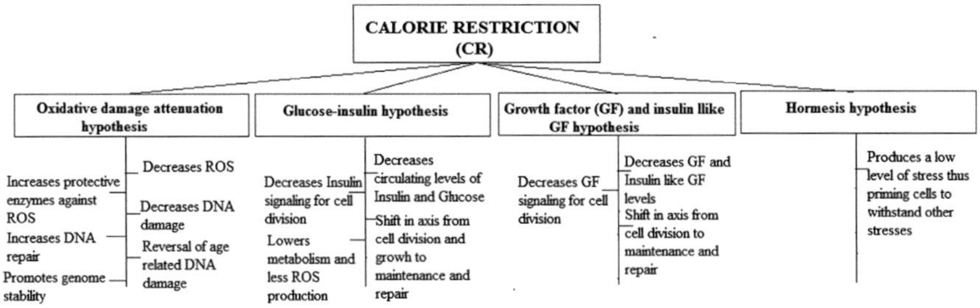

Fig. 9.3 Hypotheses of calorie restriction (CR) induced genomic stability

9.6.3 Calorie Restriction

Calorie restriction (CR) is the decreased intake of nutrients without causing malnutrition or deficiency symptoms. CR is considered to play a vital role in promoting health and increases lifespan.

CR is also thought to be a cancer prevention strategy using stress response gene activation that plays important role in the upregulation of DNA repair capacity (Fig. 9.3). Less DNA damage leads to less mutation hence reduce the incidence of cancer cells.

Four major hypotheses have been given out to clarify positive effects of CR on maintenance and stability of cells.

1. Oxidative damage attenuation hypothesis: This hypothesis suggests that oxidative damage decreases during CR in decreased production of ROS.
2. Glucose-insulin hypothesis: This hypothesis suggests that CR decreases circulating levels of both insulin and glucose, thus decreasing cell growth and division and promoting maintenance and repair.
3. Growth factor (GF) and insulin like GF hypothesis: This hypothesis suggests the same mechanism as given in Glucose-insulin hypothesis.
4. Hormesis hypothesis: CR induces a low level of stress which enables cells to counteract higher and challenging stresses through adaptive mechanisms.

CR is seen as an "intervention" that modifies the activation of particular "stress response genes" with the activation of essential enzymes in DNA repair pathways, upregulating the capacity of the cell for "DNA repair." Enhancing DNA repair minimizes DNA damage levels, which in turn lowers the incidence of mutations, maintaining genomic stability.

9.6.4 Telomerase Activation

Telomeres were discovered by American geneticist Hermann J. Muller in 1938. Telomeres are positioned at the tip of the chromosome. They are composed of non-coding repetitive sequences (TTAGGG). Telomeres undergo shortening during successive cell divisions due to the insufficiency of DNA polymerase to replicate the lagging strand of DNA till its end. In 1971 James Watson discovered that extreme termini of chromosomes are lost during DNA replication. He called it as end-replication problem. Due to this phenomenon telomere shortens by 20–40 bp per year. Critical shortening of telomere gives rise to dysfunctional telomere that initiates DNA damage responses (DDRs). DDRs may initiate oncogenic changes in cells and they continue to divide instead of going into senescence.

Telomerase enzyme which is active in highly proliferating cells such as cancer cells is able to reverse this shortening. Telomerase upregulation is found in over 90% of cancers. Telomere length is associated with genomic stability therefore inactivity of telomerase enzyme causes shortening of telomere and chromosomal instability, genetic rearrangement, and tumorigenesis. Highly active telomerase in rapidly proliferating cancer cells supports cell survival growth and metastasis. In turn Telomerase expression is regulated at transcriptional—post transcriptional and epigenetic levels. Telomere length is crucial to maintain genomic stability and cell survival. They undergo progressive shortening during successive cell divisions. Telomerase enzyme maintains telomere length hence increases the chances for cell survival. Therefore, telomere length and telomerase activity are very important for stability, propagation and survival of cancer cells. Systematic reviews and meta-analyses of the association or interaction between diet and telomerase activity or/and telomeric length or have revealed that there is an established association between certain types of nutrients and telomere length, but it is still far from fact to claim a cause-effect relationship between the two. Reasons for this ambiguity are very obvious. Variability in the type of diet used, duration and amount of diet consumed, heterogeneity of the disease, e.g. types of cancers, the presence of co-morbid like diabetes, use of tobacco are few of those factors which are supposed to affect the relationship between diet and telomere length. Nevertheless, mechanisms which are supposed to induce an association between the two are mainly oxidative stress, inflammation due to the presence of pro-inflammatory enzymes like cytokines.

Mediterranean diet is considered cancer protective diet due to polyunsaturated fatty acids that prevent telomere shortening over time. On the other hand, saturated fats, refined sugars, alcohol, tobacco are considered cancer stimulating diets as they promote telomere shortening. Diet deficiencies of vitamins, minerals, micronutrients like vitamin C, E, zinc, selenium makes cells susceptible to oxidative stress which can cause breaks in telomeric or sub-telomeric sequences.

9.6.5 Oxidative Stress

Cancer cells undergo abnormal and uncontrolled division for their rapid growth and metastasis. Their metabolism is therefore very high when compared to their normal cell counterparts. High metabolism produces oxidative stress, promoting an excess of ROS. To counter the effects of ROS many cancer cells have antioxidant defence mechanisms. A cancer preventive strategy may be aimed to enhance oxidative stress in cancer cells by selectively impairing their antioxidant mechanism. High oxidative stress promotes cell death and arrest growth and metastasis of cancer cells.

9.7 Nutrition and Epigenetics

The way nutrition affects gene regulation need to be discussed as there are various epigenetic modifications that can bring about change in gene expression. Emerging trends in the field of oncology are focusing on prevention of cancer through natural resources and a change in lifestyle pattern. An increasing body of evidence indicates that fruits and vegetables can influence epigenetic processes through dietary factors mentioned above like DNA methylation, histone modification, oxidative stress, telomerase activation, DNA damage/repair mechanism. Epigenetic modifications due to their profound impact on cell proliferation and differentiation can be regarded as dynamic hallmark of cancer [67]. The re-activation of tumour suppressor genes, initiation of apoptosis, the inhibition of oncogenes or cancer-related genes, and the activation of cell survival proteins are just a few of the activities that these bioactive nutrients are engaged in. The discovery that during carcinogenesis at least half of all tumour suppressor genes are inactivated through epigenetic mechanisms highlights the importance of epigenomic processes in cancer. Interestingly identical twins who showed the same genetic profile have almost the same epigenetic profile early in life, but with the passage of time and increasing exposure to environmental factors their epigenetic profile changes considerably and differ from each other.

During carcinogenesis processes, bioactive substances promote epigenetic alterations linked to the stimulation of tumour suppressor genes like p21WAF1/CIP1 and suppression of tumour promoting genes like the human telomerase reverse transcriptase.

These substances include sulforaphane, genistein, polyphenols, resveratrol, and curcumin, which are all found in foods like cruciferous vegetables, soybean, green tea, grapes, and turmeric, respectively. Cancer-fighting properties of dietary phytochemicals such tea polyphenols, sulforaphane (SFN), genistein, resveratrol, and curcumin have been established.

It is important to elaborate how diets interact with gene regulation through epigenetic phenomenon. Three mechanisms have been suggested for this interaction [29]. First, nutrients may act as an inhibitor of methyl group donors for SAM. Second diet may affect DNMTs hence preventing the utilization of methyl groups. Third dietary factors may involve in DNA demethylation. It is a frequently asked question how much nutrients thought to have cancer preventive elements/ mechanism should ideally be consumed. RDAs are adequate amounts of various micronutrients necessary to prevent deficiency disorders. However, for DNA repair and maintenance mechanism a higher level of such nutrients is required. Inadequate levels of cancer preventive nutrients are considered as harmful as exposure to carcinogens. The existing RDAs for dietary nutrients or some micronutrients may not be sufficient to prevent genomic instability, according to mounting evidence that greater amounts of many of these micronutrients may be required for important DNA maintenance activities. Reduced genomic stability due to suboptimal amounts of essential micronutrients required for DNA repair and maintenance will have effects akin to those of inherited genetic diseases or exposure to carcinogens. Tea polyphenols, curcumin, lycopene, genistein, sulforaphane, resveratrol, isothiocyanates, diallyl sulphide, silymarin, apigenin, rosmarinic acid, and gingerol are some of the epigenetic diet components that have demonstrated effectiveness against cancer. Moreover folate, vitamin B12, vitamin B6, choline, and methionine affect methyl groups supply in the biochemical process of DNA methylation [68].

9.7.1 Dietary Polyphenols

Plants are an abundant source of polyphenols, which are present in various food sources like fruits, vegetables, and spices. Polyphenoles are derivative of phenylalanine, which is a shikimic acid, a phenol intermediate. Based on their chemical structure they can be divided into various classes like flavonoids, phenolic acids, benzoquinones, stilbenes, liginins, xanthones, etc. Flavonoids are the largest class of polyphenols comprising of around 5000 polyphenols. Polyphenols cause change in DNMTs levels hence reducing their methylation activity and activation of tumour suppressor gene [67]. Moreover, dietary polyphenols may stimulate expression of tumour suppressing miRNAs and inhibiting expression of oncogenic micro RNAs through ROS mediated pathways [69]. Figure 9.4 shows the dietary sources of polyphenols and their effects on epigenetic processes, i.e. DNA methylation, Histone modification, and MicroRNA expression/inhibition.

9.7.2 Soybeans

Anthocyanidins is considered a sub-class of flavonoids found in soy beans and almost any type of berries. These chemical elements have been proposed as effective chemoprevention agents. They use oxidative stress induction to cause apoptosis in human leukaemia cell lines as part of their chemotherapy treatment. In the metastatic cell lines LoVo and LoVo/ADR of human colorectal cancer, delphinidin, and cyanidin are among the anthocyanidins that are thought to be lethal, causing oxidative stress via inactivating glutathione antioxidant system. Soy is also a DNMTs inhibitor by making a complex with them, reducing their methylation activity, activation of tumour suppressor genes hence playing a significant role in cancer prevention and therapy [70].

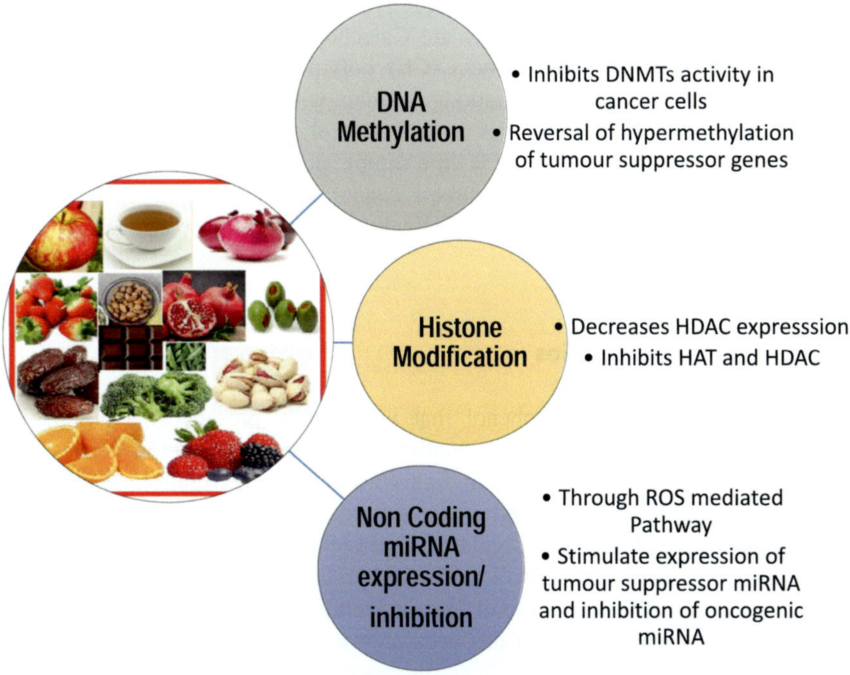

Fig. 9.4 Various dietary sources shown in the figure contain polyphenols (largest circle). These polyphenols show their anti-cancer activities through epigenetic pathways. Three epigenetic pathways are (top circle) inhibition of DNA methylation by decreased activity or inhibition of DNMTs; (middle circle) decreased HDAC activity and inhibiting both HAT and HDAC; (bottom circle) activation of tumour suppressing miRNA expression and inhibition of oncogenic miRNA expression

9.7.3 Green Tea

EGCG (2-epigallocatechin-3-gallate) is the major polyphenol found in green tea, EGCG is considered a potent demethylating agent. It inhibits methylation of *S*-adenosyl methionine (SAM) which acts as a methyl donor of catechol-*O*-amyltransferase (COMT) to inhibit catechol molecules including polyphenols [71]. Demethylation of SAM results in the formation of *S*-adenosyl L-homocysteine (SAH). SAH strongly inhibits DNMTs. In experimental research, the tea polyphenol [2]-epigallocatechin-3-gallate (EGCG) has also been hypothesized to show anti-cancer activity by inhibiting the folate pathway [72]. According to this hypothesis, if folate pathway blockage is the mechanism of EGCG's cancer preventive effects than women with low dietary folate consumption and high activity of the methylenetetrahydrofolate reductase (MTHFR) and thymidylate synthase (TYMS) genotypes would benefit more from the preventive impact of green tea against breast cancer. Epidemiological evidences provide support to the hypothesis of EGCG stimulating apoptosis and cell cycle arrest through folate pathway inhibition. However, genetic polymorphism of MTHFR and TYMS play a vital role in enhancing/lowering cancer preventive activity of EGCG. Other modifier reported for EGCG cancer preventive activity are Catechol-*O*-methyltransferase (COMT) and angiotensic converting enzyme (ACE) polymorphism. Green tea catechin protected against breast cancer among women with low activity Catechol-*O*-methyltransferase alleles. This was a case–control study which was conducted among Asian-American women [73]. In a sample population of Singaporean Chinese women, a decreased risk of breast cancer was found among those who consumed more green tea and had ACE genotype associated with the low gene activity [74].

9.7.4 Nuts and Berries

Resveratrol is a dietary polyphenol that is naturally present in a number of foods, including grape skin, peanuts, mulberries, cranberries, and blueberries. The antioxidant, anti-inflammatory, and anti-cancer effects of resveratrol are exhibited through a variety of molecular and metabolic processes. Resveratrol, for instance, affects signalling pathways that regulate cell growth, division, death, angiogenesis, and tumour metastasis. Resveratrol has been demonstrated to inhibit the proliferation of cancer cells from a variety of organs, including liver, skin, breast, prostate, lung, and colon. Additionally, it has been shown that resveratrol suppresses cell migration, adhesion, and invasion in colon cancer cells.

Resveratrol shows DNMT inhibitory activity as well as prevention of silencing BRCA 1 tumour suppressor genes. Resveratrol activation of HDAC inhibitors like SIRT-1 and p300 plays an important role in preventing tumorigenesis through histone chemical modification.

9.7.5 Spices

Spices like turmeric, cinnamon (cinnamic acid), chilli pepper, oregano, garlic, black pepper have also been claimed to show promising anti-cancer activity through epigenetic mechanisms. Many of these compounds kill cancer cells by changing the biology and physiology of cancer microenvironment.

9.8 Roles of Nutrigenomics in Upregulation of Tumour Suppressor Genes and Downregulation of Oncogenes

As the fields of genetics and nutrition come together, nutrigenomics is emerging as a new specialization. It is believed to be crucial in the early detection and prevention of tumours. Future cancer incidence is expected to rise; hence an effective preventative strategy is needed to meet this issue. The chance of developing cancer may be decreased by changing dietary habits. There is need to evaluate the effect of particular foods or any other ingredient that is biologically active and their link with cancer. As it can help in assessing the effectiveness of dietary treatments. In general, accurate and easily accessible biomarkers must be used to assess a person's susceptibility to cancer. Although the response of people to bioactive food components is dependent on both the target tissues and the effective concentration of the bioactive food components. Due to this fact, each person's reaction to food components differs from the other. Nutrigenomics is the study of how genes and diet interact in an individual and how a person's genes affect how they react to bioactive food components. It has been demonstrated that nutrients influence gene expression and alter DNA and protein molecule structure. Nutrigenomic techniques offer a chance to investigate how diet influences gene variants and epigenetic processes as well as how nutrients modulate gene expression. It may be possible to identify target molecules crucial in cancer prevention and/or symptom reduction by identifying the elements engaged in interactions between genes and nutrition in a person.

Proto-oncogenes turn become oncogenes through the process of carcinogenesis, which is the buildup of mutagens or epigenetic modifications in the genes. Resulting from chromosomal rearrangements and mutational shift, tumour suppressor genes (TP35) are silenced. Nutritional variables may influence this process through processes that encourage or impede its development. In addition to carcinogens, some foods may also include compounds that work to lessen the genetic harm produced by environmental mutagens.

Genetic research has made it feasible to comprehend how nutrients affect bodily functions at the molecular level as well as how various nutritional elements affect people differently. Nutrigenomics seeks to comprehend how each gene works and how it interacts with food in order to improve health and lower the chance of disease development [75]. Genome anomalies such as hyper or hypomethylation, mRNA downregulation, and histone deacetylation are identified as confirmed indicators in malignant cells [76]. Tumour suppressor genes are silenced by methylation within their promoter regions, and methylation inside the gene itself can result in mutational events. These pathways might be crucial in triggering the emergence of numerous different types of human malignancies. For cell differentiation and embryonic development, DNA methylation is crucial. Many studies on DNA methylation and the disease have been concentrated on cancer and tumour suppressor genes. Due to hypermethylation, tumour suppressor genes are frequently silenced in cancer cells. The genomes of cancer cells have been shown to be typically hypomethylated as compared to normal cells, with the exception of hypermethylation events at genes involved in cell cycle regulation, tumour cell invasion, DNA repair, and other activities in which silence propagates metastasis. Hypermethylation is really detectable early in some cancers, like colon cancer, and it may act as a diagnostic for the illness [77].

Over the course of five to six decades, physiologic and pathologic processes of epigenetic mechanisms are changed by nutrients. The tissue microenvironment and organizational structure of the tissue appears to have an impact on the different phases of the carcinogenesis. Prior to the clonal growth of heterogeneous populations, there are significant chances for cancer prevention in the early stages of its development. Nutrigenomics can be used as a technique in the investigation and prevention of numerous illnesses, including cancer. In the absence of changes in the DNA sequence, epigenetic processes such as DNA methylation and histone modifications control how genes are expressed and how chromatin is organized. The accumulation of epigenetic alterations that come with ageing may enhance cancer susceptibility, and this increased susceptibility could be a target for bioactive chemical therapy. The response to dietary components is mediated by nuclear receptors and transcription factors, which act as sensors for dietary components and control changes in the profile of transcripts [78].

The "Breast Cancer Type 1 Susceptibility Gene" is a tumour suppressor that performs the role of a caretaker gene, which means that it works with other oncosuppressors to repair damaged DNA [79, 80]. A few of the key processes that modulates protein are Cell cycle, transcription, genomic integrity, ubiquitination, and transcriptional control [81]. Researchers evaluated the effects of a genistein-enriched [4 and 10 ppm] diet using a murine and an in vitro cellular model. It was discovered that genistein supplementation increased BRCA1 protein levels, decreased CpG methylation levels, and lowered the affinity of BRCA1 exon 1a for the aryl hydrocarbon receptor (AHR) [82–84]. Genistein appears to have pleiotropic effects at the molecular level, activating a number of DNA damage checkpoints, causing cell cycle arrest, mitotic catastrophe, and cell death. It also causes an accumulation at G2/M, activating the chains of programmed cell death, up-regulating caspase-3 and caspase-7 as well as p38/MAPK and ATM/Chk2/Cdc25C/Cdc Genistein also fine-tunes many angiogenetic cascades [85, 86]. Genistein intake was reported to increase BRCA2 levels similarly to BRCA1 [84]. Genistein, but not daidzein, was shown to upregulate BRCA2 [87].

A number of tumour suppressor genes have been shown to be upregulated and oncogenes to be downregulated by genistein [88]. Other biological insults, such as high energy consumption, environmental pollutants, viruses, and/or bacteria, may alter the response. We may comprehend the variation in response with the aid of nutrigenomics. Nutrigenomics studies how dietary elements affect the coding and non-coding DNA segments of all the genes found in a specific species' genome in terms of its structure, function, and regulation. Food tolerance, food preference, transport, metabolism, and the effect on the target tissue are just a few of the ways that nutrigenomics might affect how the body responds to diet [5].

Regardless of intake of fat, protein, or alcohol, people with an SNP in the GLUT2 gene have a higher daily intake of sugars [89]. The Fok1 vitamin D receptor (VDR) polymorphism increases the risk of colorectal cancer in people who have the Ff or ff genotype. The risk of colon cancer rises in people with low calcium or low-fat intake in a gene-dose-dependent way, with people with the ff genotype showing an approximately 2.5-fold greater risk [90]. The relationship between lycopene and lower incidence of prostate cancer is another instance where preclinical evidence is indicative of protection. The reaction to lycopene may be affected by the XRCC1 (Arg399Gln) polymorphism [91]. Leafy green vegetables, folate, and multivitamin consumption were reported to significantly reduce the risk of methylation [92]. One key mechanism by which some foods affect gene expression patterns may include restoring correct methylation. Green tea's epigallocatechin-3-gallate, which blocks DNA methyltransferase 1's enzymatic activity, can reawaken methylation-silenced genes [28]. Additionally, in in vitro models of colorectal cancer, the Annurca polyphenol extract reversed methylation and reactivated the DNA repair mismatch gene hMLH1 [93]. Gene silencing and unsilencing may result from histone modification [94–96]. Histone acetylation, methylation, phosphorylation, ubiquitination, and biotinylation are reversible histone modifications that interact to control gene expression in addition to histone occupancy or the general recruitment and release of histones. The histone deacetylase (HDAC) enzyme can be modified to alter tumour behaviour [94, 95]. In addition to acting as an HDAC inhibitor and a powerful inducer of phase 2 detoxification enzymes, sulforaphane is a compound found in cruciferous vegetables. In humans, broccoli sprouts even in very small quantity immediately reduced HDAC activity, which remained for a considerable amount of time before returning to baseline levels within 24 h [97].

A systemic metabolic milieu that supports healthy cell replication and tissue integrity is primarily responsible for cancer protection. One of the key risk factors for a number of malignancies is dietary habits. It has been noted that certain dietary patterns, such as a diet high in sugar or meat (red meat, processed meat, fish, and processed fish), are linked to an increased risk of developing certain malignancies. Additionally, numerous lines of research showed that plant-based diets are rich in antioxidants and anti-inflammatory substances. Through a variety of mechanisms, such as hormone regulation, the downregulation of specific carcinogenic pathways, or the attenuation of inflammation, the dietary components present in vegetables and fruits work synergistically to lower the risk of cancer. These mechanisms may be suitable for the prevention of various cancers. A balanced diet that is rich in lean proteins, fruits and vegetables, whole grains, and low-fat dairy, while being low in sugar, caffeine, red meat, and alcohol, seems to be the perfect recipe. There is no evidence in the scientific community that a certain diet helps cure or treat cancer. The sufficient evidence suggests that a healthy lifestyle and dietary habits, however, can help lower the chance of acquiring some cancers.

9.9 Future Perspective

The field of genomics and nutrigenomics has made the progress at exponential rates in the recent times. However, the more effective integration of nutritional status, disease history, and genetic makeup is needed to produce more thorough phenotypic profiles for effectively using the nutrigenomic for cancer prevention and control. In order for nutrigenomics to realize its full potential, the significance of adopting a systematic approach is stressed for future research, in human subjects to fully encompass the complete range of diet interactions. More and more research is needed as the relative involvement of different genes to the emergence of chronic disease is still up for debate. Despite the fact that many genetic loci (gene variations) have been known as having a specific role in different diseases. However, they collectively account for less than 3% of fully understanding the disease. Therefore, neither our genes nor our diets can fully account for why some people are inclined to acquire specific illnesses. A person's environment and genetic makeup interact intricately to determine how their genes are expressed. It requires major research that how nutrigenomics can support individual diet and lifestyle changes by creating algorithms that integrated data on diet, phenotype, and genotype, and whether these approaches can provide greater health benefits than adhering to traditional dietary recommendations. A personalized dietary approach based on counselling and tailored approaches employing genotypic and phenotypic data were not significantly different from one another. There is still much to learn and determine in the field of combining bioinformatics, nutrition, epidemiology, molecular biology, and genomics, but nutrigenomics research in the future will undoubtedly offer more fascinating insights into both nutritional science and the human genome.

References

1. Braicu C, Mehterov N, Vladimirov B, Sarafian V, Nabavi SM, Atanasov AG et al (2017) Nutrigenomics in cancer: revisiting the effects of natural compounds. Semin Cancer Biol 46:84–106
2. German JB (2005) Genetic dietetics: nutrigenomics and the future of dietetics practice. J Am Diet Assoc 105(4):530–531
3. Lampe JW, Navarro SL, Hullar MA, Shojaie A (2013) Inter-individual differences in response to dietary intervention: integrating omics platforms towards personalised dietary recommendations. Proc Nutr Soc 72(2):207–218
4. Ordovas JM, Ferguson LR, Tai ES, Mathers JC (2018) Personalised nutrition and health. BMJ 361:k2173
5. Lampe JW, Potter JD, Costa L (2006) Eaton DJG-EIFoE. Genetic variation, diet and disease susceptibility 321–350
6. Organization WH (2014) Global status report on noncommunicable diseases 2014. World Health Organization
7. Reen JK, Yadav AK, Singh J (2015) Nutrigenomics: concept, advances and applications. Asian J Dairy and Food Res 34(3):205–212
8. Garg R, Sharma N, Jain SKJAMI (2014) Nutrigenomics and nutrigenetics: concepts and applications in nutrition research and practice 1(2):124
9. Kussmann M, Fay LB (2008) Nutrigenomics and personalized nutrition: science and concept. Pers Med 5(5):447–455
10. Panagiotou G, Nielsen J (2009) Nutritional systems biology: definitions and approaches. Annu Rev Nutr 29:329–339
11. Nelson MR, Marnellos G, Kammerer S, Hoyal CR, Shi MM, Cantor CR et al (2004) Large-scale validation of single nucleotide polymorphisms in gene regions. Genome Res 14(8):1664–1668
12. Kaput J, Rodriguez RL (2004) Nutritional genomics: the next frontier in the postgenomic era. Physiol Genomics 16(2):166–177
13. Milner JA (2004) Molecular targets for bioactive food components. J Nutr 134(9):2492s-s2498
14. Mierziak J, Kostyn K, Boba A, Czemplik M, Kulma A, Wojtasik W (2021) Influence of the bioactive diet components on the gene expression regulation. Nutrients 13(11)

15. Milner JA, McDonald SS, Anderson DE, Greenwald P (2001) Molecular targets for nutrients involved with cancer prevention. Nutr Cancer 41(1–2):1–16
16. Hardy TM, Tollefsbol TO (2011) Epigenetic diet: impact on the epigenome and cancer. Epigenomics 3(4):503–518
17. Ross SA, Davis CD (2011) MicroRNA, nutrition, and cancer prevention. Adv Nutr 2(6):472–485
18. Mirabello L, Huang WY, Wong JY, Chatterjee N, Reding D, Crawford ED et al (2009) The association between leukocyte telomere length and cigarette smoking, dietary and physical variables, and risk of prostate cancer. Aging Cell 8(4):405–413
19. Kaur S, Kumar SJIFNM (2020) Crosstalk between food components and microRNAs: role in metabolism, nutrition, health and diseases 7:1–11
20. Sanchita TR, Asif MH, Trivedi PK (2018) Dietary plant miRNAs as an augmented therapy: cross-kingdom gene regulation. RNA Biol 15(12):1433–1439
21. Lyon P, Strippoli V, Fang B, Cimmino L (2020) B vitamins and one-carbon metabolism: implications in human health and disease. Nutrients 12(9)
22. Hueda MC (2017) Functional food: improve health through adequate food: BoD—books on demand
23. McNulty H, Pentieva K (2004) Folate bioavailability. Proc Nutr Soc 63(4):529–536
24. Nasir A, Bullo MMH, Ahmed Z, Imtiaz A, Yaqoob E, Safdar M et al (2022) Nutrigenomics: epigenetics and cancer prevention: a comprehensive review 60(8):1375–1387
25. Dashwood RH, Myzak MC, Ho E (2006) Dietary HDAC inhibitors: time to rethink weak ligands in cancer chemoprevention? Carcinogenesis 27(2):344–349
26. Mendoza N, Silva EM (2018) Introduction to phytochemicals: secondary metabolites from plants with active principles for pharmacological importance. Phytochem Source Antioxid Role Dis Prev 25:1–5
27. Fang M, Chen D, Yang CS (2007) Dietary polyphenols may affect DNA methylation. J Nutr 137(1 Suppl):223s-s228
28. Fang MZ, Wang Y, Ai N, Hou Z, Sun Y, Lu H et al (2003) Tea polyphenol (−)-epigallocatechin-3-gallate inhibits DNA methyltransferase and reactivates methylation-silenced genes in cancer cell lines. Cancer Res 63(22):7563–7570
29. Ross SA (2003) Diet and DNA methylation interactions in cancer prevention. Ann NY Acad Sci 983:197–207
30. Longo VD, Fontana L (2010) Calorie restriction and cancer prevention: metabolic and molecular mechanisms. Trends Pharmacol Sci 31(2):89–98
31. Ciancarelli MGT, Di Massimo C, De Amicis D, Ciancarelli IJMRA (2017) Mediterranean diet and health promotion: evidence and current concerns. Med Res Arch 5(7)
32. Mansouri K, Rasoulpoor S, Daneshkhah A, Abolfathi S, Salari N, Mohammadi M et al (2020) Clinical effects of curcumin in enhancing cancer therapy: a systematic review. BMC Cancer 20(1):791
33. Machowetz A, Poulsen HE, Gruendel S, Weimann A, Fitó M, Marrugat J et al (2007) Effect of olive oils on biomarkers of oxidative DNA stress in Northern and Southern Europeans. FASEB J 21(1):45–52
34. Fitó M, Cladellas M, de la Torre R, Martí J, Muñoz D, Schröder H et al (2008) Anti-inflammatory effect of virgin olive oil in stable coronary disease patients: a randomized, crossover, controlled trial. Eur J Clin Nutr 62(4):570–574
35. Rossi M, Turati F, Lagiou P, Trichopoulos D, Augustin LS, La Vecchia C et al (2013) Mediterranean diet and glycaemic load in relation to incidence of type 2 diabetes: results from the Greek cohort of the population-based European Prospective Investigation into Cancer and Nutrition (EPIC). Diabetologia 56(11):2405–2413
36. Praud D, Bertuccio P, Bosetti C, Turati F, Ferraroni M, La Vecchia C (2014) Adherence to the Mediterranean diet and gastric cancer risk in Italy. Int J Cancer 134(12):2935–2941
37. Turati F, Bravi F, Polesel J, Bosetti C, Negri E, Garavello W et al (2017) Adherence to the Mediterranean diet and nasopharyngeal cancer risk in Italy. Cancer Causes Control 28(2):89–95

38. Pitsavos C, Panagiotakos DB, Tzima N, Chrysohoou C, Economou M, Zampelas A et al (2005) Adherence to the Mediterranean diet is associated with total antioxidant capacity in healthy adults: the ATTICA study. Am J Clin Nutr 82(3):694–699
39. Pérez-Jiménez J, Díaz-Rubio ME, Saura-Calixto F (2015) Contribution of macromolecular antioxidants to dietary antioxidant capacity: a study in the Spanish Mediterranean Diet. Plant Foods Human Nutr 70(4):365–370
40. Manach C, Scalbert A, Morand C, Rémésy C, Jiménez L (2004) Polyphenols: food sources and bioavailability. Am J Clin Nutr 79(5):727–747
41. Castelló A, Boldo E, Pérez-Gómez B, Lope V, Altzibar JM, Martín V et al (2017) Adherence to the Western, Prudent and Mediterranean dietary patterns and breast cancer risk: MCC-Spain study. Maturitas 103:8–15
42. Mentella MC, Scaldaferri F, Ricci C, Gasbarrini A, Miggiano GAD (2019) Cancer and Mediterranean diet: a review. Nutrients 11(9)
43. Hunter DJ, Reddy KS (2013) Noncommunicable diseases. N Engl J Med 369(14):1336–1343
44. NCD Countdown 2030 (2018) Worldwide trends in non-communicable disease mortality and progress towards Sustainable Development Goal target 3.4. Lancet 392(10152):1072–1088
45. Organization WH (2018) Noncommunicable diseases country profiles 2018
46. Sagner M, Egger G, Binns A, Rossner S (2017) Lifestyle medicine: lifestyle, the environment and preventive medicine in health and disease. Academic Press
47. Galambos L, Sturchio JL, Whitehead RC (2014) Noncommunicable diseases in the developing world: addressing gaps in Global Policy and Research. JHU Press
48. (WHO) WHO. Cancer 2018. https://www.who.int/news-room/fact-sheets/detail/cancer
49. Elsamanoudy AZ, Mohamed Neamat-Allah MA, Hisham Mohammad FA, Hassanien M, Nada HA (2016) The role of nutrition related genes and nutrigenetics in understanding the pathogenesis of cancer. J Microsc Ultrastruct 4(3):115–122
50. Patel A, Pathak Y, Patel J, Sutariya V (2018) Role of nutritional factors in pathogenesis of cancer. Food Quality Safety 2(1):27–36
51. Ferlay J, Colombet M, Soerjomataram I, Parkin DM, Piñeros M, Znaor A et al (2021) Cancer statistics for the year 2020: an overview. Int J Cancer
52. Rohan TE, Bain CJ (1987) Diet in the etiology of breast cancer. Epidemiol Rev 9:120–145
53. Chittiboyina S, Chen Z, Chiorean EG, Kamendulis LM, Hocevar BA (2018) The role of the folate pathway in pancreatic cancer risk. PLoS ONE 13(2):e0193298
54. Choi SW, Mason JB (2000) Folate and carcinogenesis: an integrated scheme. J Nutr 130(2):129–132
55. Kadayifci FZ, Zheng S, Pan YX (2018) Molecular mechanisms underlying the link between diet and DNA methylation. Int J Mol Sci 19(12)
56. Tang PK (2016) Consume, digest, and expire: the risks of domesticated carcinogens. Lancet Oncol 17(1):24–25
57. Nicastro HL, Trujillo EB, Milner JA (2012) Nutrigenomics and cancer prevention. Curr Nutr Rep 1(1):37–43
58. Vanden BW (2012) Epigenetic impact of dietary polyphenols in cancer chemoprevention: lifelong remodeling of our epigenomes. Pharmacol Res 65(6):565–576
59. Marcum JA (2019) The cancer epigenome: a review. J Biotechnol Biomed (3):67–83
60. Irimie AI, Braicu C, Pasca S, Magdo L, Gulei D, Cojocneanu R et al (2019) Role of key micronutrients from nutrigenetic and nutrigenomic perspectives in cancer prevention. Medicina 55(6)
61. Calado A, Neves PM, Santos T, Ravasco P (2018) The effect of flaxseed in breast cancer: a literature review. Front Nutr 5:4
62. De Silva SF, Alcorn J (2019) Flaxseed lignans as important dietary polyphenols for cancer prevention and treatment: chemistry, pharmacokinetics, and molecular targets. Pharmaceuticals 12(2)
63. Martín-Hernández R, Reglero G, Dávalos AJ (2018) Data mining of nutrigenomics experiments: identification of a cancer protective gene signature. J Funct Foods 42:380–386

64. Royston KJ, Paul B, Nozell S, Rajbhandari R, Tollefsbol TO (2018) Withaferin A and sulforaphane regulate breast cancer cell cycle progression through epigenetic mechanisms. Exp Cell Res 368(1):67–74
65. Kang JX (2013) Nutrigenomics and cancer therapy. J Nutrigen Nutrigenom 6(3):I-ii
66. Marcum JA (2020) Nutrigenetics/nutrigenomics, personalized nutrition, and precision healthcare. Curr Nutr Rep 9(4):338–345
67. Arora I, Sharma M, Tollefsbol TO (2019) Combinatorial epigenetics impact of polyphenols and phytochemicals in cancer prevention and therapy. Int J Mol Sci 20(18)
68. Davis CD, Uthus EO (2004) DNA methylation, cancer susceptibility, and nutrient interactions. Exp Biol Med 229(10):988–995
69. Yoshioka Y, Ohishi T, Nakamura Y, Fukutomi R, Miyoshi N (2022) Anti-cancer effects of dietary polyphenols via ROS-mediated pathway with their modulation of MicroRNAs. Molecules 27(12)
70. Xie Q, Bai Q, Zou LY, Zhang QY, Zhou Y, Chang H et al (2014) Genistein inhibits DNA methylation and increases expression of tumor suppressor genes in human breast cancer cells. Genes Chromosom Cancer 53(5):422–431
71. Link A, Balaguer F, Goel A (2010) Cancer chemoprevention by dietary polyphenols: promising role for epigenetics. Biochem Pharmacol 80(12):1771–1792
72. Inoue M, Robien K, Wang R, Van Den Berg DJ, Koh WP, Yu MC (2008) Green tea intake, MTHFR/TYMS genotype and breast cancer risk: the Singapore Chinese Health Study. Carcinogenesis 29(10):1967–1972
73. Wu AH, Tseng CC, Van Den Berg D, Yu MC (2003) Tea intake, COMT genotype, and breast cancer in Asian-American women. Cancer Res 63(21):7526–7529
74. Yuan JM, Koh WP, Sun CL, Lee HP, Yu MC (2005) Green tea intake, ACE gene polymorphism and breast cancer risk among Chinese women in Singapore. Carcinogenesis 26(8):1389–1394
75. Wajed SA, Laird PW, DeMeester TR (2001) DNA methylation: an alternative pathway to cancer. Ann Surg 234(1):10–20
76. Ardekani AM, Jabbari S (2009) Nutrigenomics and cancer. Avicenna J Med Biotechnol 1(1):9–17
77. Nepomuceno JC (2013) Nutrigenomics and cancer prevention. In: Cancer treatment. IntechOpen, pp 391–416
78. Fujii T, Medeiros RT, Yamada R (eds) (2010) Nutrigenomics and nutrigenetics: important concepts for the nutrition science
79. Jhanwar-Uniyal M (2003) BRCA1 in cancer, cell cycle and genomic stability. Front Biosci 8:s1107–s1117
80. De la Torre C, Pincheira J, López-Sáez JF (2003) Human syndromes with genomic instability and multiprotein machines that repair DNA double-strand breaks. Histol Histopathol 18(1):225–243
81. Walsh MF, Nathanson KL, Couch FJ, Offit K (2016) Genomic biomarkers for breast cancer risk. Adv Exp Med Biol 882:1–32
82. Donovan MG, Selmin OI, Doetschman TC, Romagnolo DF (2019) Epigenetic activation of BRCA1 by genistein in vivo and triple negative breast cancer cells linked to antagonism toward aryl hydrocarbon receptor. Nutrients 11(11)
83. Cabanes A, Wang M, Olivo S, DeAssis S, Gustafsson JA, Khan G et al (2004) Prepubertal estradiol and genistein exposures up-regulate BRCA1 mRNA and reduce mammary tumorigenesis. Carcinogenesis 25(5):741–748
84. Bernard-Gallon DJ, Satih S, Chalabi N, Rabiau N, Bosviel R, Fontana L et al (2010) Phytoestrogens regulate the expression of genes involved in different biological processes in BRCA2 knocked down MCF-7, MDA-MB-231 and MCF-10a cell lines. Oncol Rep 23(3):647–653
85. Varinska L, Gal P, Mojzisova G, Mirossay L, Mojzis J (2015) Soy and breast cancer: focus on angiogenesis. Int J Mol Sci 16(5):11728–11749
86. Křížová L, Dadáková K, Kašparovská J, Kašparovský T (2019) Isoflavones 24(6):1076

87. Vissac-Sabatier C, Bignon YJ, Bernard-Gallon DJ (2003) Effects of the phytoestrogens genistein and daidzein on BRCA2 tumor suppressor gene expression in breast cell lines. Nutr Cancer 45(2):247–255
88. Hilakivi-Clarke L, Andrade JE, Helferich W (2010) Is soy consumption good or bad for the breast? J Nutr 140(12):2326s-s2334
89. Eny KM, Wolever TM, Fontaine-Bisson B, El-Sohemy A (2008) Genetic variant in the glucose transporter type 2 is associated with higher intakes of sugars in two distinct populations. Physiol Genomics 33(3):355–360
90. Wong H-L, Seow A, Arakawa K, Lee H-P, Yu MC, Ingles SAJC (2003) Vitamin D receptor start codon polymorphism and colorectal cancer risk: effect modification by dietary calcium and fat in Singapore Chinese. Carcinogenesis 24(6):1091–1095
91. Goodman M, Bostick RM, Ward KC, Terry PD, van Gils CH, Taylor JA et al (2006) Lycopene intake and prostate cancer risk: effect modification by plasma antioxidants and the XRCC1 genotype. Nutr Cancer 55(1):13–20
92. Stidley CA, Picchi MA, Leng S, Willink R, Crowell RE, Flores KG et al (2010) Multivitamins, folate, and green vegetables protect against gene promoter methylation in the aerodigestive tract of smokers. Cancer Res 70(2):568–574
93. Fini L, Selgrad M, Fogliano V, Graziani G, Romano M, Hotchkiss E et al (2007) Annurca apple polyphenols have potent demethylating activity and can reactivate silenced tumor suppressor genes in colorectal cancer cells. J Nutr 137(12):2622–2628
94. Glozak MA, Seto E (2007) Histone deacetylases and cancer. Oncogene 26(37):5420–5432
95. Myzak MC, Dashwood RH (2006) Histone deacetylases as targets for dietary cancer preventive agents: lessons learned with butyrate, diallyl disulfide, and sulforaphane. Curr Drug Targets 7(4):443–452
96. Holloway AF, Oakford PC (2007) Targeting epigenetic modifiers in cancer. Curr Med Chem 14(24):2540–2547
97. Dashwood RH, Ho E (2007) Dietary histone deacetylase inhibitors: from cells to mice to man. Semin Cancer Biol 17(5):363–369

Cancer Prevention and Treatment Based on Lifestyles

10

Deeba Amraiz, Aysha Karim Kiani, Uzma Azeem Awan, Tayyaba Amraiz, Bushra Azeem Awan, and Muhammad Irfan

Contents

D. Amraiz (✉) · A. K. Kiani · U. A. Awan
Department of Biological Sciences, National University of Medical Sciences, Rawalpindi, Pakistan
e-mail: deeba.amraiz@numspak.edu.pk

U. A. Awan
School of Chemistry and Biochemistry, Georgia Institute of Technology, Atlanta, USA

T. Amraiz
Department of Biosciences, COMSATS University Islamabad, Islamabad, Pakistan

B. A. Awan
Department of Physiotherapy, University of Lahore, Lahore, Pakistan

M. Irfan
Department of Zoology Wildlife and Fisheries, PMAS-Arid Agriculture University Rawalpindi, Rawalpindi, Pakistan

R. F. Saeed and S. ul. Shaheed (eds.), *Nutrition and Dietary Interventions in Cancer*, Cancer Treatment and Research 191, https://doi.org/10.1007/978-3-031-55622-7_10

Abbreviations

AEs	Adverse events
BCC	Basal cell carcinoma
BHB	β-Hydroxybutyrate
BMI	Body mass index
CAM	Complementary and alternative medicine
CDKs	Cyclin-dependent kinases
CHO	Carbohydrate
CRC	Colorectal cancer
CRF	Cancer-related fatigue
DSR	Differential stress resistances
DSS	Differential stress sensitization
EGFR	Epidermal growth factor receptor
FMD	Fasting mimicking diet
GFs	Growth factors
GLUTs	Glucose transporters
Hcar2	Hydroxycarboxylic acid receptor 2
HNC	Head and neck cancer
ICNIRP	International commission on non-ionizing radiation protection
IF	Intermittent fasting
IGF-1	Insulin-like growth factor-1
IGFBPs	IGF-1-binding proteins
KD	Ketogenic diet
mTOR	Mammalian target of rapamycin
NMDA	N-methyl-D-aspartate
OCC	Oral cavity cancer
OPC	Oropharyngeal cancer
OxPhos	Oxidative phosphorylation
PAHs	Polycyclic aromatic hydrocarbons
PC	Pharyngeal cancer
QOL	Quality of life
RF	Radio frequency

RNS	Reactive nitrogen species
ROS	Reactive oxygen species
STF	Short-term fasting
Tregs	T-regulatory cells
VDR	Vitamin D receptor
VOCs	Volatile organic compounds

10.1 Introduction

The burden of cancer is unlikely to be totally eliminated despite advancements in cancer therapies and detection techniques. A logical approach to controlling cancer is primary prevention while also looking for novel treatments and earlier detection. The implementation of lifestyle changes aimed at enhancing primary prevention and reducing the risk of cancer involves various strategies. These strategies encompass opting for a healthy diet that primarily comprises plant-based foods, maintaining a healthy weight throughout one's lifetime, engaging in regular physical activity, limiting or completely eliminating the consumption of tobacco/alcohol, avoiding exposure to radiation and other carcinogens. These strategies for cancer prevention are anticipated to exert a significant influence on the occurrence of various cancers, including melanoma, breast cancer, colorectal cancer, oesophageal cancers, liver cancers, and head and neck cancers [1]. The routine use of sunscreen, wearing protective clothes, finding shade, minimizing outdoor activities between 10 am and 2 pm, and refraining from indoor tanning are all part of the lifestyle recommendations for melanomas [2]. The association of cancer risk, including lung cancer, with the intake of carotenoids has been studied, and it was found that increased consumption of β-carotene and vitamin A was notably linked to a decreased risk of developing cancer [3]. Approximately 90% of individuals diagnosed with lung cancer are smokers, and the combination of alcohol consumption with cigarette smoking can increase the risk of cancer development. Globally, smokeless tobacco usage accounts for 400,000 cases of oral cancer, constituting 4% of all cancer types [4]. Therefore, avoiding tobacco products and limiting alcohol use would probably have a significant impact on the incidence of cancer. A strong correlation between diet, obesity, and metabolic syndrome and different types of cancer has been found. These factors may contribute to approximately 30–35% of cancer-related deaths, suggesting that a considerable proportion of such fatalities can be prevented by making dietary modifications and including them in the standard cancer treatment regimes. These include fasting and fasting mimicking diets, ketogenic diets, calorie restriction, etc. [5]. In this chapter, we discuss lifestyle intervention strategies to improve cancer prevention and risk reduction while promoting the health of cancer patients. The therapeutic role of some dietary regimens and supplements, along with complementary and alternative health approaches, in cancer treatment has also been discussed here.

10.2 Fasting and Fasting Mimicking Diet

Fasting, a practice rooted in religious customs, involves voluntarily refraining from consuming any food or specific types of food for an allocated time. Extended periods of fasting (long-term fasting), lasting for a few consecutive weeks or months, may not be suitable for cancer patients in the field of oncology due to the possibility of causing unintended weight loss, which is undesirable. Nevertheless, shorter-term fasting approaches, conducted over a span of weeks or months, incorporating fasting durations ranging from 12 to 72 h with unrestricted eating during designated feeding hours, could potentially be manageable and appropriate for individuals with cancer [6]. Due to the potential of Intermittent fasting (IF) to alter nutrient metabolism and energy balance, promote better health, and influence the onset of various diseases in the field of oncology in particular, IF is gaining significant attention globally. IF is a dietary pattern represented by alternating periods of eating and fasting and involves a calorie-restricted eating regimen for 1–3 days per week. Fasting mimicking diet (FMD), which consists of a low calorie and protein, plant-based diet for a period of three to five days within each chemotherapy cycle, is a less intense dietary approach than fasting [7]. The types of various fasting regimens are given in Table 10.1.

10.2.1 Signalling Pathways in Cancer and the Role of Nutritional Interventions

Tumour cells exhibit a range of characteristics that contribute to their malignant behaviour. These include augmented proliferation rates, loss or disruption of tumour suppressor mechanisms, the capacity of invading and metastasizing other tissues and organs, induction of angiogenesis, evasion of apoptosis and immune destruction, and changes in metabolic pathways. The presence of sugars and amino

Table 10.1 Types and definitions of various fasting regimens

Fasting regimen	Definition	Reference
Fasting	Voluntarily refraining from consuming any food or specific types of food for a certain period of time	[13]
Intermittent fasting	A calorie restricted eating regimen or water-only fasting that alternates between periods of eating and fasting for 1–3 days per week	[13, 14]
Periodic fasting	A severely calorie-restricted diet or water-only fasting lasting for 48 h and, in some cases, 1 week or longer	[17]
Short term fasting	A temporary fasting period, usually lasting from 12 to 72 h, for example alternate day fasting	[18]
Fasting mimicking diet	Cycles of fasting or low-calorie diet which is low in carbohydrates, proteins, and high in unsaturated fats	[16, 19]

acids has an impact on several key characteristics associated with cancer, and this impact is, in part, mediated through the regulation of signalling pathways such as insulin-like growth factor-1 (IGF-1), Rat sarcoma (Ras), protein kinase A (PKA), and phosphatidylinositol-3 kinase (PI3K)–AKT [8]. The constitutive activation of these signalling pathways can also arise from mutations in oncogenes. To fulfil the heightened bioenergetic and biosynthetic requirements, these pathways often stimulate glycolysis, resulting in upregulated expression of glycolytic enzymes and glucose transporters within cancer cells. Consequently, various types of tumour cells rely on the enhancement of glucose or specific amino acid supply [9]. Hyperglycaemia has been linked to decreased progression-free survival or overall survival in patients suffering from cancer [10]. This highlights the significance of altered metabolic demands and glucose utilization in cancer progression and patient outcomes, thus indicating the effectiveness of nutritional interventions in the regulation of cancer cells growth and survival. Fasting in this regard, has been shown to enhance lifelong health by slowing aging, promoting longevity, reducing oxidative stress and inflammation, initiating cellular repair, and improving the functions of the brain and heart [11]. Fasting exhibits promising potential for both preventing and treating cancer by augmenting the effectiveness and tolerability of anticancer therapeutics. Furthermore, fasting appears to enhance the quality of life in individuals with cancer through multiple adaptive biological mechanisms induced by the fasting regimen [12].

10.2.2 Effects of Various Fasting Regimens on Cancer Cells

Recent studies have demonstrated that the modification of cancer cells energy metabolism, can further lead to the inhibition of tumour growth and strengthen the immune defence system against tumours. Moreover, IF has been shown to reduce the side effects of chemotherapy and radiotherapy while increasing the susceptibility of cancer cells to these conventional cancer treatments. Consequently, IF is increasingly being recognized as a promising approach in the realm of clinical cancer therapy [13, 14]. The administration of fasting or an FMD can result in low levels of blood glucose and insulin-like growth factor-1 (IGF1). These modifications influence several cellular signalling pathways, encompassing Akt, Ras, and the mammalian target of rapamycin (mTOR), which leads to the inhibition of cell multiplication and growth [15]. This is crucial because cancer cells primarily rely on glucose metabolism, making them more susceptible to the effects of chemotherapy when exposed to FMD (Fig. 10.1). This process, known as differential stress sensitization (DSS), enhances the effectiveness of cancer treatment. Fasting also triggers a response known as differential stress resistance (DSR) to nutritional stress. During DSR, healthy cells allocate their resources towards protection and internal repair, potentially resulting in reduced toxicity from chemotherapy. Recent preclinical studies demonstrated that fasting or FMD not only promotes the protection of healthy cells but also has the potential to benefit effector T cells, thus improving the body's immune response against tumours [16].

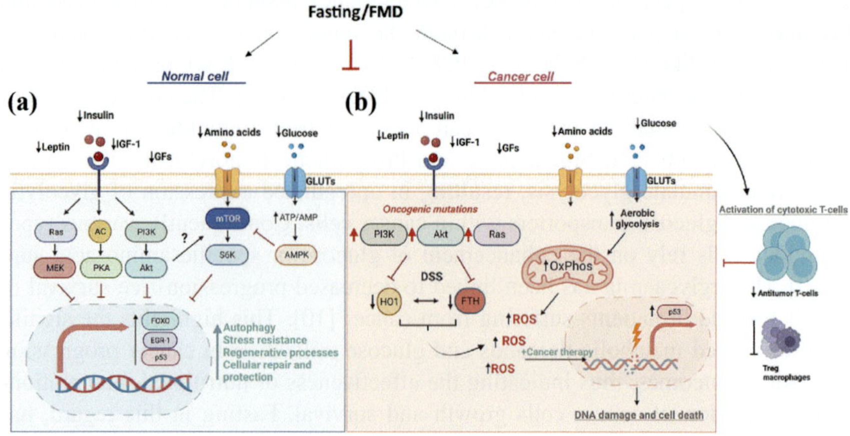

Fig. 10.1 Mechanistics of fasting or fasting mimicking diet in the prevention and treatment of cancer

Intermittent fasting (IF); periodic fasting (PF), short-term fasting (STF), fasting mimicking diet (FMD).

IGF-1, insulin like growth factor-1; GFs, growth factors, GLUTs, glucose transporters; OxPhose, oxidative phosphorylation; ROS, reactive oxygen species; Treg, T regulatory cells; PI3K/Akt, Ras/PKA and mTOR/S6K are the signalling molecules that are downregulated as a result of decreased insulin, leptin, and IGF-1 levels; FOXO, EGR-1, and P53 are the transcription factors that are then activated. Adapted from Blazevits et al. [20].

10.2.3 Fasting in Pre-clinical Studies of Cancer

The advantages of including fasting in cancer therapy have been clearly demonstrated in pre-clinical investigations. These include protecting healthy cells from the toxic effects of chemotherapy while simultaneously enhancing the vulnerability of tumour cells to chemotherapy and also boosting the chemotherapy induced intratumoural infiltration of CD8 + T cells, thereby delaying the advancement of the disease [21]. In mouse models of colon cancer, short-term fasting (STF) leads to glucose and amino acid deficiencies, resulting in the anti-Warburg effect. This effect is characterized by elevated oxygen consumption but an inability to produce ATP, leading to oxidative stress and apoptosis [22]. Recent studies in mice have shown that intermittent fasting cycles, involving refraining from food for 12–72 h followed by a period of refeeding, exhibit useful effects on lifespan, age-related diseases, health indicators, stress levels, metabolic response, and tissue regeneration [23, 24]. In experiments involving xenograft mouse models of breast cancer, melanoma, and neuroblastoma, the combination of fasting and high-dose chemotherapy offered protection to healthy cells against oxidative stress, DNA damage, and treatment-associated endometrial hyperplasia [21]. Furthermore, it was suggested in this study that two rounds of 48 h fasting alone proved to be equally effective as two rounds of chemotherapy in reducing the advancement of tumours [21]. These effects may result from a decrease in glucose levels, insulin, IGF-1, and inflammatory markers in the blood, along with an increase in IGF-1-binding proteins (IGFBPs) and ketone bodies [25]. These results indicate that the nonpharmacological management of diet along with standard therapies may play a significant role in enhancing survival rates for certain types of cancer.

10.2.4 Fasting in Clinical Studies of Cancer

Until now, only a limited number of small-scale clinical trials have been carried out to evaluate the significance of different forms of intermittent fasting along with chemotherapy in relation to cancer development and prognosis by assessing metabolic and hormonal factors. The design and findings of some of the studies are summarized in Table 10.2. These clinical studies demonstrated that incorporating fasting as a supplementary approach to chemotherapy is both safe and well-tolerated. Additionally, fasting may potentially decrease the toxicity associated with chemotherapy [15, 26–28]. A clinical trial was conducted to assess the safety, immunomodulatory, and metabolic effects of a cyclic, five-day fasting-mimicking diet (FMD) combined with conventional cancer treatments. Among a group of 101 patients, the FMD proved to be well-tolerated and feasible, with a consistent decrease in levels of blood glucose and growth factors. These observed metabolic changes reflect the metabolic alterations that contribute to the tumour suppressing effects of fasting/FMD, as observed in preclinical experiments. Furthermore, the FMD modifies both the overall immune response and the immune activity within tumours, ultimately triggering multiple anti-tumour immune mechanisms [29]. In a series of clinical trials, a cohort of over 300 cancer patients experienced FMD cycles in conjunction with other treatment modalities, and the incidence of adverse reactions linked to FMD cycles has been exceptionally low [26, 29, 30]. Furthermore, in clinical trials, FMDs have demonstrated numerous favourable effects on factors associated with cancer progression, including enhanced insulin sensitivity, decreased levels of glycaemia, insulin, and leptin, as well as diminished systemic inflammation [20].

Research is currently underway to investigate short-term, controlled, and flexible fasting regimens as a potentially powerful and affordable complement to standard cancer treatment protocols. Studies on preclinical models indicate that fasting targeted around chemotherapy or radiation may decrease the side effects of treatment and improve its effectiveness. Human trials are currently being conducted to assess the safety, tolerance, and underlying mechanisms of this approach.

Table 10.2 Clinical trials of various fasting regimens combined with conventional therapies

NCT number	Name of the study	Phase	Treatment	Tumour type	Study results
NCT04833439	The effect of a fasting mimicking diet on the immune system: an exploratory study	Not applicable	A plant-based diet low in calories, proteins for 3 days	Non-cancer, healthy subjects	Changes in the pattern of gene expression in peripheral blood mononuclear cells (PBMCs) was observed after an overnight period of fasting and upon completion of two cycles of a FMD, as compared to the initial condition
NCT03340935	Safety, feasibility and metabolic effects of the fasting mimicking diet (FMD) in cancer patients	Not applicable	Fasting Mimicking Diet (or FMD) consists in a 5-day plant-based, low-calorie (600 kcal on day 1, followed by 300 kcal/day on days 2 to 5), low-protein, low carbohydrate diet PLUS standard anti-tumour treatments	Malignant neoplasm	Ongoing
NCT03700437	Randomized controlled pilot study to evaluate fasting-mimicking diet in patients receiving chemo-immunotherapy for treatment of metastatic non-small-cell lung cancer	Not applicable	Chemo-immunotherapy + FMD (fast-mimicking diet)	Non-small cell lung cancer	Not available

(continued)

Table 10.2 (continued)

NCT number	Name of the study	Phase	Treatment	Tumour type	Study results
NCT03595540	Phase II clinical study of a fasting-mimicking diet in patients undergoing oncologic treatment	Phase II	FMD (Prolon, by L-Nutra) in patients undergoing active cancer treatment	Solid or hematologic tumours	The FMD showed a decrease in fat mass, insulin production as well as levels of circulating IGF1 and leptin. As a result, incorporating periodic cycles of FMD alongside conventional cancer treatments is both safe and feasible
NCT02126449	Dietary restriction as an adjunct to neoadjuvant chemotherapy for HER2 negative breast cancer	Phase II	Short term fasting using FMD around neoadjuvant chemotherapy (AC > T)	Breast cancer	Patients using FMD exhibited either a complete or partial response as observed through radiological examination. Additionally, a significant tumour-cell reduction of 90–100% tumour cell loss was observed, based on the Miller&Payne 4/5 pathological response
NCT05503108	DIRECT-2: fasting mimicking diet program to improve chemotherapy in HR+, HER2 breast cancer	Phase III	The FMD by L-Nutra is vegetarian diet with low calorie and low protein intake to be followed for four consecutive days starting 3 days prior to and the day of neoadjuvant chemotherapy administration	Breast cancer	Ongoing

(continued)

Table 10.2 (continued)

NCT number	Name of the study	Phase	Treatment	Tumour type	Study results
NCT03700437	Randomized controlled pilot study to evaluate fasting-mimicking diet in patients receiving chemo-immunotherapy for treatment of metastatic non-small-cell lung cancer	Not applicable	Chemo-immunotherapy + FMD (fast-mimicking diet) Chemolieve®, involves a plant-based FMD that provides approximately 300 cal per fasting day and includes all the necessary food and supplements to be consumed during the dietary intervention	Non-small-cell lung cancer	Not available
NCT00936364	Short-term fasting prior to platinum-based chemotherapy: feasibility and impact on toxicity	Not applicable	Short-term starvation prior to chemotherapy administration	Malignant solid tumours	Implementation of a 72 h fasting period before undergoing chemotherapy is both safe and feasible in patients diagnosed with cancer

10.3 Ketogenic Diet

A ketogenic diet (KD) refers to a diet that is extremely low in carbohydrates (CHO) and does not primarily focus on calorie restriction or fasting. The macronutrient distribution of the KD typically involves obtaining around 90% of calories from fat, with carbohydrate and protein contributing only 2 and 8%, respectively. These proportions are attained by adhering to the established ratio of 4:1 for fat to carbohydrate and 3:1 for fat to protein [31]. KD has been found to effectively generate ketone bodies (β-hydroxybutyrate and acetoacetate), and these ketone bodies have the ability to suppress appetite and low plasma glucose levels in individuals without cancer [32]. These diets, which are chronically high in fatty acids and low in carbohydrates, force the body to transition from CHO to fatty acid metabolism because enhanced FA oxidation elevates ketone bodies in the blood [33]. KDs is based on the Warburg effect, a biochemical process in which the metabolic characteristics of cancer cells are altered to enhance cellular growth, proliferation, and sustained maintenance over the long-term. This transformation often involves an increase in glucose uptake and the conversion of glucose into lactate through fermentation. Therefore, KDs aid in reducing the levels of blood glucose, which in turn leads to a reduction in circulating insulin and IGF-1. Due to the reliance of most cancer cells on glycolysis for their survival, restricting carbohydrate intake can result in the depletion of the ATP source specifically for cancer cells. In contrast, normal cells have the ability to employ ketone bodies as an alternative energy source to sustain their survival [34]. Among the ketone bodies, β-hydroxybutyrate has shown distinct anti-inflammatory properties. The mechanisms behind this effect include the suppressed expression of interleukin-1b (IL-1b) in bone marrow-derived macrophages and the enhanced expression of uncoupling protein 2 in mitochondria, contributing to the overall protective effect of β-hydroxybutyrate against oxidative stress and therefore an expansion of lifespan [35]. Furthermore, a decreased expression of pro-inflammatory cytokines such as tumour necrosis factor-α (TNF-α) and interferon-γ (IFN-γ) has been linked with the utilization of KD. These anti-inflammatory properties of KD could potentially improve the effectiveness of cancer treatment and prevention [36]. Research has also indicated the beneficial effects of KD in preventing the progression of colon cancer by promoting intra-tumour oxidative stress, leading to the inhibition of matrix metalloproteinase-9 (MMP-9) expression and enhancement of M2 to M1 tumour-associated macrophages (TAMs) [37]. MMPs are associated with cancer progression, metastasis, and angiogenesis in addition to their involvement in the breakdown of extracellular matrix proteins [38].

The potential therapeutic use of low CHO diet regimens is being investigated in the management of cancers due to the higher glucose consumption often exhibited by cancer cells in contrast to normal cells. Studies done in cellular and animal models have examined the effects of KD on cancer prevention and therapy; however, clinical evidence indicating the safety and efficacy of these reduced carbohydrate diets is still in its infancy [39].

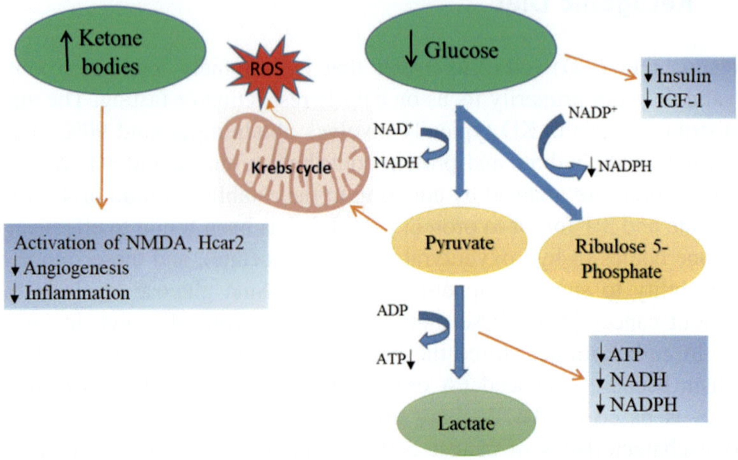

Fig. 10.2 Molecular targets of ketogenic diet. NMDA, N-methyl-D-aspartate; Hcar2, hydroxycarboxylic acid receptor 2; ROS, reactive oxygen species; NAD, nicotinamide adenine dinucleotide; NADH, nicotinamide adenine dinucleotide hydrogen; ADP, adenosine diphosphate; ATP, adenosine triphosphate; NADP, nicotinamide adenine dinucleotide phosphate; NADPH, nicotinamide adenine dinucleotide phosphate hydrogen; IGF1, insulin-like growth factor1

10.3.1 Ketogenic Diet in Preclinical Studies of Cancer

In various preclinical studies using mouse models, ketogenic diets have shown effective anti-tumour activities against various cancers, including colon, gastric, prostrate, head and neck, brain, and thyroid, when used alongside chemotherapy or radiotherapy as an adjuvant treatment [39]. A recent study demonstrated the inhibitory potential of KDs on tumourigenesis in autochthonous animal models of colorectal cancer (CRC). The tumour-inhibitory properties of KDs resulted from the ketone body β-hydroxybutyrate by effectively reducing the growth of colonic cryptic cells and strongly suppressing the growth of intestinal tumours. It was further suggested that BHB exerts its effects through hydroxycarboxylic acid receptor 2 (HCAR2) and activates the transcriptional regulator homeodomain-only protein homeobox (HOPX), leading to modifications in gene expression and cell proliferation inhibition [40]. BHB and acetone have been identified as regulators of N-methyl-D-aspartate (NMDA), which holds physiological significance due to the presence of NMDA receptors in different cancer types [41, 42]. The molecular targets associated with the consumption of a ketogenic diet for the management of cancer are given in Fig. 10.2.

10.3.2 Ketogenic Diet in Clinical Studies of Cancer

A few clinical trials have evaluated the impact of ketogenic diet on cancer alongside chemotherapy, radiotherapy, or other antiangiogenic treatments, yielding diverse outcomes. Based on the results of these case reports and small trials, the utilization of KD has demonstrated safety and tolerability among patients diagnosed with cancer. As an example, a four-week small scale preliminary study was undertaken to assess the safety and feasibility of a KD among ten individuals diagnosed with different cancer types. It was found that within the group of patients who experienced either stable disease or partial remission, their average levels of BHB were three times higher in comparison to the patients with progressive disease [43]. Similarly, Schmidt et al. carried out a pilot study in which they administered KD along with oil-protein shakes as snacks to a subgroup of 7 out of 16 patients diagnosed with different advanced stage metastatic cancers. The study revealed a statistically significant average weight loss, while blood lipid or cholesterol levels remained stable. Additionally, certain measures of quality of life (QOL) showed improvement, and no severe adverse events (AEs) were reported [44]. A retrospective study assessed 53 patients getting treated for high-grade glioma with adequate levels of glucose. Among the 53 patients, six of them followed a ketogenic diet while undergoing treatment, which consisted of a micronutrient composition of 77% fat, 8% CHO, and 15% protein. The researchers observed an average blood glucose level of 122 mg/dl for patients following a standard diet, whereas those on a KD had an average blood glucose level of 84 mg/dl, which reflected a decrease from the average pre-diet blood glucose level of 142.5 mg/dl [44]. A randomized controlled trial involving breast cancer patients found that the use of a medium-chain triglyceride (MCT)-based KD resulted in reduction of fasting blood sugar (FBS) levels and an increase in blood ketone levels within the intervention group. The study also indicated a significant downward trend in body weight, BMI, and the percentage of body fat among the intervention group suggesting a favourable impact of the MCT based KD in patients with breast cancer [45]. Based on the results of some studies, the KD was found to have a notable impact on insulin levels, demonstrating a significant decrease. Moreover, there was an observed inverse correlation between concentrations of BHB and IGF-1 [46]. Recent literature on the trials conducted in adult patients (18 years of age and older) diagnosed with different cancer types, including glioblastomas, breast cancer, liver, lungs and pancreatic, colorectal, and head and neck cancer suggests promising outcomes such as improved survival rate, increased progression-free survival, higher response rates to conventional treatments and enhanced quality of life [47]. Although the limited studies and small trials on KD demonstrate safety and tolerance in cancer patients, further research is required to comprehensively assess the effectiveness of KD in treating cancer. There is also a need to investigate and explore a wider range of combination therapies involving the utilization of KD in human subjects.

10.4 Dietary Supplements

Dietary supplements are any vitamin, herbal product, mineral, or other ingestible product that provides additional health benefits to the diet. Dietary supplements are consumed worldwide and comprise a broad range of ingestible products distinguishable from other conventional food products and drugs [48].

10.4.1 Vitamins

Several dietary components, as well as vitamins, are reported to inhibit signalling pathways and molecular events that lead to various developmental stages of cancer.

For several years, the role of vitamins like vitamin B and D has been comprehensively studied in the reduction of cancer incidence as well as subsequent death [49]. Furthermore, scientists are also focused on vitamin D role in prevention of various types of cancer. In liver, vitamin D_2 as well as D_3 are changed into the circulating vitamin D, i.e. 25(OH)D (25-hydroxyvitamin D: calcidiol), which is then altered into the hormonally active vitamin D, also known as $1{,}25(OH)_2D$ (1,25-dihydroxyvitamin D: calcitriol), in the kidneys [48, 50, 51].

According to the results of numerous *in vitro* research studies, vitamin D prevents the differentiation and proliferation of various tumour cells as well as initiating apoptosis in certain tumour cells [52]. Similarly, vitamin B and its corresponding vitamins are universally essential for the human body and are considered to significantly influence cancer risk [53].

10.4.1.1 Breast Cancer

Vitamin D has a significant influence on multiple organ functions in our body, such as the mammary glands. Vitamin D affects mammary gland development through the actions of vitamin D receptor (VDR), as most of the antiproliferative, pro-apoptotic, and pro-differentiating functions of vitamin D are carried out by VDR [54]. Abe et al. and Colston et al. were the initial researchers to report the anti-cancerous activities of vitamin D [55, 56]. Many clinical and observational research have disclosed the vitamin D ability to regulate the induction as well as the progression of cancer [57–59]. These observational and clinical trials highlighted the VDR role as well as its subsequent proteins like CYP27B1 (cytochrome P450 family 27 subfamily B member 1) and CYP24A1 (family 24 subfamily A member 1) in breast cancer (BC) progression [60].

Additionally, many research studies have also shown that patients with TNBC (triple-negative breast cancer) have the lowest concentration of vitamin D in all types of BC, thus proposing that vitamin D might be responsible for some protective effect against TNBC [60].

Moreover, according to Bauer et al., a meta-analysis including nine analytical studies comprising 5206 patients and 6450 control subjects reported a nonlinear inverse association between breast cancer risk among postmenopausal females and plasma Vit D levels [60, 61]. Also, several *in vitro* and *in vivo* studies have established 1,25(OH)2D3 and its structural analogues effect on various functions within breast cancer, like proliferation, apoptosis, differentiation, epithelial–mesenchymal transition, and autophagy. The latest research has also shown the effect of 1,25(OH)2D3 treatment on cell metabolism and cancer stem cells population [62].

Similarly, an *in vitro* case control prostate cancer study that used the MCF-7 (breast cancer) cell line in comparison with the MCF10A (non-tumourigenic epithelial) cell line presented a significant reduction in cell proliferation after various thiamine dosage treatment (1–2 mg/mL for 24 h) in the MCF7 cell line alone, thus revealing a positive association of B12 and holohaptocorrin levels with cancer risk. Additionally, during a NCC (nested case–control) study, vitamin B12 levels in the blood showed a positive association with overall lung cancer risk [53].

10.4.1.2 Colorectal Cancer (CRC)

Vitamin D has also been comprehensively studied for its protective effect against colorectal cancer (CRC 14–19). Increased vitamin D intake is stated to be linked with decreased risks of early-onset of CRC as well as its precursors. Possible mechanisms that explain this inverse relation of vitamin D intake with CRC risk involve inhibition of mechanisms like proliferation, invasiveness, migration, and colon cancer cells' angiogenesis, and regulation of the immune cells of the intestine [63]. Moreover, patients suffering from CRC having an increased prediagnostic 25(OH)D levels showed lower cancer associated mortality risk [64]. The COLON study (colorectal cancer) showed that the supplementation of vitamin D (more than 50 nmol/L) accompanied by the higher intake of magnesium (median split), decreases the mortality among colorectal cancer (CRC) patients [65, 66].

Ng et al., during a randomized trial related to chemotherapy, analyzed serum 25(OH)D levels among 515 patients suffering from stage 4 colorectal cancer and revealed that the Vitamin D deficiency (<20–30 ng/mL) was very predominant among all stage 4 colorectal cancer patients [65, 67]. Recently, a large cohort study performed by Yuan et al. established that the deficiency of vitamin D (less than 20–30 ng/mL) among 1041 patients with a previous history of untreated metastatic or advanced colorectal cancer [65, 68].

10.4.1.3 Lung Cancer

In the last few decades, defects in vitamin D levels, or VDR, showed an association with the pathogenesis of various cancers like lung cancer [52].

Epidemiological research has revealed the significant role of suitable Vitamin D levels in lung cancer prevention. Similarly, several investigative studies have also exposed the relationship between serum levels of Vitamin D and lung cancer risk [52].

A research study revealed linkage between higher circulating VitD concentrations with decreased mortality rate and increased survival rates among patients with lung cancer [69]. Furthermore, another cohort study performed in Finland, involving lung cancer patients reported a negative association of VitD levels with lung cancer among female patients and also in younger patients [52, 70].

Moreover, variations in Vitamin D signalling genes might affect susceptibility to lung cancer and the quantity and quality of different treatment responses [52, 71]. Vitamin D upregulates p53, a tumour suppressor gene expression and downregulates the expression of pro-apoptotic Bcl-2 (B-cell lymphoma 2) in human lung carcinoma cell line (A549) [52, 71].

Additionally, vitamin D therapy has been reported to enhance the suppressive effect of VDR on the epidermal growth factor receptor (EGFR) gene. Research studies have reported a significant influence of vitamin D on the EGFR signalling pathway in lung cancer cell lines; therefore, they proposed that VitD/VDR therapy might be an effective treatment option for lung cancer through EGFR signalling modulation [52, 72, 73]. Similarly, a NCC (nested case–control) research study, has also shown positive association of blood vitamin B12 levels with the overall risk of lung cancer [53].

10.4.1.4 Ovarian Cancer

Several studies on sun exposure have exposed negative correlation of vitamin D levels with the risk of ovarian cancer. Furthermore, ovarian cancer research in cell lines, human xenograft models, and mouse models has provided strong evidence of VitD role in the reduction of proliferation, enhanced apoptosis, as well as suppression of tumour progression. Likewise, during Mendelian randomization studies, genetically reduced 25(OH)D levels were linked with a statistically significant increased ovarian cancer risk, hence validating the vitamin D effect on ovarian cancer [50, 74].

In an Australian cohort study, researchers have correlated the higher serum levels of 25D3 at the diagnostic stage with a longer survival of females with invasive ovarian cancer [75]. Similarly, a Mendelian randomized research study carried out in the European population has reported inverse association between genetically reduced 25D3 levels and increased ovarian cancer susceptibility [76]. Furthermore, on the basis of certain GWAS (genome wide association studies), a higher 25D3 concentration was expected to be linked with a reduced Epithelial ovarian cancer (EOC) risk [64, 77].

In another case–control study including 1631 females with epithelial ovarian cancer (EOC), elevated 25(OH)D concentrations showed association with the extended patients survival rates [78]. Other studies have also explored VDR genetic variants, which mediates 1,25(OH)D activity, and suggested the influence of VitD on ovarian cancer risk and survival rate [79–83]. Further advanced research on the anti-cancer effect of VitD is required in future to comprehensively understand the personalized response to VDR agonist treatment [50]. For this purpose, various omics approaches, including epigenomic, metabolomic, genomic, proteomic, as well as transcriptomic should be combined for the comprehension and prediction of the particular sensitivity or susceptibility to each of these compounds [49, 84].

10.4.2 Carotenoids and Cancer

The carotenoids are the antioxidants present in fruits and vegetables, and have immuno-regulatory and anti-mutagenic functions. Several studies have established an association of various carotenoids with protection against different types of cancers. Though such associations could not directly suggest causal relationships, they still depict significant patterns that lead to decreased cancer incidence. In addition to the aesthetic properties of carotenoids, they are also considered as strong antioxidants and are considered to be involved in the production of various nutrients like vitamin A [85, 86]. Certain carotenoids because of their antioxidant activities reduce the harmful effects of ROS (reactive oxygen species). Reactive oxygen species (ROS) are linked with various diseases such as cancer, cardiovascular and neurodegenerative diseases, and aging.

Scientific literature has widely reported the significant role of carotenoids in apoptosis, gene regulation, angiogenesis, as well as immune regulation [86, 87]. In addition to that, the pathways related to the antioxidant function are considered to be modified with the consumption of carotenoid [88].

10.4.2.1 Head and Neck Cancer

Head and neck cancer (HNC) includes oral cavity cancer, laryngeal cancer, and pharyngeal cancer. Carotenoids, due to their antioxidant properties, have been known to have anti-mutagenic as well as immune regulatory activities. Therefore, several research studies have reported a link between carotenoid intake and decreased risk of head and neck cancer (HNC), however, the mechanism through which carotenoids affect HNC risk is yet to be explored further [87].

In two meta-analyses published by Leoncini et al., they have discussed the relationship of all carotenoids with HNC [85, 89]. The meta-analysis comprised of sixteen epidemiological studies related to specific carotenoids dietary consumption, and they reported a reduced risk of HNC in association with β-carotene intake, similarly, 46% decreased oropharyngeal cancer (OPC) risk as well as 57% reduced risk of laryngeal cancer (LC).

Similarly, β-cryptoxanthin and lycopene were linked with reduced laryngeal cancer (LC) risk by 59 and 50%, respectively. Also, α-carotene, β-cryptoxanthin, and lycopene had been reported to cause 26% reduced risk of oral cavity cancer (OCC) and pharyngeal cancer (PC) [85, 87].

In another collective analysis involving 10 case–control studies, comprising 18,207 patients and 12,248 controls and carried out in North America, Japan, and Europe, the researchers reported the reduction in cancer risk linked with the total carotenoid consumption, i.e. 39% decreased risk of OCC (oral cavity cancer) and PC (pharyngeal cancer), and 39% reduced risk of LC (laryngeal cancer) [89].

10.4.2.2 Breast Cancer

Research studies have proposed a significant role of carotenoids against prostate and breast cancers. A recent cell culture study has proposed that the intake of 1 μM of β-carotene is enough to reduce anti-apoptotic proteins like PARP and Bcl-2 expression. Similarly, studies on the MCF-7 breast cancer cell line have revealed that the intake of 2 or more μM of lycopene results in reduced proliferation as well as increased apoptosis among cells. Lycopene consumption also considerably increases the p53 and Bax mRNA expression [90, 91].

Fulan Hu et al., in their meta-analysis investigated the association of carotenoids with breast cancer, along with the quantitative estimation of their dose–response relationships [92]. Their meta-analysis results have shown significant decrease in breast cancer risk associated with the dietary consumption of α-carotene, while the link of dietary and total β-carotene consumption with the risk of breast cancer has to be further investigated [92].

Another research study has focused on the analysis of certain vegetables, fruits, carotenoids, and vitamins association with breast cancer risk in a large case–control study comprising 5707 females with invasive breast cancer and 6389 controls, both patients and controls belong to pre-menopausal and post-menopausal stages from the states of Wisconsin, Massachusetts, and New Hampshire. The results have insinuated that high carotenoids consumption might decrease the breast cancer risk among premenopausal females while no such effect was observed in postmenopausal subjects, specifically among smokers [93]. Collectively, carotenoids exhibit the potential to reduce the growth of breast cancer cells [90, 91].

10.4.2.3 Colorectal Cancer

According to many epidemiological and clinical studies, the CRC risk is linked with dietary as well as serum carotenoids, as well as retinol. A cell culture study has reported that two or more μM of lycopene caused a substantial reduction in the proliferation of HT-29 human colorectal cancer cell lines. This decrease in proliferation of cancer cells might be caused by PI3K/Akt signalling pathway inhibition [94]. Lycopene consumption also enhances the expression of p21 and PCNA while suppressing the expression of PGE2, COX-2, and phosphorylated ERK1/2 proteins in cancer mouse models. Similarly, plasma MMP-9 concentrations were observed to have inverse association with the dietary lycopene [95].

Xiaoyong Han et al. performed a meta-analysis to establish the link of colorectal cancer (CRC) risk with serum as well as dietary carotenoids and retinol [96]. In this meta-analysis, they have included 22 relevant studies, and their results revealed that higher concentrations of β-cryptoxanthin, lycopene, α- and β-carotene reduce the risk of CRC, thus ascertaining the significant inverse association of concentrations of serum carotenoid with CRC [96]. Collectively, these results proposed that lycopene as well as other carotenoids could decrease tumour growth and progression in CRC [95].

10.4.2.4 Lung Cancer

Carotenoids protect the lungs from early cancer development by using their antioxidant properties at different concentrations achieved by diet. In different studies, β-carotene has shown a linear dose–response association with lung cancer in such a way that the risk of lung cancer was observed to be decreased by 2% after the intake of each additional milligram of β-carotene per day. Similarly, 1% reduction was observed in the lung cancer risk after each extra 10 μg of β-cryptoxanthin consumption per day or 3% reduction after the consumption of each extra milligram of lycopene per day [97].

Lately, in a case–control study of lung cancer in Hawaii, scientists have observed an inverse association between lung cancer risk and vegetable consumption that have high concentrations of different carotenoids. The resultant data from this study proposed a protective effect of carotenoids against lung cancer [98]. Similarly, in a random-effects meta-analysis carried out by Lisa Gallicchio et al., including six clinical trials as well as 25 observational studies, they evaluated the link of carotenoids with the lung cancer and suggested an inverse association between carotenoids consumption and lung cancer risk, although the decrease in the risk of lung cancer is usually small and cannot be considered statistically significant [97].

10.4.2.5 Prostate Cancer

Carotenoids, due to its antioxidant role, might decrease tumour-promoting inflammation. α-carotene, β-carotene, and lycopene are studied extensively for their association with prostate cancer. More than seventy research studies have assessed these carotenoids associations with prostate cancer and their results have shown that higher consumption of lycopene as well as its concentrations in blood are linked with the reduced risk of prostate cancer. Two other cell culture studies have also established that the lycopene-treated cells show significant reduction in cell proliferation and cell cycle progression [90, 99].

Similarly, a nested case–control study has reported the associations of plasma *cis*-lycopene, *trans*-lutein, β-*trans*-carotene, and dihydrolycopene with prostate cancer risk after multiple comparison adjustments. Also, the study showed that mostly in African Americans, *Trans* β-carotene isomers have positive association with prostate cancer risk, irrespective of their smoking status or multivitamin use [100].

Moreover, another case–control study including 65 patients of prostate cancer as well as 132 controls has investigated the impact of plasma lycopene along with other carotenoids and vitamins like retinol, α- and γ-tocopherols on prostate cancer. Results have disclosed substantial inverse relationship of prostate cancer with plasma carotenoids like lycopene and zeaxanthin concentrations while β-cryptoxanthin and lutein have also shown some borderline associations with prostate cancer [101].

10.5 Physical Activity

Currently, smoking is the most significant modifiable factor of risk for cancer; however, inadequate physical activity is quickly overtaking smoking as the second-most prevalent cause of cancer [102]. Over 25% of the adult population, or 1.4 billion people, participate in inadequate physical exercise, according to data collected by the World Health Organization (WHO) [103]. As obesity develops at earlier ages, the risk factors are now exposed to more people across their lifetimes. In comparison to low income nations, high-income affluent countries have double the levels of inadequate activity. Over time, the levels of physical inactivity have been increasing drastically, which has detrimental effects on the environment, economy, quality of life, and community well-being [104, 105]. It is widely known that regular physical activity can prevent and control non-communicable diseases like cardiovascular diseases, hypertension, type II diabetes mellitus, stroke, and many different cancers. Physical activity has been linked by decades of epidemiologic studies to a reduced risk of developing various common malignancies. According to estimates from 2012, increased BMI was observed in 3.6% of all new cancer cases worldwide [106].

10.5.1 Physical Activity in Cancer Prevention

Any skeletal muscle-powered movement that requires energy expenditure is considered physical activity. While exercise is only one aspect of it; however, it can be performed at different intensities and is accumulated through work, household duties, travel, or leisure activities like walking, cycling, active play, and sports [107]. Appropriate physical activity alters the body's metabolism to make it less susceptible to various malignancies. The type and intensity of physical exercise can have an impact on the body's metabolic state and overall energy requirements, which can then have an impact on the amount of food (and nutrients) that can be consumed without causing the body to store excess energy as fat. A surplus of calories consumed without being offset by exercise results in an increased energy balance, which causes weight gain and higher body fatness [107]. Despite the fact that physical activity might be predominantly significant in weight-loss management, it has some additional beneficial result on lowering cancer risk through multiple mechanisms, like immune-regulatory system modulation [108–110], reductions in circulating oestrogen levels [111], decreased oxidative stress [112], insulin resistance [113], inflammation [114], epigenetic alterations [115], decreased telomere attrition [116], and enhance DNA repair mechanism [109]. All of these factors are connected with the development and progression of cancers at different anatomical sites.

Regardless of physical activity effect on obesity, it is inversely connected with colon and breast cancer, according to a 2020 Mendelian randomization (MR) study that used data from the UK Biobank. It was also shown that the relationship between cancer prevalence and physical activity was unrelated to BMI [117].

Additionally, the incidence of kidney cancer, bladder cancer, and CRC is inversely connected with strength training, which increases the mass of skeletal muscle [118, 119]. Increases in glucose homeostasis and insulin sensitivity brought on by aerobic workout [120], may lower the incidence of malignancies such as colon, liver, pancreatic, and endometrial cancers that are linked to insulin resistance (and the related cellular signalling pathways) [121]. Different types of cancer respond differently to exercise's ability to lower cancer risk. Despite the lack of evidence linking exercise to a lower chance of developing cancer, studies have demonstrated that altering one's lifestyle can lower cancer incidence [122]. Heavy housework is one example of a high intensity activity that is advantageous to women and is thought to reduce the chance of developing breast cancer. For instance, getting 3 to 5 h of exercise each week can lower your risk of getting cancer [123].

A study found that people who exercised had a 15% to 20% minimize the breast cancer risk and about 24% decreased risk of colon cancers [124]. Exercise therapy has been demonstrated to reduce post-menopausal women's chance of developing breast cancer and to shield breast cancer patients from autonomic nerve dysfunction [125, 126]. Exercise-induced lifestyle modifications are helpful for minimizing the risk of CRC. In 126 research studies evaluating the association between exercise and CRC, people who engaged in more exercise had a 19% decreased chance of developing the disease [127]. The incidence of cancer was 19% lower among those who exercised compared to those who performed less exercise, according to an analysis of studies on stomach cancer that comprised 10 cohorts with twelve case–control studies [128]. Previous studies have shown that one of the key risk factors for endometrial cancer is obesity. Exercise lowered obesity, and women who exercised frequently had a 20% lower risk of developing endometrial cancer than those who did not, according to a review of 33 research [129]. Similarly, a review study on oesophageal cancer revealed that individuals who exercised the most had a 21% reduced chance of developing the disease than those who exercised the least [130]. Exercise done in the free time of participants decreased their chance of bladder cancer development by 13% and renal cancer by 23% in research with more than 1 million participants [131]. A review of 25 research indicated that, while there was no difference between nonsmokers who exercised and those who didn't in terms of acquiring lung cancer, there was a difference between smokers who exercised and those who didn't [132].

10.5.2 Physical Activity in Cancer Treatment

Besides cancer prevention, exercise also lessens the negative effects of cancer therapy. Cancer therapies, including chemotherapy and targeted therapy, can have side effects including fatigue, memory loss, depression, loss of muscle, and bone mass, cardiac toxicity, and others. Poor treatment outcomes and poor quality of life outcomes could result from these adverse responses [122]. The fact that certain cancer patients are unable to adhere or tolerate treatment, due to adverse reactions, means that the course of the disease may be affected by the treatment. Nevertheless, numerous studies have shown that continuing physical activity might mitigate some treatment-related side effects. Exercise training can impact the specificity of cancer and the physiological and emotional outcomes of cancer treatment. Exercise not merely lessens the adverse effects of treatment procedures, but also enhances its therapeutic effect. This is why it is beneficial to incorporate exercise into the treatment process [133]. The therapeutic advantages and associated negative side effects of cancer treatment can both be tempered by exercise. However, the main concern for medical professionals is whether exercise may impact cancer survival and prognosis. According to research, exercise does not directly increase one's likelihood of surviving gastric cancer, non-Hodgkin lymphoma and several other malignancies [134].

In order to affect cancer metabolism and stop anaerobic glycolysis, exercise can be targeted as cancer-suppressor gene therapy. The link between cancer metabolism and the host is influenced by the frequency, frequency, intensity, and kind of physical activity during exercise. Vasoconstriction is reduced in a hypoxic environment, increasing cancer perfusion and decreasing cancer hypoxia [135, 136]. Exercise makes cancer cells more docile. Exercise is hypothesized to diminish the hypoxic microenvironment in cancer, which is necessary for the features of cancer cells and the invasiveness of the cancer microenvironment [135].

Immune aging is characterized by an increase in cells that are getting older and losing their ability to function, a decrease in NK cell activity, an increase in inflammation, damage to dendritic and monocyte cells that take up and present antigens, and reduction in the number of immature T cells that react to cancer cells that are still forming. The increased risk of cancer in older individuals is actually brought on by immunological aging [137]. Exercise can partially slow immunological aging due to its capacity to boost immune cell activity [115]. Exercise thus acts as a preventative measure against immune-related malignant tumours. In conclusion, research-based data have demonstrated that physical exercise can minimize the risk of cancer. It can lessen the development and spread of cancer, lessen the negative effects of cancer therapy, increase patients' toleration of the medication, and enhance their quality of life (Fig. 10.3).

10.6 Weight Management

A body that is overweight or obese (very overweight) contains more fat than other tissues like muscle and bone. Unhealthy levels of excess weight increase the chance of developing some cancers as well as the likelihood that they may return following treatment. According to the WHO, more than 340 million children and adolescents, along with 1.9 billion adults, were lived with overweight or obesity in 2016 and that figure is expected to climb [138]. The worldwide burden of cancer is predicted to continue to hike as a result of existing trends towards decreasing

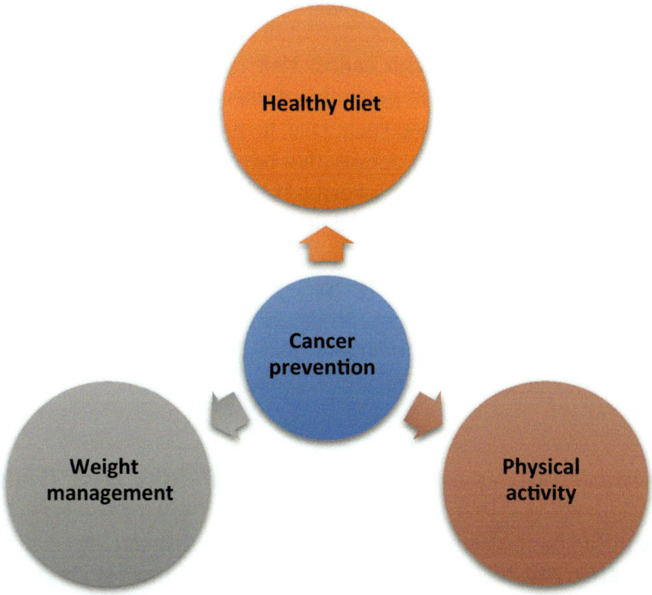

Fig. 10.3 Schematic representation of cancer prevention associated with healthy diet, physical activity, and weight management

physical activity and body fatness, especially given estimates of an aging world population. If current trends continue, obesity and overweight will likely surpass smoking as the leading cause of cancer.

10.6.1 Relationship Between Obesity and Cancer

Since the beginning of the twentieth century, reports and discussions on the link between fat and cancer have appeared in the literature since 1987 [139]. The prevalence of common malignancies associated with excess body fat would increase along with the prevalence of overweight and obesity in the population. As a result, future cancer therapies will become more and more expensive, and the long-term therapeutic management of related comorbidities would strain health-care systems financially. One of the key strategies for preventing cancer is to maintain a healthy weight. It is critical to consider the significance of excess body fat in infancy because it has been shown to affect the chance of developing a number of diseases, including cancer, as an adult. Hidayat et al. found connections between early body fatness and the later emergence of eight different malignancies [140]. Weight growth increases the chance of being overweight and obese as well as postmenopausal breast cancer (6% every 5 kg rise in adult weight) [141]. Even while it seems that there is a growing connection between cancer and obesity in adults, the importance of weight increase throughout the course of adulthood tends to be generally overlooked.

Body fatness is associated with cancer risk factors due to growing evidence that being overweight or obese in general is a major contributing factor to numerous malignancies during the past year. Due to higher fasting insulin levels and inflammatory mediators linked to obesity that have proliferative effects (Hallmark: persistent proliferative signalling), obesity is linked to a number of metabolic and endocrine disorders [142]. Normal cells undergo the mechanism of apoptosis, which plays a role in downregulating apoptosis and survival after DNA damage (*Hallmark: resisting cell death*) [143]. As we know, cancer cells spread through the bloodstream or lymphatic system (*Hallmarks: activating invasion and metastasis*). Hence, many abnormalities in endocrine and metabolic are link with obesity including insulin levels, inflammatory mediators.

10.6.2 Opportunities and Difficulties in Weight Loss Trials

Irrespective of the method employed to lose weight, research is necessary to ascertain whether programs that are successful in achieving modest short-term weight loss and maintain it over time can effectively reduce the risk of cancer. The persistence of overweight and obesity, as well as any potential consequences of the delayed risk reduction following weight loss, must be completely taken into consideration in the study design. Determining whether any weight gain following weight loss cancels out any favourable effects is also crucial. An emphasis on weight control enables the adoption and testing of a lifestyle pattern that includes meal size and quality, alcohol consumption, and physical activity. Even though there are still many unanswered questions about lifestyle interventions, such as dosage, time span, type (for physical activity), caloric composition, and dietary value (regarding food intake), as well as strategies for ensuring long-term compliance, extensive knowledge can be gained from longer-term lifestyle trials, such as those highlighting diabetes prevention.

10.6.3 Weight Management Recommendations

Measures should be taken to maintain body weight, here are a few recommendations:

- Eat a lot of fruits, vegetables, lean proteins, and whole grains.
- Maintaining a healthy body weight
- Eat meals like fish, almonds, and healthy fats like olive oil and nuts.
- Avoid packaged foods with lots of artificial additives, white breads, cookies, and other highly processed meals.
- Reduce the intake of red meat and processed meat.

- Avoid sugary beverages including soda, fruit juice, and other high-sugar beverages. Check the sugar and calorie content of any alcoholic beverages and your coffee.
- Plan to do 30–60 min of exercise most days of the week. Moderate or vigorous exercise are both acceptable. Go for a run, a brisk stroll, or enrol in a fitness class. Do what you can if you can't get 30–60 min, your risk of cancer is reduced even by a few extra minutes every day.

10.7 Avoiding Tobacco and Radiation

10.7.1 Tobacco as Carcinogen

Tobacco as well as tobacco smoke comprise a mixture of more than 9500 chemical compounds, and several of these compounds have been identified by regulatory agencies as being harmful for human health. In 2012, the FDA (Food and Drug Administration, USA) formulated a list of hazardous or potentially hazardous constituents of tobacco smoke and unburned tobacco, of which 79 are considered to have carcinogenic properties [144]. Tobacco smoke is reported to increase cancer risk through its carcinogenic contents, like nitrosamines, acrylamines, polycyclic aromatic hydrocarbons (PAHs), cadmium, and volatile organic compounds (VOCs) [145, 146].

A well-established causal relationship between lung cancer risk and smoking exists [145]. Strong experimental and observational evidence has shown that smoking is amongst the major risk factors for various cancers, including kidney, bladder, gastrointestinal tract, head and neck, colorectum, oesophagus, pancreas, stomach, liver, uterine cervix, and myeloid leukaemia [144, 145, 147–149].

Several carcinogens present in tobacco smoke have been found to cause tumours in mammary glands among lab animals. While human studies have established that various constituents of tobacco could reach the breast tissue. Moreover, the uptake as well as metabolic activation of the carcinogens involved in breast cancer, such as 4-aminobiphenyl and polycyclic aromatic hydrocarbons (PAHs) is mostly raised among smokers than in nonsmokers [148].

Similarly, head and neck squamous cell carcinoma (HNSCC) is one of the types of cancer that has a strong association with tobacco consumption. The HNSCC risk among smokers is almost ten times greater than that among nonsmokers, and nearly 70–80% of the new HNSCC diagnosed cases are linked with tobacco as well as alcohol consumption [149].

Tobacco smoke mostly acts by the action of chemicals, like ROS and RNS (reactive oxygen- and nitrogen species), and others, that could damage the target macromolecules like nucleic acids, lipids, and proteins. Scientific evidence shows that in cancer as well as inflammation, smoking-induced ROS and the resultant oxidative stress play a significant role. This smoking induced oxidative stress leads to inflammation, which in turn results in more ROS production, which causes further oxidative damage to the macromolecules that might trigger carcinogenesis [150].

10.7.2 Radiation as Carcinogen

Radiofrequency EMF (electromagnetic fields) exposure in humans mostly occurs from the utilization of various personal devices (like cell phones, bluetooth, cordless phones, and amateur radios), occupational sources (like induction heaters, high-frequency dielectrics, and high-powered pulsed radars), and environmental sources (like medical applications, broadcast antennae, and mobile-phone base stations). In the general population, the most substantial exposure is received from those transmitters that are close to the body, like hand-held devices, including mobile phones. Moreover, a large number of workers from different fields are also exposed, like radar operators, security and military personnel operating walkie-talkie devices, television and radio antenna repair and maintenance workers, welders doing plastic sealing and dielectric welding, workers utilizing radio frequency (RF) radiation for testing or drying operations, as well as physiotherapists using medical diathermy equipment [151].

Stang et al. have performed hospital as well as population-based case–control research studies on uveal melanoma development in context with occupational exposures of electromagnetic radiation like RF radiation, from different occupational sources [152]. Similarly, Karipidis et al. performed a case–control study among five main population centres of Victoria, Australia, and showed association of glioma risk with occupational exposure of radio frequency (RF) radiation [153].

In addition to that ultraviolet (UV) radiation, an invisible part of the electromagnetic spectrum, with shorter wavelengths as compared to visible light, also has carcinogenic effects. The main UV source is sunlight, though some industrial processes like electric arc welding might also emit UV radiation. The ICNIRP (International Commission on Non-Ionizing Radiation Protection) have provided a guideline limit of artificial UV radiation exposure on the eyes and unprotected skin that is 30 J/m^2 within 8 h time period [154]. UV radiation is one of an important risk factor of basal cell carcinoma (BCC). It is reasonably assumed that those workers that have a prolonged outdoor work-related exposure to UV radiations have increased risk of basal cell carcinoma (BCC) development. 19 case–control as well as five cohort studies have reported a significant association of occupational exposure of UV radiation and the risk of basal cell carcinoma (BCC) [155].

10.8 Complementary and Alternative Therapies

The term "complementary and alternative medicine" (CAM) encompasses a diverse range of medical and health care products and practices that lie outside the purview of conventional or mainstream medicine. CAM may be used by cancer patients alongside conventional medical approaches to assist them in finding comfort and relief from cancer treatment-related stress and anxieties, and also help them cope with the side effects, including nausea, pain, and fatigue. Complementary and alternative therapies in cancer care include herbal medicine, acupuncture, mind–body techniques (meditation and yoga), nutritional supplements, energy healing practices, and massage therapies [156]. The utilization of CAM among cancer patients has been steadily on the rise. According to estimates, complementary, alternative, or integrative therapies are used in cancer therapy by 33–47% of cancer patients worldwide [157]. Cancer-related fatigue (CRF) significantly influences the patient's quality of life as it disturbs many different aspects of life, such as basic daily tasks, social activities, work responsibilities, recreational activities, and relationships with family and friends. CRF can also influence a patient's ability to comply with their cancer treatments. Thus, most cancer patients seek out alternative or complementary care options in an effort to restore their well-being and effectively manage their symptoms [158, 159]. Although some of these therapies may help in relieving symptoms and improving the life quality of individuals with cancer, their effectiveness in the treatment process may vary and require additional research to incorporate these modalities into the cancer treatment regime.

10.9 Conclusion

In conclusion, lifestyle modifications play a crucial role in both cancer prevention and therapy. These primary preventive strategies include adhering to a balanced and healthy diet, getting regular exercise, abstaining from alcohol and tobacco use, maintaining a healthy body weight, and avoiding exposure to radiation and other carcinogens. It has been emphasized that incorporating lifestyle changes has a tremendous influence on lowering the incidence of cancer and also improving patient outcomes after a cancer diagnosis. Lifestyle changes can support conventional cancer treatment by raising cancer patient's general quality of life and enhancing treatment outcomes while lowering the adverse effects of the standard therapies. The lifestyle interventions discussed here are the most cost-effective strategies for controlling various cancers, including melanoma, breast cancer, colorectal cancer, oesophageal cancer, liver cancer, and head and neck cancer. Adopting a healthy lifestyle to improve the overall health of cancer patients is a priority in international strategies nowadays. Despite the effectiveness of these lifestyle factors on the wellbeing of cancer patients, uncertainty still prevails due to the limited clinical data on the safety and efficacy of complementary therapies.

The research challenges in this area need to be addressed along with immediate policy measures to encourage and foster healthy lifestyles in an effort to effectively reduce the burden of cancer and cancer-related deaths.

References

1. LoConte NK, Gershenwald JE, Thomson CA, Crane TE, Harmon GE, Rechis R (2018) Lifestyle modifications and policy implications for primary and secondary cancer prevention: diet, exercise, sun safety, and alcohol reduction. Am Soc Clin Oncol Educ Book 38:88–100
2. Tripp MK, Watson M, Balk SJ, Swetter SM, Gershenwald JE (2016) State of the science on prevention and screening to reduce melanoma incidence and mortality: the time is now. CA: A Cancer J Clin 66(6):460–480
3. Sun Y, Wu J, Yoon H-S, Buchowski MS, Cai H, Deppen SA et al (2022) Associations of dietary intakes of carotenoids and vitamin a with lung cancer risk in a low-income population in the southeastern United States. Cancers 14(20):5159
4. Anand P, Kunnumakara AB, Sundaram C, Harikumar KB, Tharakan ST, Lai OS et al (2008) Cancer is a preventable disease that requires major lifestyle changes. Pharm Res 25:2097–2116
5. Vernieri C, Nichetti F, Raimondi A, Pusceddu S, Platania M, Berrino F et al (2018) Diet and supplements in cancer prevention and treatment: clinical evidences and future perspectives. Crit Rev Oncol Hematol 123:57–73
6. Doyle C, Kushi LH, Byers T, Courneya KS, Demark-Wahnefried W, Grant B et al (2006) Nutrition and physical activity during and after cancer treatment: an American Cancer Society guide for informed choices. CA a Cancer J Clin 56(6):323–353
7. Brandhorst S, Choi IY, Wei M, Cheng CW, Sedrakyan S, Navarrete G et al (2015) A periodic diet that mimics fasting promotes multi-system regeneration, enhanced cognitive performance, and healthspan. Cell Metab 22(1):86–99
8. Levine ME, Suarez JA, Brandhorst S, Balasubramanian P, Cheng C-W, Madia F et al (2014) Low protein intake is associated with a major reduction in IGF-1, cancer, and overall mortality in the 65 and younger but not older population. Cell Metab 19(3):407–417
9. Schiliro C, Firestein BL (2021) Mechanisms of metabolic reprogramming in cancer cells supporting enhanced growth and proliferation. Cells 10(5):1056
10. Lin X, Xiao Z, Chen T, Liang SH, Guo H (2020) Glucose metabolism on tumor plasticity, diagnosis, and treatment. Front Oncol 10:317
11. Mattson MP, Longo VD, Harvie M (2017) Impact of intermittent fasting on health and disease processes. Ageing Res Rev 39:46–58
12. Tiwari S, Sapkota N, Han Z (2022) Effect of fasting on cancer: a narrative review of scientific evidence. Cancer Sci 113(10):3291–3302
13. Patterson RE, Sears DD (2017) Metabolic effects of intermittent fasting. Ann Rev Nutri 37
14. Longo VD, Mattson MP (2014) Fasting: molecular mechanisms and clinical applications. Cell Metab 19(2):181–192
15. Safdie FM, Dorff T, Quinn D, Fontana L, Wei M, Lee C et al (2009) Fasting and cancer treatment in humans: a case series report. Aging 1(12):988
16. Brandhorst S (2021) Fasting and fasting-mimicking diets for chemotherapy augmentation. Geroscience 43(3):1201–1216
17. Longo VD, Di Tano M, Mattson MP, Guidi N (2021) Intermittent and periodic fasting, longevity and disease. Nature aging 1(1):47–59
18. Turbitt WJ, Demark-Wahnefried W, Peterson CM, Norian LA (2019) Targeting glucose metabolism to enhance immunotherapy: emerging evidence on intermittent fasting and calorie restriction mimetics. Front Immunol 1402

19. Wei M, Brandhorst S, Shelehchi M, Mirzaei H, Cheng CW, Budniak J et al (2019) Fasting-mimicking diet and markers/risk factors for aging, diabetes, cancer, and cardiovascular disease. Sci Transl Med 9(377):eaai8700
20. Blaževitš O, Di Tano M, Longo VD (2023) Fasting and fasting mimicking diets in cancer prevention and therapy. Trends Cancer
21. Lee C, Raffaghello L, Brandhorst S, Safdie FM, Bianchi G, Martin-Montalvo A et al (2012) Fasting cycles retard growth of tumors and sensitize a range of cancer cell types to chemotherapy. Sci Translat Med 4(124):124ra27–ra27
22. Bianchi G, Martella R, Ravera S, Marini C, Capitanio S, Orengo A et al (2015) Fasting induces anti-Warburg effect that increases respiration but reduces ATP-synthesis to promote apoptosis in colon cancer models. Oncotarget 6(14):11806
23. De Cabo R, Mattson MP (2019) Effects of intermittent fasting on health, aging, and disease. N Engl J Med 381(26):2541–2551
24. Longo VD, Cortellino S (2020) Fasting, dietary restriction, and immunosenescence. J Allerg Clinic Immunol 146(5):1002–1004
25. Vernieri C, Casola S, Foiani M, Pietrantonio F, de Braud F, Longo V (2016) Targeting cancer metabolism: dietary and pharmacologic interventionsanticancer metabolic therapies. Cancer Discov 6(12):1315–1333
26. de Groot S, Vreeswijk MP, Welters MJ, Gravesteijn G, Boei JJ, Jochems A et al (2015) The effects of short-term fasting on tolerance to (neo) adjuvant chemotherapy in HER2-negative breast cancer patients: a randomized pilot study. BMC Cancer 15(1):1–9
27. Dorff TB, Groshen S, Garcia A, Shah M, Tsao-Wei D, Pham H et al (2016) Safety and feasibility of fasting in combination with platinum-based chemotherapy. BMC Cancer 16(1):1–9
28. Bauersfeld SP, Kessler CS, Wischnewsky M, Jaensch A, Steckhan N, Stange R et al (2018) The effects of short-term fasting on quality of life and tolerance to chemotherapy in patients with breast and ovarian cancer: a randomized cross-over pilot study. BMC Cancer 18:1–10
29. Vernieri C, Fucà G, Ligorio F, Huber V, Vingiani A, Iannelli F et al (2022) Fasting-mimicking diet is safe and reshapes metabolism and antitumor immunity in patients with cancer. Cancer Discov 12(1):90–107
30. de Groot S, Lugtenberg RT, Cohen D, Welters MJ, Ehsan I, Vreeswijk MP et al (2020) Fasting mimicking diet as an adjunct to neoadjuvant chemotherapy for breast cancer in the multicentre randomized phase 2 DIRECT trial. Nat Commun 11(1):3083
31. Allen BG, Bhatia SK, Anderson CM, Eichenberger-Gilmore JM, Sibenaller ZA, Mapuskar KA et al (2014) Ketogenic diets as an adjuvant cancer therapy: history and potential mechanism. Redox Biol 2:963–970
32. Yancy WS Jr, Olsen MK, Guyton JR, Bakst RP, Westman EC (2004) A low-carbohydrate, ketogenic diet versus a low-fat diet to treat obesity and hyperlipidemia: a randomized, controlled trial. Ann Intern Med 140(10):769–777
33. Dhamija R, Eckert S, Wirrell E (2013) Ketogenic diet. Can J Neurol Sci 40(2):158–167
34. Choi J-W, Hua TN (2021) Impact of lifestyle behaviors on cancer risk and prevention. J Lifestyle Med 11(1):1
35. Shimazu T, Hirschey MD, Newman J, He W, Shirakawa K, Le Moan N et al (2013) Suppression of oxidative stress by β-hydroxybutyrate, an endogenous histone deacetylase inhibitor. Science 339(6116):211–214
36. Talib WH, Mahmod AI, Kamal A, Rashid HM, Alashqar AMD, Khater S et al (2021) Ketogenic diet in cancer prevention and therapy: molecular targets and therapeutic opportunities. Curr Issues Mol Biol 43(2):558–589
37. Zhang N, Liu C, Jin L, Zhang R, Wang T, Wang Q et al (2020) Ketogenic diet elicits antitumor properties through inducing oxidative stress, inhibiting mmp-9 expression, and rebalancing m1/m2 tumor-associated macrophage phenotype in a mouse model of colon cancer. J Agric Food Chem 68(40):11182–11196
38. Said AH, Raufman JP, Xie G (2014) The role of matrix metalloproteinases in colorectal cancer. Cancers 6(1):366–375

39. Elisia I, Krystal G (2021) The pros and cons of low carbohydrate and ketogenic diets in the prevention and treatment of cancer. Front Nutr 8:634845
40. Dmitrieva-Posocco O, Wong AC, Lundgren P, Golos AM, Descamps HC, Dohnalová L et al (2022) β-Hydroxybutyrate suppresses colorectal cancer. Nature 605(7908):160–165
41. Pflanz NC, Daszkowski AW, James KA, Mihic SJ (2019) Ketone body modulation of ligand-gated ion channels. Neuropharmacology 148:21–30
42. Mundi MS, Mohamed Elfadil O, Patel I, Patel J, Hurt RT (2021) Ketogenic diet and cancer: fad or fabulous? J Parenter Enter Nutr 45(S2):S26–S32
43. Fine EJ, Segal-Isaacson C, Feinman RD, Herszkopf S, Romano MC, Tomuta N et al (2012) Targeting insulin inhibition as a metabolic therapy in advanced cancer: a pilot safety and feasibility dietary trial in 10 patients. Nutrition 28(10):1028–1035
44. Schmidt M, Pfetzer N, Schwab M, Strauss I, Kammerer U (2011) Effects of a ketogenic diet on the quality of life in 16 patients with advanced cancer: a pilot trial. Nutr Metab (Lond) 8(1):54
45. Khodabakhshi A, Akbari ME, Mirzaei HR, Mehrad-Majd H, Kalamian M, Davoodi SH (2020) Feasibility, safety, and beneficial effects of mct-based ketogenic diet for breast cancer treatment: a randomized controlled trial study. Nutr Cancer 72(4):627–634
46. Plotti F, Terranova C, Luvero D, Bartolone M, Messina G, Feole L et al (2020) Diet and chemotherapy: the effects of fasting and ketogenic diet on cancer treatment. Chemotherapy 65(3–4):77–84
47. Lane J, Brown NI, Williams S, Plaisance EP, Fontaine KR (2021) Ketogenic diet for cancer: critical assessment and research recommendations. Nutrients 13(10)
48. Bonetti G, Herbst KL, Donato K, Dhuli K, Kiani AK, Aquilanti B et al (2022) Dietary supplements for obesity. J Prev Med Hyg 63(2 Suppl 3):E160–E168
49. Munoz A, Grant WB (2022) Vitamin D and cancer: an historical overview of the epidemiology and mechanisms. Nutrients 14(7)
50. L'Esperance K, Datta GD, Qureshi S, Koushik A (2020) Vitamin D exposure and ovarian cancer risk and prognosis. Int J Environ Res Public Health 17(4)
51. Kiani AK, Medori MC, Dhuli K, Donato K, Caruso P, Fioretti F et al (2022) Clinical assessment for diet prescription. J Prev Med Hyg 63(2 Suppl 3):E102–E124
52. Wang W, Hu W, Xue S, Chen Q, Jiang Y, Zhang H et al (2021) Vitamin D and lung cancer; association, prevention, and treatment. Nutr Cancer 73(11–12):2188–2200
53. Peterson CT, Rodionov DA, Osterman AL, Peterson SN (2020) B vitamins and their role in immune regulation and cancer. Nutrients 12(11)
54. Hossain S, Beydoun MA, Beydoun HA, Chen X, Zonderman AB, Wood RJ (2019) Vitamin D and breast cancer: a systematic review and meta-analysis of observational studies. Clin Nutr ESPEN 30:170–184
55. Abe E, Miyaura C, Sakagami H, Takeda M, Konno K, Yamazaki T et al (1981) Differentiation of mouse myeloid leukemia cells induced by 1 alpha,25-dihydroxyvitamin D3. Proc Natl Acad Sci U S A 78(8):4990–4994
56. Colston K, Colston MJ, Feldman D (1981) 1,25-dihydroxyvitamin D3 and malignant melanoma: the presence of receptors and inhibition of cell growth in culture. Endocrinology 108(3):1083–1086
57. Welsh J (2018) Vitamin D and breast cancer: past and present. J Steroid Biochem Mol Biol 177:15–20
58. Narvaez CJ, Matthews D, LaPorta E, Simmons KM, Beaudin S, Welsh J (2014) The impact of vitamin D in breast cancer: genomics, pathways, metabolism. Front Physiol 5:213
59. Feldman D, Krishnan AV, Swami S, Giovannucci E, Feldman BJ (2014) The role of vitamin D in reducing cancer risk and progression. Nat Rev Cancer 14(5):342–357
60. Blasiak J, Pawlowska E, Chojnacki J, Szczepanska J, Fila M, Chojnacki C (2020) Vitamin D in triple-negative and brca1-deficient breast cancer-implications for pathogenesis and therapy. Int J Mol Sci 21(10)

61. Bauer SR, Hankinson SE, Bertone-Johnson ER, Ding EL (2013) Plasma vitamin D levels, menopause, and risk of breast cancer: dose-response meta-analysis of prospective studies. Medicine (Baltimore) 92(3):123–131
62. Vanhevel J, Verlinden L, Doms S, Wildiers H, Verstuyf A (2022) The role of vitamin D in breast cancer risk and progression. Endocr Relat Cancer 29(2):R33–R55
63. Kim H, Lipsyc-Sharf M, Zong X, Wang X, Hur J, Song M et al (2021) Total Vitamin D intake and risks of early-onset colorectal cancer and precursors. Gastroenterology 161(4):1208–1217
64. Guo H, Guo J, Xie W, Yuan L, Sheng X (2018) The role of vitamin D in ovarian cancer: epidemiology, molecular mechanism and prevention. J Ovarian Res. 11(1):71
65. Na SY, Kim KB, Lim YJ, Song HJ (2022) Vitamin D and colorectal cancer: current perspectives and future directions. J Cancer Prev 27(3):147–156
66. Wesselink E, Kok DE, Bours MJ, De Wilt JH, Van Baar H, Van Zutphen M et al (2020) Vitamin D, magnesium, calcium, and their interaction in relation to colorectal cancer recurrence and all-cause mortality. Am J Clin Nutr 111(5):1007–1017
67. Ng K, Sargent DJ, Goldberg RM, Meyerhardt JA, Green EM, Pitot HC et al (2011) Vitamin D status in patients with stage IV colorectal cancer: findings from intergroup trial N9741. J Clin Oncol 29(12):1599
68. Yuan C, Sato K, Hollis BW, Zhang S, Niedzwiecki D, Ou F-S et al (2019) Plasma 25-hydroxyvitamin D levels and survival in patients with advanced or metastatic colorectal cancer: findings from CALGB/SWOG 80405 (Alliance). Clin Cancer Res 25(24):7497–7505
69. Pilz S, Tomaschitz A, Obermayer-Pietsch B, Dobnig H, Pieber TR (2009) Epidemiology of vitamin D insufficiency and cancer mortality. Anticancer Res 29(9):3699–3704
70. Kilkkinen A, Knekt P, Heliövaara M, Rissanen H, Marniemi J, Hakulinen T et al (2008) Vitamin D status and the risk of lung cancer: a cohort study in Finland. Cancer Epidemiol Biomark Prev 17(11):3274–3278
71. Maj E, Filip-Psurska B, Switalska M, Kutner A, Wietrzyk J (2015) Vitamin D analogs potentiate the antitumor effect of imatinib mesylate in a human A549 lung tumor model. Int J Mol Sci 16(11):27191–27207
72. Verone-Boyle AR, Shoemaker S, Attwood K, Morrison CD, Makowski AJ, Battaglia S et al (2016) Diet-derived 25-hydroxyvitamin D3 activates vitamin D receptor target gene expression and suppresses EGFR mutant non-small cell lung cancer growth in vitro and in vivo. Oncotarget 7(1):995
73. McGaffin KR, Chrysogelos SA (2005) Identification and characterization of a response element in the EGFR promoter that mediates transcriptional repression by 1, 25-dihydroxyvitamin D3 in breast cancer cells. J Mol Endocrinol 35(1):117–133
74. Qin B, Moorman PG, Alberg AJ, Barnholtz-Sloan JS, Bondy M, Cote ML et al (2016) Dairy, calcium, vitamin D and ovarian cancer risk in African-American women. Br J Cancer 115(9):1122–1130
75. Garland CF, Mohr SB, Gorham ED, Grant WB, Garland FC (2006) Role of ultraviolet B irradiance and vitamin D in prevention of ovarian cancer. Am J Prev Med 31(6):512–514
76. Boscoe FP, Schymura MJ (2006) Solar ultraviolet-B exposure and cancer incidence and mortality in the United States, 1993–2002. BMC Cancer 6:264
77. Tran B, Jordan SJ, Lucas R, Webb PM, Neale R (2012) Australian Ovarian Cancer Study G. Association between ambient ultraviolet radiation and risk of epithelial ovarian cancer. Cancer Prev Res (Phila) 5(11):1330–1336
78. Webb PM, de Fazio A, Protani MM, Ibiebele TI, Nagle CM, Brand AH et al (2015) Circulating 25-hydroxyvitamin D and survival in women with ovarian cancer. Am J Clin Nutr 102(1):109–114
79. Laczmanski L, Lwow F, Osina A, Kepska M, Laczmanska I, Witkiewicz W (2017) Association of the vitamin D receptor FokI gene polymorphism with sex- and non-sex-associated cancers: a meta-analysis. Tumour Biol 39(10):1010428317727164

80. Christakos S, Dhawan P, Verstuyf A, Verlinden L, Carmeliet G (2016) Vitamin D: metabolism, molecular mechanism of action, and pleiotropic effects. Physiol Rev 96(1):365–408
81. Gnagnarella P, Raimondi S, Aristarco V, Johansson HA, Bellerba F, Corso F et al (2020) Vitamin D receptor polymorphisms and cancer. Sunlight Vit D Skin Cancer 53–114
82. Laczmanski L, Lwow F, Osina A, Kepska M, Laczmanska I, Witkiewicz W (2017) Association of the vitamin D receptor FokI gene polymorphism with sex-and non-sex-associated cancers: a meta-analysis. Tumor Biol 39(10):1010428317727164
83. Mostowska A, Sajdak S, Pawlik P, Lianeri M, Jagodzinski PP (2016) Polymorphic variants in the vitamin D pathway genes and the risk of ovarian cancer among non-carriers of BRCA1/BRCA2 mutations. Oncol Lett 11(2):1181–1188
84. Carlberg C, Haq A (2018) The concept of the personal vitamin D response index. J Steroid Biochem Mol Biol 175:12–17
85. Leoncini E, Nedovic D, Panic N, Pastorino R, Edefonti V, Boccia S (2015) Carotenoid intake from natural sources and head and neck cancer: a systematic review and meta-analysis of epidemiological studies. Cancer Epidemiol Biomarkers Prev 24(7):1003–1011
86. Chew BP, Park JS (2004) Carotenoid action on the immune response. J Nutr 134(1):257S-S261
87. Brewczynski A, Jablonska B, Kentnowski M, Mrowiec S, Skladowski K, Rutkowski T (2021) The association between carotenoids and head and neck cancer risk. Nutrients 14(1)
88. Serebryakov PV, Pankova VB, Fedina IN, Rushkevich OP (2021) Coverage of issues of professional malignant neoplasms of the respiratory tract in modern clinical guidelines of the Ministry of Health of Russia. Vestn Otorinolaringol 86(5):48–53
89. Leoncini E, Edefonti V, Hashibe M, Parpinel M, Cadoni G, Ferraroni M et al (2016) Carotenoid intake and head and neck cancer: a pooled analysis in the international head and neck cancer epidemiology consortium. Eur J Epidemiol 31(4):369–383
90. Rowles JL 3rd, Erdman JW Jr (2020) Carotenoids and their role in cancer prevention. Biochim Biophys Acta Mol Cell Biol Lipids 1865(11):158613
91. Peng SJ, Li J, Zhou Y, Tuo M, Qin XX, Yu Q et al (2017) In vitro effects and mechanisms of lycopene in MCF-7 human breast cancer cells. Genet Mol Res 16(2)
92. Hu F, Wang Yi B, Zhang W, Liang J, Lin C, Li D et al (2012) Carotenoids and breast cancer risk: a meta-analysis and meta-regression. Breast Cancer Res Treat 131:239–253
93. Mignone LI, Giovannucci E, Newcomb PA, Titus-Ernstoff L, Trentham-Dietz A, Hampton JM et al (2009) Dietary carotenoids and the risk of invasive breast cancer. Int J Cancer 124(12):2929–2937
94. Tang FY, Shih CJ, Cheng LH, Ho HJ, Chen HJ (2008) Lycopene inhibits growth of human colon cancer cells via suppression of the Akt signaling pathway. Mol Nutr Food Res 52(6):646–654
95. Tang FY, Pai MH, Wang XD (2011) Consumption of lycopene inhibits the growth and progression of colon cancer in a mouse xenograft model. J Agric Food Chem 59(16):9011–9021
96. Han X, Zhao R, Zhang G, Jiao Y, Wang Y, Wang D et al (2022) Association of retinol and carotenoids content in diet and serum with risk for colorectal cancer: a meta-analysis. Front Nutr 9:918777
97. Gallicchio L, Boyd K, Matanoski G, Tao XG, Chen L, Lam TK et al (2008) Carotenoids and the risk of developing lung cancer: a systematic review. Am J Clin Nutr 88(2):372–383
98. Le Marchand L, Hankin JH, Kolonel LN, Beecher GR, Wilkens LR, Zhao LP (1993) Intake of specific carotenoids and lung cancer risk. Cancer Epidemiol Biomark Prevent Publ Am Assoc Cancer Res Cospon Am Soc Prevent Oncol 2(3):183–187
99. Rafi MM, Kanakasabai S, Reyes MD, Bright JJ (2013) Lycopene modulates growth and survival associated genes in prostate cancer. J Nutr Biochem 24(10):1724–1734
100. Lee SA, Cai Q, Franke AA, Steinwandel M, Wu J, Wen W et al (2021) Associations of subtype and isomeric plasma carotenoids with prostate cancer risk in low-income African and European Americans. Cancer Epidemiol Biomarkers Prev 30(10):1846–1857

101. Lu Q-Y, Hung J-C, Heber D, Go VLW, Reuter VE, Cordon-Cardo C et al (2001) Inverse associations between plasma lycopene and other carotenoids and prostate cancer. Cancer Epidemiol Biomark Prev 10(7):749–756
102. Anderson AS, Renehan AG, Saxton JM, Bell J, Cade J, Cross AJ et al (2021) Cancer prevention through weight control—where are we in 2020? Br J Cancer 124(6):1049–1056
103. Guthold R, Stevens GA, Riley LM, Bull FC (2018) Worldwide trends in insufficient physical activity from 2001 to 2016: a pooled analysis of 358 population-based surveys with 1· 9 million participants. Lancet Glob Health 6(10):e1077–e1086
104. Bull FC, Al-Ansari SS, Biddle S, Borodulin K, Buman MP, Cardon G et al (2020) World Health Organization 2020 guidelines on physical activity and sedentary behaviour. Br J Sports Med 54(24):1451–1462
105. WHO (2022) Global status report on physical activity 2022. World Health Organization. Licence: CC BY-NC-SA 3.0 IGO
106. Arnold M, Pandeya N, Byrnes G, Renehan AG, Stevens GA, Ezzati M et al (2015) Global burden of cancer attributable to high body-mass index in 2012: a population-based study. Lancet Oncol 16(1):36–46
107. Jackson A (2018) Diet, nutrition, physical activity and cancer: a global perspective.continuous update project expert report 2018. World cancer research fund/american institute for cancer research. Available at dietandcancerreportorg
108. McTiernan A (2008) Mechanisms linking physical activity with cancer. Nat Rev Cancer 8(3):205–211
109. Friedenreich CM, Neilson HK, Lynch BM (2010) State of the epidemiological evidence on physical activity and cancer prevention. Eur J Cancer 46(14):2593–2604
110. Hojman P (2017) Exercise protects from cancer through regulation of immune function and inflammation. Biochem Soc Trans 45(4):905–911
111. Oh H, Arem H, Matthews CE, Wentzensen N, Reding KW, Brinton LA et al (2017) Sitting, physical activity, and serum oestrogen metabolism in postmenopausal women: the Women's Health Initiative Observational Study. Br J Cancer 117(7):1070–1078
112. de Sousa CV, Sales MM, Rosa TS, Lewis JE, de Andrade RV, Simões HG (2017) The antioxidant effect of exercise: a systematic review and meta-analysis. Sports Med 47:277–293
113. Gunter MJ, Xie X, Xue X, Kabat GC, Rohan TE, Wassertheil-Smoller S et al (2015) Breast cancer risk in metabolically healthy but overweight postmenopausal women. Can Res 75(2):270–274
114. Clemente-Suárez VJ, Martín-Rodríguez A, Redondo-Flórez L, Ruisoto P, Navarro-Jiménez E, Ramos-Campo DJ et al (2023) Metabolic health, mitochondrial fitness, physical activity, and cancer. Cancers 15(3):814
115. Ferioli M, Zauli G, Maiorano P, Milani D, Mirandola P, Neri LM (2019) Role of physical exercise in the regulation of epigenetic mechanisms in inflammation, cancer, neurodegenerative diseases, and aging process. J Cell Physiol 234(9):14852–14864
116. Nomikos NN, Nikolaidis PT, Sousa CV, Papalois AE, Rosemann T, Knechtle B (2018) Exercise, telomeres, and cancer:"the exercise-telomere hypothesis." Front Physiol 9:1798
117. Papadimitriou N, Dimou N, Tsilidis KK, Banbury B, Martin RM, Lewis SJ et al (2020) Physical activity and risks of breast and colorectal cancer: a Mendelian randomisation analysis. Nat Commun 11(1):597
118. Mazzilli KM, Matthews CE, Salerno EA, Moore SC (2019) Weight training and risk of 10 common types of cancer. Med Sci Sports Exerc 51(9):1845
119. Rezende LF, Lee DH, Keum N, Wu K, Eluf-Neto J, Tabung FK et al (2020) Resistance training and total and site-specific cancer risk: a prospective cohort study of 33,787 US men. Br J Cancer 123(4):666–672
120. Bird SR, Hawley JA (2017) Update on the effects of physical activity on insulin sensitivity in humans. BMJ Open Sport Exerc Med 2(1):e000143
121. Inoue M, Tsugane S (2012) Insulin resistance and cancer: epidemiological evidence. Endocr Relat Cancer 19(5):F1–F8

122. Wang Q, Zhou W (2021) Roles and molecular mechanisms of physical exercise in cancer prevention and treatment. J Sport Health Sci 10(2):201–210
123. Magné N, Melis A, Chargari C, Castadot P, Guichard J-B, Barani D et al (2011) Recommendations for a lifestyle which could prevent breast cancer and its relapse: physical activity and dietetic aspects. Crit Rev Oncol Hematol 80(3):450–459
124. Desnoyers A, Riesco E, Fülöp T, Pavic M (2016) Physical activity and cancer: update and literature review. La Revue de medecine interne. 37(6):399–405
125. Gonçalves AK, Florêncio GLD, de Atayde Silva MJM, Cobucci RN, Giraldo PC, Cote NM (2014) Effects of physical activity on breast cancer prevention: a systematic review. J Phys Act Health 11(2):445–454
126. JB SG, Silva-Filho A, Dias C, Leite R, Mostarda C (2017) Effect of exercise training and detraining in autonomic modulation and cardiorespiratory fitness in breast cancer survivors. J Sports Med Physic Fit 57(7–8):1062–1068
127. Liu L, Shi Y, Li T, Qin Q, Yin J, Pang S et al (2016) Leisure time physical activity and cancer risk: evaluation of the WHO's recommendation based on 126 high-quality epidemiological studies. Br J Sports Med 50(6):372–378
128. Psaltopoulou T, Ntanasis-Stathopoulos I, Tzanninis I-G, Kantzanou M, Georgiadou D, Sergentanis TN (2016) Physical activity and gastric cancer risk: a systematic review and meta-analysis. Clin J Sport Med 26(6):445–464
129. Schmid D, Behrens G, Keimling M, Jochem C, Ricci C, Leitzmann M (2015) A systematic review and meta-analysis of physical activity and endometrial cancer risk. Eur J Epidemiol 30:397–412
130. Behrens G, Jochem C, Keimling M, Ricci C, Schmid D, Leitzmann MF (2014) The association between physical activity and gastroesophageal cancer: systematic review and meta-analysis. Eur J Epidemiol 29:151–170
131. Moore SC, Lee I-M, Weiderpass E, Campbell PT, Sampson JN, Kitahara CM et al (2016) Association of leisure-time physical activity with risk of 26 types of cancer in 1.44 million adults. JAMA Int Med 176(6):816–825
132. Schmid D, Ricci C, Behrens G, Leitzmann MF (2016) Does smoking influence the physical activity and lung cancer relation? A systematic review and meta-analysis. Euro J Epidemiol 31:1173–1190
133. Christensen JF, Simonsen C, Hojman P (2011) Exercise training in cancer control and treatment. Compr Physiol 9(1):165–205
134. Patel AV, Friedenreich CM, Moore SC, Hayes SC, Silver JK, Campbell KL et al (2019) American College of Sports Medicine roundtable report on physical activity, sedentary behavior, and cancer prevention and control. Med Sci Sports Exerc 51(11):2391
135. Koelwyn GJ, Quail DF, Zhang X, White RM, Jones LW (2017) Exercise-dependent regulation of the tumour microenvironment. Nat Rev Cancer 17(10):620–632
136. McCullough DJ, Stabley JN, Siemann DW, Behnke BJ (2014) Modulation of blood flow, hypoxia, and vascular function in orthotopic prostate tumors during exercise. JNCI: J Nat Cancer Inst 106(4)
137. Bigley AB, Spielmann G, LaVoy EC, Simpson RJ (2013) Can exercise-related improvements in immunity influence cancer prevention and prognosis in the elderly? Maturitas 76(1):51–56
138. WHO (2020) Obesity estimates. Geneva, World Health Organisation. https://www.hoint/news-room/fact-sheets/detail/obesity-and-overweight
139. Simopoulos AP (1987) Obesity and carcinogenesis: historical perspective. Am J Clinic Nutri 45(1):271–276
140. Hidayat K, Du X, Shi BM (2018) Body fatness at a young age and risks of eight types of cancer: systematic review and meta-analysis of observational studies. Obes Rev 19(10):1385–1394
141. Research WC (2023) Diet, nutrition, physical activity and cancer: a global perspective. body fatness and weight gain and the risk of cancer. https://www.crforg/dietandcancer/exposures/body-fatness. Accessed on 22, March 2023

142. Ellulu MS, Patimah I, Khaza'ai H, Rahmat A, Abed Y (2017) Obesity and inflammation: the linking mechanism and the complications. Arch Med Sci 13(4):851–863
143. Harris BHL, Macaulay VM, Harris DA, Klenerman P, Karpe F, Lord SR et al (2022) Obesity: a perfect storm for carcinogenesis. Cancer Metastasis Rev 41(3):491–515
144. Li Y, Hecht SS (2022) Carcinogenic components of tobacco and tobacco smoke: A 2022 update. Food Chem Toxicol 165:113179
145. Larsson SC, Carter P, Kar S, Vithayathil M, Mason AM, Michaelsson K et al (2020) Smoking, alcohol consumption, and cancer: A mendelian randomisation study in UK Biobank and international genetic consortia participants. PLoS Med 17(7):e1003178
146. Secretan B, Straif K, Baan R, Grosse Y, El Ghissassi F, Bouvard V et al (2009) A review of human carcinogens–Part E: tobacco, areca nut, alcohol, coal smoke, and salted fish. Lancet Oncol 10(11):1033–1034
147. Wei P-L, Chang Y-J, Ho Y-S, Lee C-H, Yang Y-Y, An J et al (2009) Tobacco-specific carcinogen enhances colon cancer cell migration through α7-nicotinic acetylcholine receptor. Ann Surg 249(6):978–985
148. Hecht SS (2002) Tobacco smoke carcinogens and breast cancer. Environ Mol Mutagen 39(2–3):119–126
149. Jethwa AR, Khariwala SS (2017) Tobacco-related carcinogenesis in head and neck cancer. Cancer Metastasis Rev 36:411–423
150. Caliri AW, Tommasi S, Besaratinia A (2021) Relationships among smoking, oxidative stress, inflammation, macromolecular damage, and cancer. Mutat Res Rev Mutat Res 787:108365
151. Humans IWGotEoCRt (2013) Non-ionizing radiation, Part 2: Radiofrequency electromagnetic fields. IARC Monogr Eval Carcinog Risks Hum 102(Pt 2):1–460
152. Stang A, Anastassiou G, Ahrens W, Bromen K, Bornfeld N, Jockel KH (2001) The possible role of radiofrequency radiation in the development of uveal melanoma. Epidemiology 12(1):7–12
153. Karipidis KK, Benke G, Sim MR, Kauppinen T, Giles G (2007) Occupational exposure to ionizing and non-ionizing radiation and risk of glioma. Occup Med (Lond) 57(7):518–524
154. Gupta S, Sharma RS, Singh R (2022) Non-ionizing radiation as possible carcinogen. Int J Environ Health Res 32(4):916–940
155. Bauer A, Diepgen TL, Schmitt J (2011) Is occupational solar ultraviolet irradiation a relevant risk factor for basal cell carcinoma? a systematic review and meta-analysis of the epidemiological literature. Br J Dermatol 165(3):612–625
156. Institute NC (2023) Complementary and alternative medicine: national cancer institute. https://www.cancer.gov/about-cancer/treatment/cam
157. Horneber M, Bueschel G, Dennert G, Less D, Ritter E, Zwahlen M (2012) How many cancer patients use complementary and alternative medicine: a systematic review and metaanalysis. Integr Cancer Ther 11(3):187–203
158. Frenkel M, Slater R, Sapire K, Sierpina V (2018) Complementary and integrative medicine in lung cancer: questions and challenges. J Altern Complement Med 24(9–10):862–871
159. David A, Hausner D, Frenkel M (2021) Cancer-related fatigue-is there a role for complementary and integrative medicine? Curr Oncol Rep 23(12):145

Nutrition and Dietary Intervention in Cancer: Gaps, Challenges, and Future Perspectives

11

Falak Zeb, Aqsa Mehreen, Huma Naqeeb, Muneeb Ullah, Afraa Waleed, Uzma Azeem Awan, Adnan Haider, and Muhammad Naeem

Contents

F. Zeb
Research Institute for Medical and Health Sciences, University of Sharjah, Sharjah, United Arab Emirates
e-mail: fzeb@sharjah.ac.ae

A. Mehreen · A. Waleed · U. A. Awan · A. Haider · M. Naeem (✉)
Department of Biological Sciences, National University of Medical Sciences, Rawalpindi, Pakistan
e-mail: m.naeem@numspak.edu.pk

A. Mehreen
e-mail: aqsamehreenstudent@numspak.edu.pk; aqsamehreen36@gmail.com

A. Waleed
e-mail: afraawaleed_student@numspak.edu.pk

U. A. Awan
e-mail: uzma.awan@numspak.edu.pk

A. Haider
e-mail: adnan.haider@numspak.edu.pk

H. Naqeeb
Department of Clinical Nutrition, Shaukat Khanum Memorial Cancer Hospital, and Research Center, Peshawar, Pakistan
e-mail: huma.naqeeb@skm.org.pk

M. Ullah
College of Pharmacy, Pusan National University, Busan, South Korea
e-mail: munibdawar72@gmail.com

R. F. Saeed and S. ul. Shaheed (eds.), *Nutrition and Dietary Interventions in Cancer*, Cancer Treatment and Research 191, https://doi.org/10.1007/978-3-031-55622-7_11

11.1 Introduction

According to the National Cancer Institute of the National Institutes of Health, the term cancer refers to a category of diseases in which normal cells get mutated and transform into abnormal cells. These abnormal cells divide uncontrollably and are capable of invading other tissues ultimately leading to the destruction of normal body tissues [1]. Cancer has reportedly become one of the leading causes of death all around the globe and approximately 10 million people died because of cancer in 2020 [2]. Cancerous cells follow the process of metastasis by which these can spread to different parts of the body. Cancerous cells break off from their original site of development and use blood and the lymphatic system as a transport medium to spread across distant regions and organs of the body [3]. It is multifactorial diseases and numerous internal as well as external factors contribute to its pathogenesis. It is mainly a genetic disease but a combination of various external factors contributes in its onset [4]. This malicious disease develops at the cellular level mainly because of somatic mutation in DNA because of exposure to certain mutagenic factors. These mutations then trigger the expression of various oncogenic genes and the repression in the activity of tumor suppressive genes hence leading to uncontrolled cell duplication sequences [5, 6]. An increase in oxidative stress inside the body triggers the tumor formation [7–9]. A number of phytochemicals present in our food can be used to scavenge those free radicals present inside of our body thus resulting in modulation and suppression in tumor expansion in body [9, 10]. Based on pathophysiology, cancer can be classified as into different types as shown in Fig. 11.1. Further classification of different types of cancers is done according the type of organ and cell where the cancer begins. For example, if the onset of cancer is in the colon that cancer is named as colon

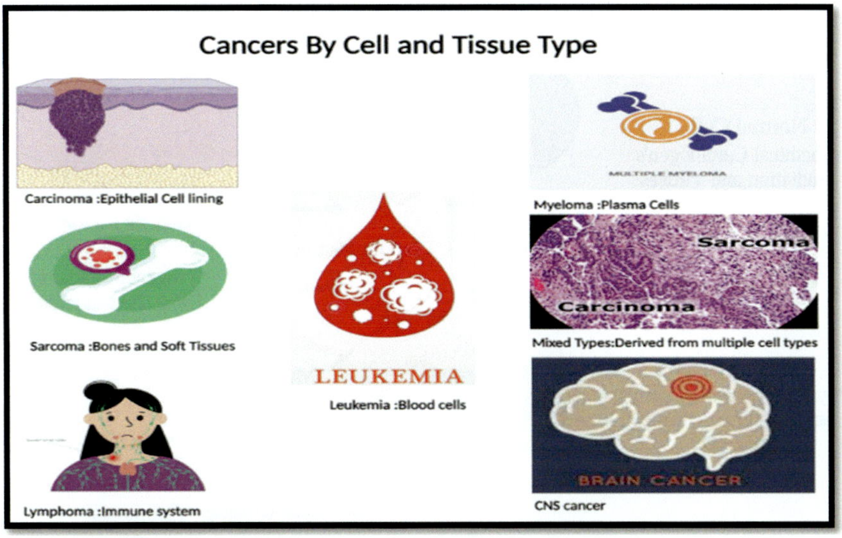

Fig. 11.1 Types of cancers based on cell types (created in BioRender.com)

cancer; or the cancer of the melanocyte of the skin is referred as melanoma [11]. Process of development of cancer, its progression and its incidence does not occur suddenly, it can take several years of its manifestation (Fig. 11.2).

An unhealthy diet may raise cancer risk, and malnutrition can reduce the effectiveness of cancer therapy, making food and nutrition crucial in both preventing and treating the disease. Recent epidemiological studies have shown genetic and behavioral variables in cancer prevention, and the discovery of innovative molecular agents has revolutionized cancer care. Since cancer treatment success rates have increased, nutrition and food have become focal points in post-treatment care for survivors [12].

Preventative studies have received the lion's share of attention in the field of cancer and nutrition research, while studies focusing on treatment and care have lagged far behind. Cancer patients and their doctors may benefit greatly from understanding the link between diet and therapy. In this regard, some promising insights on the roles of diet and nutrition in cancer prevention [13, 14], and treatment [15–17] are reported; it is possible that food and nutrition might have a major effect on health. New strategies for treating triple-negative breast tumors have been explored in two recent trials [15, 17]. Targeted treatments, such as a hormone or HER-2 targeted therapy, are typically ineffective against triple-negative breast cancer, leading to a poor prognosis for patients. According to Hossain et al., mycobiome and folate are two areas of particular interest [17]. Although these investigations are in the preclinical stages, they present us with innovative options to enhance outcomes in patients with this subtype of breast cancer, for whom the use of chemotherapy and molecular medicines is restricted [12].

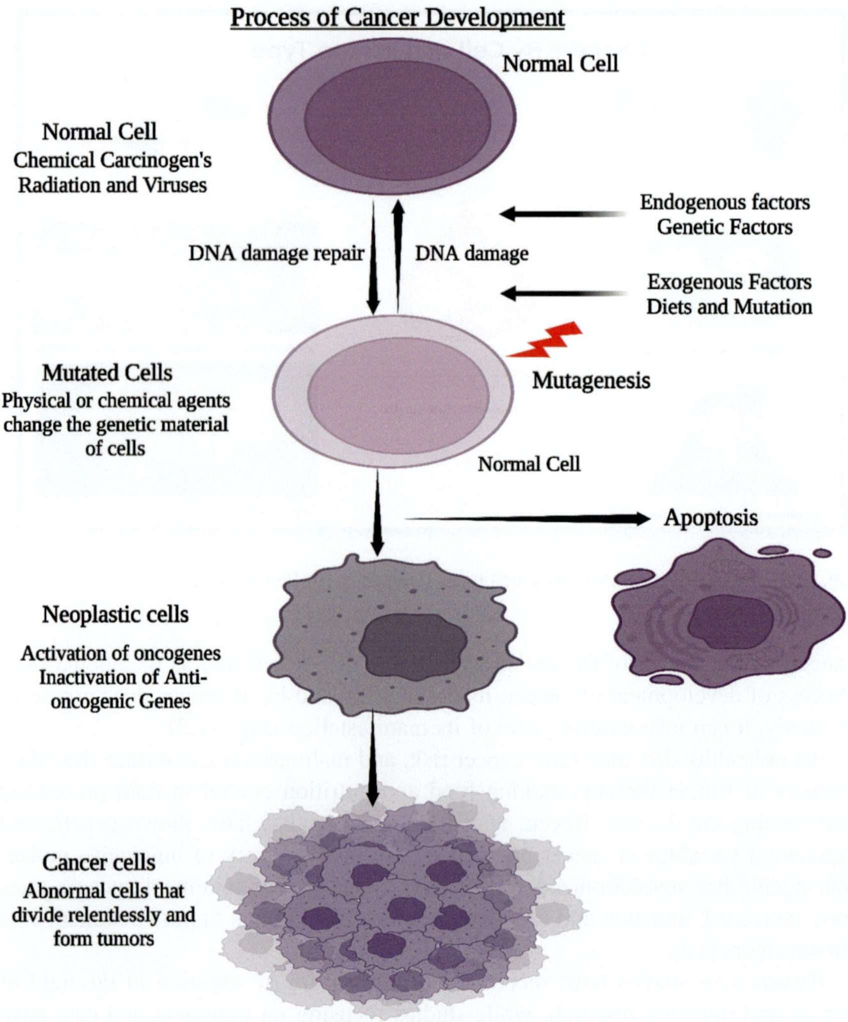

Fig. 11.2 Process of cancer development (created in BioRender.com)

Diet quality was revealed to lower the incidence of lung cancer, highlighting the importance of a balanced diet in cancer prevention [14]. Finkeldey's comprehensive evaluation of 18 randomized controlled trials including premenopausal and postmenopausal women found no conclusive evidence that isoflavones lower breast cancer risk [13, 18, 19]. In addition to medical or pharmaceutical intervention, cancer patients and survivors often need nutritional assistance. Even for malignancies with a poor prognosis, like pancreatic cancer, this may enhance both qualities of life and treatment results [20]. In the future, we expect to see more studies on nutritional care to avoid undernutrition and loss of quality of life in cancer patients, which would boost the efficacy of therapy [12].

11.2 Nutritional Needs of Cancer Patient

Cancer patients are highly susceptible to malnutrition because of change in the metabolic activities and difficulty in absorption of nutrients. Previously conducted studies have proven that about 40–80% of the cancer patients suffer from malnutrition [21]. The elevated range of malnutrition is dependent on various factors such as type and stage of cancer and the treatment nature being opted for cancer treatment [22]. During the treatment tenure for cancer, the patients have to go through a lot of physical and psychological stress and better nutrition is necessary to provide enough strength to patient to withstand the therapy and to enhance their quality of life. During nutritional therapy of cancer patient's dietary choices are made which are not normally recommended when a person is healthy. Patients having cancer need better diet such as intake of high energy food, high protein intake to maintain healthy weight and increased consumption of fluids to prevent dehydration (Table 11.1). All the dietary interventions are made according to the individual nutritional assessment, but the general recommendations are kept same [23, 24].

i. **Energy**

   Cancer patients require more energy as cancer induces hypermetabolic state in the body. In addition, increased energy is required during healing of tissue in cancer patients [24]. In cancer the energy intake of patient is affected which ultimately leads toward change in the total energy expenditure. Total energy expenditure is quite difficult to be measured directly, resting energy expenditure is used to determine about the nutritional requirements of cancer patients. Energy requirements vary in different types of cancer [25]. Calculation of energy needs follows determination of the resting energy expenditure (REE) and additional needs for activity and tissue healing, in accordance with practice guidelines for the type of cancer. Macronutrient composition should be apportioned to allow sufficient protein for tissue healing and maintenance. Energy intake levels should be ranging from 20 to 35 kcal/kg of body weight

Table 11.1 Nutritional goals in cancer treatment

Nutritional intakes	Amount
Energy	20–30 kcal/kg/d for cancer patients
Proteins	1–1.5 g/kg/d
Vitamins and minerals	Vitamins and minerals must be supplied in sufficient amount according to the recommended dietary allowance

depending on the age, gender and activity level of the patient [26]. Carbohydrates comprise most of the calorie intake, with fat providing about 30% of the total calories. Overfeeding must be avoided to minimize the risk of refeeding syndrome [27].

ii. **Protein**

Proteins are the ultimate source to keep our muscles strong and to keep immune system in healthy condition. During cancer due to insufficient intake of protein in diet the body starts breaking down the muscles to keep the protein requirements in balance which leads to muscle loss. To prepare the body to respond to cancer therapy efficiently it is necessary to maintain proper nutritional intake of essential amino acids as well as nitrogen. If the protein requirements are completely fulfilled it helps the body to respond more efficiently toward the treatment and also maintenance of a healthy body weigh due to reduced tissue catabolism [28]. For cancer patient protein intake of about 1.2–1.5 g/kg per day is recommended as per the nutritional requirements. Proteins supplements can also be used in case of severe malnutrition condition such as cachexia [24].

iii. **Vitamins and Minerals**

Vitamins are necessary for proper utilization of energy present in the food because a lot of enzymes are there which require vitamins as cofactors in metabolic pathways [29]. During cancer treatment, patients are usually unable to eat properly ultimately leading to deficiency of vitamins and minerals in body. Uptake of vitamins is usually recommended by the medical PR actioners depending upon nutritional requirement of the individual. A healthy immune system depends on healthy intake of vitamins and minerals [30]. The best way to maintain balanced vitamin and minerals levels is by enhanced consumption of fruits and vegetables [24, 31].

iv. **Fluids**

In cancer fluids intake is as crucial as balanced food intake. In cancer, due to side effects of cancer treatments patients might suffer from diarrhea and vomiting which leads to dehydration [32]. It is especially important to maintain the proper hydration level in body to keep electrolytes balance and removal of toxins from the body. During cancer treatment, cancerous cells are destroyed leading to production of toxic metabolites. Thus, adequate fluid intake is necessary to remove those toxic metabolites from body. On average most of the adults need 35 mL/kg of fluid intake each day [31–33].

11.3 Pharmacological Depletion of Nutrients

A lot of times, cancer cells are deficient in nutrients that regular cells don't need. This highlights a weakness of cancer cells that may be addressed by dietary changes and pharmaceutical strategies alike. Despite the possibility that dietary depletion of some of the nutrients described here may be preferable, the literature exclusively discusses pharmaceutical depletion. Improvements in nutritional depletion and responses to cancer treatment are predicted to occur from combining dietary restriction with pharmaceutical targeting of certain selectively critical nutrients, such as amino acids and vitamin folate [34].

11.3.1 Asparagine

Improved survival has been linked to lower asparagine concentrations in the plasma of leukemia patients [35]. Asparagine's importance in tumor development is highlighted by the ability of asparaginase to deplete it from the diet, suggesting the enzyme's therapeutic potential. Because asparagine serves as both an amino acid exchange factor (primary for the amino acids serine, histidine, and arginine) and as a metastasis-promoting metabolite, it is absolutely necessary for a number of different anabolic pathways [36, 37]. Regrettably, pharmacologic asparagine reduction is often associated with toxicity [35]. Asparagine depletion due to a poor diet is a topic of little research at present. A published study found that a diet low in asparagine was sufficient to prevent metastasis in a mouse model of breast cancer. This dietary-mediated depletion was found to be sufficient to prevent metastasis. However, there is a possibility that the levels of asparagine in the blood of mice who were fed an asparagine-deficient diet would be decreased [37]. To evaluate the anti-tumor therapeutic potential of dietary-mediated asparagine depletion, further study is required, particularly for leukemia, where the abnormal cells are typically asparagine auxotrophic [34, 35].

11.3.2 Arginine

As a result of the downregulation of the enzyme argininosuccinate synthetase 1, hepatocellular carcinomas, some melanomas, and prostate carcinomas are arginine auxotrophs. These tumors are unable to produce arginine from citrulline (as part of the urea cycle), despite the fact that quiescent cells may do so [38]. Depriving cancer cells of arginine by diet or treating them with the arginine-degrading enzyme arginine deiminase may combat their reliance on the amino acid (ADI) [39, 40]. Studies on melanoma and hepatocellular cancer models in vitro and in vivo, as well as a clinical study including patients with hepatocellular carcinoma, have shown the efficacy of arginine depletion by AD [41]. In mice that already have melanoma, inhibiting autophagy in the liver leads hepatocytes to release the enzyme arginase 1 (ARG1), which lowers overall levels of arginine in the body and, as a result, slows the progression of the cancer [42].

Because it serves as the substrate for the enzyme that produces nitric oxide (NO), arginine has an effect on NO levels throughout the body [43]. Although it is known that NO has a function in immunity, and it has an effect that is carcinogenic in conditions characterized by persistent inflammation, whether dietary arginine restriction may lower NO levels and so bypass this effect is uncertain [44]. If nitric oxide's function in activating immune cells is critical for tumor immunity, then NO and arginine, which is its precursor, are not effective therapy targets for cancer [34].

11.3.3 Cystine

Considering that cystine is a step along the path to cysteine an antioxidant that is a component of glutathione, it plays a significant role in keeping cellular redox equilibrium. Higher concentration of Cystine is found in the plasma and cystine utilizes specific cysteine-glutamate antiporter known as xCT (SLC7A11) for entry with in the cells. In three animal models of tumor development, cystine deprivation has been found to reduce tumor growth and increase patient survival. Mutations in the epidermal growth factor receptor in non-small-cell lung cancer (NSCLC) xenografts [45]; prostate xenografts; and a genetic leukemia (*TCL1*-Tg:*Trp53*−/−)model [46]. Cystine depletion by pharmacological enzymatic breakdown was utilized in these investigations, although a comparable effect might be produced with dietary restriction [34].

The loss of cystine causes a shortage of the amino acid cysteine and, by extension, the antioxidant glutathione (GSH). These cells die through ferroptosis because their ability to react to oxidative damage is compromised, and oxidative damage is especially severe in cancer cells. Lack of damage in healthy tissues after chronic cystine depletion in mice supports the tumor-specific impact (up to 50 days) [46].

11.3.4 Folate

Folate, a form of vitamin B9, is needed to produce nucleotides and is therefore vital for the functioning of all cells. Rapidly dividing cells including enterocytes, hematopoietic cells, and tumor cells need copious amounts of folate for the synthesis of new nucleotides used in DNA replication and gene expression. It has been known for over seventy years that adding more folic acid to one's diet speeds up the progression of acute lymphoblastic leukemia (ALL) [47]. With this knowledge, anti-folate cancer therapies might be created [48] and highlight the importance of folate in tumor development [48, 49]. Anti-folate methotrexate is now the gold standard for the treatment of childhood leukemia and is also used in the management of a variety of other cancers, most often hematological malignancies. Anti-folates interfere with the production of nucleotides, which are in great demand by rapidly replicating cancer cells [50].

Considering that anti-folate cancer therapy is mostly pharmacologic, it is challenging to predict how much dietary folate restriction might contribute to tumor inhibition. Intestinal tumor development and progression in Apcmin/+ mice were suppressed by a combination of dietary uridine supplementation and folate restriction [51]. In order to determine whether or not dietary folate restriction alone has an anti-tumorigenic effect, it is necessary to assess the relative risks of cancer in both the normal and folate-free diet groups [34].

11.3.5 Glutamine and Glutamate

The amino acid glutamine and its immediate metabolite, glutamate, both have roles in the proliferation of cancer cells via different metabolic pathways. The tricarboxylic acid (TCA) cycle uses them to produce energy molecules ATP and NADH [52]. Glutamine is an essential component for nucleotide biosynthesis as during pyrimidine and purines biosynthesis one and two nitrogen atoms are contributed by glutamine. To maintain the cellular redox balance and facilitate glutathione synthesis, glutamine is essential [53]. Last but not least, glutamine and glutamate both have a role in the synthesis of lipids in hypoxic conditions [54]. Both preclinical and clinical researches have indicated that inhibiting the enzyme glutaminase, which is the first enzyme in the process of glutamine catabolism, may reduce the growth of tumors. On the other hand, if an excessive amount of glutamate is present, the inhibition may be circumvented [55]. As a result, asparagine may be able to prevent glutamine depletion; nevertheless, limiting glutamine in one's diet without also limiting glutamate consumption is not expected to have a significant impact on the metabolic processes of cancer cells. The dependency of tumors on glutamine in vivo is not as well established as it is for cancer cells in vitro. In vivo studies have not been as conclusive [53]. Transformed and non-transformed rapidly replicating cells alike are thought to have a conditional need for glutamine [56]. As a result, it would be useful to zero down on how glutamine is used by cancer cells specifically. Cancer cells, for instance, are more vulnerable to oxidative stress [57], and cancer cells may be more vulnerable to the effects of glutamine deficiency and reduced antioxidant defense [58]. Blocking mTOR or aspartate transporters may prevent the metabolic rewiring that permits glutamine-deprived cancer cells to survive and so boost the specificity of glutamine deprivation's inhibitory impact on tumors [34, 59].

Limiting glutamine in the diet as a therapy option should take into account glutamine levels in the tumor microenvironment as shown in Fig. 11.3. There was no significant decrease in tumor load when glutamine levels were lowered in the blood but not the cerebellum of mice with glioblastoma [60]. Mice with medulloblastoma fared better when their glutamine levels were restricted by their diets. This includes a significant drop in cerebellar and CSF glutamine levels [61]. Since glutamine is secreted by stromal cells, it is extremely challenging to reduce glutamine levels in the microenvironment of brain tumors [60]. Measurements of glutamine at the tumor site are crucial for interpreting in vivo studies using glutamine depletion in these tumor models [62]. Aspartate transaminase (GOT1) (L-aspartate + 2-oxoglutarate oxaloacetate + L-glutamate) is an enzyme located in the cytoplasm that prevents glutamate from being converted to -ketoglutarate

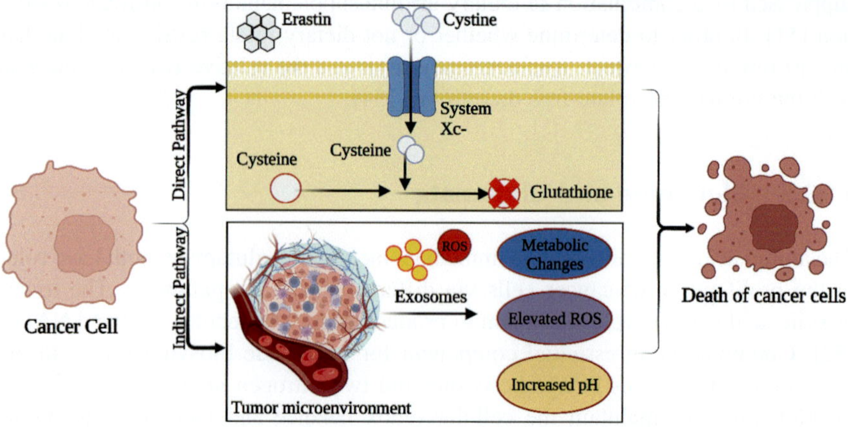

Fig. 11.3 Pharmacological depletion of glutamine (glutathione) in cancer therapy. Glutathione plays a major role in tumorigenesis, because of direct pathway inhibition of glutathione ferroptosis and by indirect pathways the tumor microenvironment is susceptible to immune response of immune system

in proliferating mammary epithelial cells and cancer cells harboring the oncogene KRAS [58]. Human pancreatic ductal adenocarcinoma (PDAC) cells benefit from this because it promotes their proliferation and redox stability [58]. Directly contributing to glutathione formation, and indirectly through cystine import via the glutamate-cystine antiporter xCT, glutamate helps maintain intracellular antioxidant levels high in lung cancer [63]. Because of the xCT antiporter, glioma cells are able to generate glutamate, which protects them from oxidative damage caused by the cystine they import. An increase in glutamate levels in the peritumoral fluid is the root cause of seizures in glioma patients; this glutamate is created by the glioma itself and is poisonous to the healthy neurons in the tumor environment [62]. Although inhibiting xCT transporter has therapeutic success and glutamate was shown to have a role in the development of gliomas [60, 62], to what extent limiting glutamate intake in the diet may lower peritumoral glutamate levels are not yet known [34].

11.3.6 Aspartate

Aspartate plays a role in protein synthesis, nucleic acid synthesis, the urea cycle, and the malate-aspartate shuttle. Since aspartate synthesis is reliant on cellular respiration, low levels of aspartate may be growth-limiting under hypoxic conditions—which are widespread in malignancies. As it turns out, hypoxic cells don't produce much aspartate [64, 65]. Additionally, aspartate is a limiting metabolite in tumors when they are studied in vivo [64]. Aspartate production may be inhibited by electron transport chain inhibitors through the respiration-dependent mitochondrial enzyme aspartate aminotransferase (GOT2). As a result of these circumstances, the cytosolic enzyme GOT1 is used by the cell to produce aspartate, which then enables the protein and nucleic acid production pathways. Increasing the amounts of aspartate inside cells by the overexpression of exogenous asparaginase, which transforms asparagine into aspartate [64], or SLC1A3, the aspartate transporter, increases the likelihood that cancer cells would survive in vivo despite the presence of low oxygen levels [65]. Remarkably, recovery of reduced de novo aspartate synthesis in hypoxic cells by nucleoside supplementation highlights the fact that aspartate contributes to pyrimidine and purine production rather than TCA cycle flux under hypoxia circumstances [65].

Aspartate restriction may be used as adjunctive therapy for the treatment of solid tumors, which are often hypoxic due to poor vascularization. In addition to a reduced ability to manufacture aspartate, hypoxia also causes numerous other cellular vulnerabilities that may be addressed in a reasonably focused way. Because of the importance of aspartate in nucleotide synthesis in hypoxic tumors, it may be beneficial to combine aspartate restriction with medicines that target nucleotide biosynthesis, such as methotrexate and fluorouracil [34].

11.3.7 Alanine

However, despite alanine's potential to replace glucose and glutamine as a significant TCA cycle substrate in pancreatic ductal adenocarcinoma (PDAC), it is not likely to be a nutrient that can be targeted by diet [66, 67]. Using alanine produced by stromal cells, PDAC cells become less reliant on blood-borne nutrition. It is very unlikely that a dietary strategy would be helpful in this scenario since dietary alterations alter food availability in the bloodstream without affecting the capacity of stromal cells to generate non-essential amino acids like alanine [34, 66].

11.3.8 Fatty Acids

Fatty acid oxidation (FAO) is a far more efficient means of producing ATP than either glucose fermentation or amino acid catabolism. Establishing whether cancer cells can use fatty acids as a substrate when glucose is scarce, or even as a preferred substrate regardless of glucose availability, is crucial for understanding if fatty acid deprivation could affect cancer progression. FAO is the primary source of ATP synthesis in several types of malignancies. Under conditions of metabolic stress, some breast cancer tumors turn on a transcription factor called fatty acid oxidase [68, 69], or in the setting of excessive expression of MYC or carnitine palmitoyl transferase (CPT1C) [70, 71]. OxPhos-DLBCL is a subtype of diffuse large B cell lymphoma (DLBCL) that may oxidize fatty acids as its primary energy source and is susceptible to pharmacologic disruption of this pathway [72]. A low-fat diet increases the longevity of obese mice with leukemia, highlighting the importance of fatty acids to the formation of malignant malignancies and hinting that adipocytes are unlikely to compensate for the lack of fatty acids [73].

By the excessive consumption of high-fat diet, activity and quantity of the intestinal stem cells also increases which ultimately leads to raised incidence of adenomas and carcinomas in the gut. Consumption of diet having higher fat content leads to activation of PPARδ which then permits the progenitor cells to facilitate the in vivo proliferation and colony formation in vitro in comparison to the intestinal stem cells [74]. However, it has not yet been decided if limiting fatty acids would have the reverse effect, i.e., decrease the number of spontaneous adenomas or carcinomas in the gut. FAO also promotes cancer cells by supplying NADPH. NADPH is an essential modulator of redox equilibrium and a growth-limiting metabolite. FAO inhibition induces the buildup of ROS and inhibits glioma cell growth [75], and AMPK signaling promotes NADPH generation and cancer cell survival in response to FAO activation [76].

These data, taken together, point to the possibility that there is therapeutic promise in depriving patients of essential fatty acids to starve some forms of cancer [77]. These results also raise the idea that a high-fat ketogenic diet can have detrimental consequences that promote the growth of tumors in some types of malignancies. Therefore, it is not apparent which forms of cancer or which people (with different dietary habits) would benefit the most from either a diet low in fat or a diet rich in fat [34].

11.4 Medical Nutrition Therapy for Cancer Patients

Cancer treatment can disturb the normal metabolic function of the body. Cancer patients face different problems such as loss of appetite, disturbance in metabolism of different nutrients as well as creates disturbance in absorption of nutrients from food which leads to malnutrition among the cancer patients. So along with other treatments available for cancer patients' nutritional assistance is necessary to speed up the recovery process. Nutritional treatment in cancer patients follows the Nutrition Care Process (NCP). The NCP is specifically designed with intricacy, and all the steps in the entire process are related to each other so that all the aspects in the nutritional therapy are covered [78].

i. **Nutrition assessment**: Nutritional assessment is the first step in the nutritional care process. It is a systematic process which involves the collection of data regarding the dietary consumptions of the patients. This step is performed to develop a basic insight toward the patients baseline nutritional status [79]. The information regarding the food intake is collected from either patient themselves or family members of the patient who are the keen observer of the nutritional profile of the patients. Body Mass Index (BMI) is also determined, but it is not the main criteria as the BMI can be changed because of various other factors such as genetics [80]. Nutritional assessment is the systematic process which involves continual reassessments and analysis of the nutritional status of patients in comparison to the standard criterion [24, 81].

ii. **Nutrition diagnosis**: It involves the identification of any existing nutritional problem in the patients. Cancer patients suffer from malnutrition because of problem in absorption of nutrients and inability of consume food [24]. Nutritional diagnosis focuses on the physical state, baseline nutritional status of the patient and the common symptoms of the nutritional deficiency associated diseases such as anorexia, sarcopenia, and cachexia. After the nutritional diagnosis, it is solely the responsibility of the nutritional professional to treat the nutritional problem [82].

iii. **Nutrition intervention**: It involves the development of the nutritional plan keeping in view the nutritional status of the patient as cancer patients suffer a lot during the treatment. So after the nutritional assessment and nutritional diagnosis of the cancer patient nutritional interventions are planned [83]. Nutritional interventions are done to assist and to provide nutritional support to the patients to enhance the impact of their cancer therapy. Nutritional interventions are planned according to the nutritional behavior of the respective patient, nutritional deficiencies, susceptibility of patient to be at risk to malnourishment and environmental condition. Nutritional Intervention is the direct measure opted to resolve any diseases detected during nutritional diagnosis [84, 85]. Nutritional interventions are the main supportive approaches opted to protect the patient from being critically malnourished and to enhance the quality of life among them [86, 87].

iv. **Nutrition monitoring and evaluation**: Nutritional monitoring and assessment is a continued process. Main aim of nutritional monitoring and evaluation is to determine whether the goals to eliminate the problems associated with nutritional deficiencies are being met or not [88]. Nutritional monitoring and evaluation evaluate the expected outcomes in response to the nutritional interventions with the outcomes being achieved. This provides with the clear inter relationship for outcomes of nutritional intervention.

Each of these steps must be designed according to the following guidelines:

a. The plan must be designed targeting the specific nutritional deficiencies and with measurable outcomes for nutritional evaluation.
b. An effective nutritional plan will only be development using a holistic approach for continuous reassessment of the nutritional status of respective patients along with collaboration by the healthcare team [24].
c. The plan must be devised keeping an eye over the signs and symptoms associated with the improvement in quality of life of the cancer patient due to nutritional interventions.

11.5 Role of Nutrition in Cancer Prevention and Management

Nutrition plays a critical role in the prevention and management of various diseases. In the modern era, people are nowadays more susceptible to diseases because of changes in lifestyle and dietary practices [89]. Nutrigenomics is one of the leading emerging fields that also emphasizes on the importance and impact of dietary practices on the development of various diseases more prominently cancer [90]. Studies have proven the importance of dietary modifications in different fundamental metabolic processes which lead to onset and prevention of cancer. Different fundamental process within the cell such as the process of differentiation of cells, their proliferation, apoptosis and necrosis as well as expression of oncogenes and tumor suppressive genes are influenced by the diet. Bioactive components in food interact synergistically with all the cellular processes mentioned above [91]. Previously conducted studies have proven that 30–40% of all types of cancers can be cured by adaptation of better dietary practices and lifestyle modifications [92]. It goes both ways healthy lifestyle and healthy diet leads to activation of metabolic pathways ultimately leading to cancer prevention and suppression of oncogenes. However bad nutritional practices such as enhanced intake of sugars, refined flour, red meat and imbalance between omega 3 and omega 6 fatty acids leads to more susceptibility toward cancer. Different nutritional interventions based on type of cancer have been proven effective in previous research. For example, in colorectal cancer, enhanced uptake of dietary fibers and calcium has been proven to effective in its prevention.

11.5.1 Role of High-Fat Diets

Unquestionably, the dietary therapies for cancer in mice that have received the most investigation are those that explore the connection between Western-style diets or high-fat diets and the development, progression, and mortality of cancer. These commercially accessible diets are notorious for their high-fat content (up to 60%), which leads to fast weight gain [93]. High-fat diets have been linked to an increased risk of colorectal and breast cancer in mice, according to the majority of this research [94–97]. Transgenerational effects of maternal exposure to high-fat diets are also of interest, with multiple mice studies reporting an increase in the incidence and development of breast and prostate cancer in children [98–101].

Some of the explanations for the association between high-fat diets and the development of cancer in these animal models include inflammatory pathways, adipokines, gut microbiota, estrogen metabolism, and metabolic factors and/or signaling [102, 103]. Increased consumption of dietary fat has been linked to an increased risk of developing cancer in animals however, the translational significance of this research is hampered by methodological shortcomings in the published literature. Diets used in many rodent studies include abnormally high amounts of dietary fat (40–60% of energy from fat), which is much higher than the average human diet (30–40% of energy from fat) [93, 104]. There is just one source of fat in these diets, and that source is either beef tallow, coconut oil, or milk fat; there is no other supply of fat (for instance, the omega-6 fatty acid to omega-3 fatty acid ratio, the monounsaturated fatty acid to polyunsaturated fatty acid ratio, or the proportion of proteins, carbohydrates, and fats). In rats, diets high in fat have been associated to an increased risk of getting cancer; however, the mechanisms that underlie this relationship need to be investigated in more depth [104].

11.5.2 Role of the Ketogenic Diet

Multiple preclinical studies are finding that the ketogenic diet has anticancer effects. A meta-analysis of animal experiments ($n = 12$) found that mice fed a ketogenic diet were less likely to acquire cancer than mice on a high-carbohydrate diet [105]. A 2019 review found that the ketogenic diet for cancer reduced tumor growth, improved survival, delayed tumor onset, and reversed cancer-induced cachexia in the great majority of preclinical mouse studies [106]. In addition, both a mouse model of neuroblastoma and mice with xenografts in their lungs have shown that the ketogenic diet makes cancer cells more vulnerable to chemotherapy and radiation, respectively [107, 108]. Cancer treatment settings account for the vast majority of animal investigations on the ketogenic diet and cancer, with a focus on brain tumor and colorectal cancer models [104, 109, 110].

Ketogenic diets have been shown to reduce cancer risk, although it's not clear how. Nevertheless, various possible methods have been hypothesized, such as modulating gene expression, inhibiting angiogenesis, targeting mitochondrial, glucose, and amino acid metabolism in cancer cells, and preventing the production of reactive oxygen species (ROS) [106]. Small sample numbers, varied contexts, and a lack of established processes complicate the translation of results from mice models to the clinic, despite the mainly favorable preclinical findings. In addition, preliminary studies have shown that the anticancer effectiveness of ketogenic diets may vary depending on the specific kind of cancer being treated and the patient's genetic history [111]. In order to facilitate adaptation and clinical recommendation of ketogenic diet for prevention and treatment of cancer large scale experimentation is required with range of mouse models along with preventative models. This will make it easier for any recommendations to be implemented into clinical practice [104].

11.5.3 Role of the Mediterranean Diet

Only one study has ever been done to see what effect eating foods from different parts of the Mediterranean has on the likelihood of cancer developing in mice. It has been shown that eicosatetraenoic acid, which is a kind of omega-3 polyunsaturated fatty acid, together with a mixture of bioactive phytochemical extracts that are similar to the primary categories that make up the Mediterranean diet, may suppress colon cancer in mice. The regulation of apoptosis and intestinal dysbiosis was shown to be associated to this impact [112]. Further animal experiments that properly duplicate the dietary patterns that are described in the epidemiological literature are necessary in order to determine whether or not the Mediterranean diet reduces the risk of cancer and to characterize the mechanisms that are involved in this determination [104, 112].

11.6 Nutritional Status and Surgery Oncology Patient

Nutritional status of the patient for successful surgical outcome is necessary. Better nutritional status better the postoperative recovery of patient. Balanced nutrition plays the prime role behind the better metabolic function, better nutrients absorption and stronger immune system ultimately leading to improved quality of life [113]. Preoperative optimization of basal nutritional status of cancer patient is the most thriving aspect for faster healing postoperatively [114, 115]. Designing of nutritional interventions which result in faster healing, stronger immune system is necessary both pre and post operatively. Postoperative nutritional care can be modified depending upon the surgery. Like in any of postoperative healing period of any surgery performed on GI tract the patients are unable to digest food properly. So, the nutritional interventions must be done accordingly keeping an eye over the patient compliance [116].

These challenges are characteristic of the portion of the GI tract involved rather than to the cancer itself, as seen in the following:

i. **Head and neck surgery**

   During head and neck surgery, the most affected area is oropharyngeal area. Due to this, the patient feel difficulty in consumption of food so the postoperative nutritional care must be designed accordingly [117]. During the process of healing in surgeries involving the oropharyngeal area, different dietary modifications are being made which most commonly include diets with textural modifications such as maximum intake of fluids or in serious conditions may require modifications in feeding modalities by use of feeding tubes [118, 119].

ii. **Gastric or intestinal resections**

   After gastrointestinal resections, different problems may occur which require proper nutritional evaluation. Because after intestinal resections improper digestion and absorption of food becomes the limiting factor behind slower healing process and weight loss [120]. So special nutritional interventions are necessary regarding nutrients composition, food texture and feeding timing as well. Consumption of fat soluble nutrients and electrolytes is usually preferred in such condition [121].

iii. **Pancreatectomy**

Pancreatectomy comes with more critical postoperative complications as removal of pancreas leads to loss of digestive enzymes causing poor absorption of food and loss of nutrients. The patients may need to take digestive enzymes and insulin to prevent further complications [122].

11.7 Nutritional Status and Radiation Oncology Patient

Radiation therapy has side effects, but these are less prevalent in comparison to the chemotherapeutic agents. Patients who receive radiation therapy in head and neck region and in the abdominal cavity are more susceptible nutrition related signs and symptoms [123]. Medical nutritional therapy has been proven to improve quality of life among patients having radiation therapy by enhanced protein and calorie intake [124].

i. **Head and neck radiation therapy**

   Radiation therapy in head and neck region affects the mucosal and salivary secretions which influence the sensation of food taste and sensitivity toward temperature and texture of food. Mucositis, Xerostomia and dyssomnia (loss of smell) are enlisted among the top side effects of radiation therapy. Medical Nutrition Therapy in such cases emphasize over modification in food aroma and appearances [125]. Common treatment options that negatively impact the saliva secretions can be reverted completely via emphasizing on use of specific medi-ation as well inclusion of foods and chewing gums which ultimately stimulates saliva production [126, 127].

ii. **Abdominal cavity radiation therapy**

   Radiation therapy in the abdominal cavity can lead to production of denuded bowl mucosa, loss of villi, ulceration, and inflammation. Medical nutrition therapy in such cases emphasizes over macronutrient composition, electrolytes and fluids in diet [128].

11.8 Nutritional Status and Chemotherapy Patient

Chemotherapeutic agents adversely affect normally reproducing cells, which is more evident in cells of gastrointestinal tract, bone marrow and hair follicles [129]. Chemotherapeutic agents adversely affecting the bone marrow interfere with production of blood cells such as red and white blood cells as well platelets. In such cases, medical nutritional therapy suggests enhanced uptake of vitamins and minerals involved in formation of red blood cells as well as platelets [130]. Medical nutritional therapy suggests the use of neutropenic diet in which foods having high microbial count such as raw fruits and vegetables are restricted. Moreover, along with these different medicines can also be prescribed that stimulate these blood cells production. Most common side effects of chemotherapy in cancer are as follows:

i. Gastrointestinal effects of chemotherapy induce nausea, vomiting and ulcers. Among the gastrointestinal effects nausea and vomiting are on top and effects approximately 50% of the patients at some point during the treatment process [131].
ii. Inadequate control of chemotherapy-induced emesis can cause malabsorption and electrolytes imbalance. Dietary intervention must be done under consideration of registered dietitian to control chemotherapy-induced emesis to improve quality of life in cancer patients [132].
iii. Due to side effects of chemotherapy, diseases such as colostomies and ileostomies are caused which require proper guidance for medical nutritional therapy. Mainly in order to relive such sort of gastrointestinal distress medical nutritional therapy emphasizes on alteration in food texture, macronutrients composition of food as well as timing of feeding [133] (Table 11.2).

11.9 Nutritional-Based Gaps and Challenges

i. **Alternations in Nutritional Status**

Malnutrition is commonly diagnosed in cancer patients as during the cancer treatment, food intake and absorption of nutrients from food are compromised. Malnutrition in cancer patients causes the immune system to be less responsive and weaker which leads to inferior quality of life, short survival time [26]. These three basic systemic effects are common in association to the disease, like Anorexia, change in Metabolic state and Negative Nitrogen Balance due to poor dietary consumption of protein ultimately leading to muscle loss from body [139]. All these effects vary from person to person depending upon the type and stage of cancer the patient is. More than 50% of deaths are caused due to extreme forms of cachexia in cancer patients [140, 141]. Anorexia is an eating disorder which is accompanied by feeling of discomfort in normal eating of food as well negative thoughts which in serious conditions may develop into depression. Due the course of cancer treatment, the patient is already going through a lot both on mental and physical grounds [142]. At such time, when a healthy and balanced nutrition is necessary anorexic patients are unable to consume healthy diet which lead weight loss and poor response toward therapy. It may develop into cachexia if left untreated [143].

ii. **Cachexia**

Cachexia is caused due to systemic metabolic effects, and its etiology is not clearly understood till date. In cachexia, extreme weight loss occurs associated due to alteration in whole metabolism of body during cancer treatment [144].

Table 11.2 Dietary modification for dealing food-related complications in cancer patients

Side effect	Dietary modifications	Reference
Anorexia	Small portion of high nutrient meals Foods with unpleasant odor must be avoided	[134]
Changed taste and odor perception	Use of organic food and seasonings to enhance food flavor Use of protein rich food such as fish, milk and cheese Restricted use of red meat	[135]
Stomatitis and mucositis	Use of food in liquid in semisolid form and in form of puree Restricted use of citrus, spicy and acidic food Use of food with sauces and gravies Carbonated beverages are avoided	[136]
Xerostomia	Increased fluid intake Increased use of soft and moist food and alcohols must be avoided	[137]
Dysphagia	Use of high protein and high calorie food Encourage use of commercially available nutritional supplements	[138]
Nausea and vomiting	Small and frequent meals Use of dry food without added fats and sauces Foods with pungent smells are restricted	[137]
Diarrhea	Increased fluid consumption it prevents dehydration Restricted use of greasy, fried and high-fat food Avoid caffeine	[137]

iii. **Malnutrition across the course of cancer treatment**

Malnutrition is one of the leading and frequent complication faced by cancer patients which causes hindrance in normal recovery process during therapy. But tackling down of cancer patients with malnutrition is one of the most challenging task [145]. The main aim while nutritional assessment and diagnosis of cancer patients is to detect early signs of malnutrition to help patients in surviving against this brutal disease [140]. Role of nutritional status in cancer patients is stressed out a lot for a successful therapy still its consideration is lacking in clinical practice [145, 146].

Malnutrition is one of the leading cause behind the increased mortality rate in cancer patient as it hinders the normal process of healing, poor quality of life and worst postoperative outcomes and complications. Severe cases of malnutrition in cancer patients is an independent predictor for short survival rate [147–149] (Fig. 11.4).

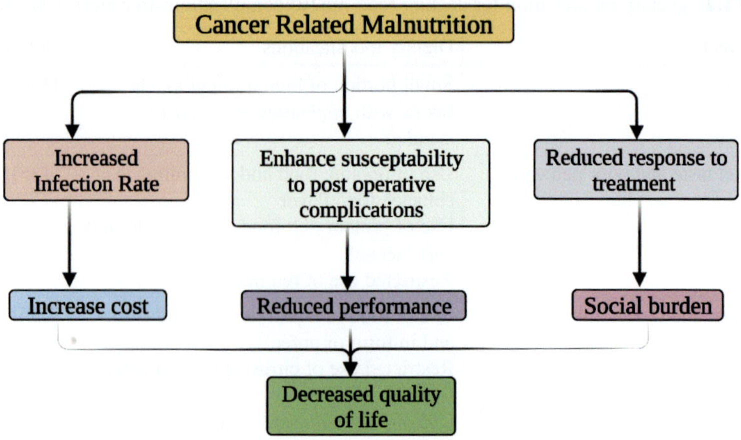

Fig. 11.4 Flowchart of cancer-related malnutrition [151]

11.10 Implementation Research to Test Programs and Policies

Despite the efforts being put in implementation of cancer prevention strategies, still a lot of substantial gaps are left. It is evident that just by educating people about importance of better dietary practices and preventative and management strategies for cancer is insufficient for obtaining sustained and substantial behaviors. Proper implementation of cancer prevention and management strategies needs development of proper public health policies encouraging the healthy lifestyle. To ensure long-term implementation of such heath policies need development of proper frame work for evaluation and assessment of effectiveness of such policies and programs [150].

i. One of the main barriers in implementation of nutritional therapy in cancer patients is lack of information and awareness in healthcare professionals regarding positive impact of nutritional interventions in cancer patients.
ii. Another challenge in the treatment of digestive cancer that most of the patients are reluctant toward use of multivitamins and oral supplements because of higher prices and in case of some patient's lifelong supplementation is required as well. So in such cases it is important to develop policies to make total reimbursement for these supplements to save lives of such patients.
iii. Correct prescription and constant monitoring of at home artificial nutrition for patients must be provided using the standardized quality criteria without any additional cost. Integration of proper protocols to easily access the rehabilitation programs must be ensured for patients with digestive cancer.
iv. For better detection of malnutrition in cancer patients CT scan and bioimpedance must be used.

v. New nutritional guidelines must be designed in accordance with the new treatment strategy used for treatment of cancer such as immunotherapy.
vi. Proper programs must be organized to increase awareness in health professionals and public regarding importance of nutrition in cancer treatment.
vii. Proper training must be provided to healthcare professionals for nutritional assessment and counseling of cancer patients.
viii. Collection and analysis of data regarding the impact of nutritional therapy in cancer
ix. Increase in research must be encouraged in order to identify the nutritional and other loopholes in treatment of conditions such as malnutrition, sarcopenia and cancer.

There is a dire need to spread the word regarding the importance of nutrition in cancer treatment in public as well as the healthcare professionals to save the lives people suffering from cancer. Development of new strategies for nutritional assessment, its evaluation and implementation must be done to improve quality of life in cancer patients. Proper health policies must be developed with specific framework to check the impact of nutritional interventions and make amendments accordingly to ensure better quality of thousands of people.

11.11 Conclusion and Future Perspective

The nutritional therapies are cost-effective and might be available by patients regardless of their socioeconomic situation, but pharmacologic interventions can be expensive, increase the drug load, and be less flexible to a broad variety of malignancies and treatments. In addition, these interventions allow the patient to participate in their treatment in a way that could significantly impact outcomes and encourages patient engagement and adherence.

In the future, we expect to see more studies on nutritional care to avoid undernutrition and loss of quality of life in cancer patients, which would boost the efficacy of therapy. In immunological cause of cancer genetic, proteomic, and molecular approach are used in identification of pathways associate in cancer development.

Acknowledgements The author would like to acknowledge the National University of Medical Sciences (NUMS).

Conflict of Interest The authors declared that they have no competing or conflict of interest.

References

1. Suresh S (2007) Biomechanics and biophysics of cancer cells. Acta Biomater 3(4):413–438
2. Ferlay J et al (2021) Cancer statistics for the year 2020: an overview. Int J Cancer
3. Fares J et al (2020) Molecular principles of metastasis: a hallmark of cancer revisited. Signal Transduct Target Ther 5(1):28

4. Anand P et al (2008) Cancer is a preventable disease that requires major lifestyle changes. Pharm Res 25(9): 2097–2116
5. Gupta C, Prakash D (2014) Phytonutrients as therapeutic agents. J Complement Integr Med 11(3):151–169
6. Moorthy B, Chu C, Carlin DJ (2015) Polycyclic aromatic hydrocarbons: from metabolism to lung cancer. Toxicol Sci 145(1):5–15
7. Key TJ et al (2004) Diet, nutrition and the prevention of cancer. Public Health Nutr 7(1a):187–200
8. Calle EE et al (2003) Overweight, obesity, and mortality from cancer in a prospectively studied cohort of US adults. New Engl J Med 348(17):1625–1638
9. Garcia M et al (2007) Global cancer facts & figures 2007 1(3):52
10. World Cancer Reasearch Fund, American Institute for Cancer Research (2018) Diet, nutrition, physical activity and cancer: a global perspective
11. Estanqueiro M et al (2015) Nanotechnological carriers for cancer chemotherapy: the state of the art. Colloids Surf B Biointerfaces 126:631–648
12. Narimatsu H, Yaguchi YT (2022) The role of diet and nutrition in cancer: prevention, treatment, and survival. MDPI, p 3329
13. Alegria-Lertxundi I et al (2020) Gene–diet interactions in colorectal cancer: survey design, instruments, participants and descriptive data of a case-control study in the Basque country. Nutrients 12(8):2362
14. Park S-Y et al (2021) Diet quality and risk of lung cancer in the multiethnic cohort study. Nutrients 13(5):1614
15. Coleman MF et al (2021) Metabolic response of triple-negative breast cancer to folate restriction. Nutrients 13(5):1637
16. Maiuolo J et al (2021) Nutraceuticals and cancer: potential for natural polyphenols. Nutrients 13(11):3834
17. Hossain F et al (2021) Obesity modulates the gut microbiome in triple-negative breast cancer. Nutrients 13(10):3656
18. Finkeldey L, Schmitz E, Ellinger S (2021) Effect of the intake of isoflavones on risk factors of breast cancer—a systematic review of randomized controlled intervention studies. Nutrients 13(7):2309
19. Manolio TA, Bailey-Wilson JE, Collins FS (2006) Genes, environment and the value of prospective cohort studies. Nat Rev Genet 7(10):812–820
20. Rovesti G et al (2021) Clinical implications of malnutrition in the management of patients with pancreatic cancer: introducing the concept of the Nutritional Oncology Board. Nutrients 13(10):3522
21. Muscaritoli M et al (2017) Prevalence of malnutrition in patients at first medical oncology visit: the PreMiO study. Oncotarget 8(45):79884
22. Bozzetti F et al (2012) The nutritional risk in oncology: a study of 1,453 cancer outpatients. Support Care Cancer 20(8):1919–1928
23. Rivadeneira DE et al (1998) Nutritional support of the cancer patient. CA Cancer J Clin 48(2):69–80
24. Arends J et al (2019) ESPEN guidelines on nutrition in cancer patients. Clin Nutr 36(1):11–48
25. Bulmuş Tüccar T, Acar Tek N (2021) Determining the factors affecting energy metabolism and energy requirement in cancer patients. J Res Med Sci 26:124
26. Arends J et al (2017) ESPEN expert group recommendations for action against cancer-related malnutrition. Clin Nutr 36(5):1187–1196
27. Kreymann G, Adolph M, Mueller MJ (2009) Energy expenditure and energy intake—guidelines on parenteral nutrition, chapter 3. Ger Med Sci 7:Doc25
28. Doyle C et al (2006) Nutrition and physical activity during and after cancer treatment: an American Cancer Society guide for informed choices. CA Cancer J Clin 56(6):323–353
29. Huskisson E, Maggini S, Ruf (2007) The role of vitamins and minerals in energy metabolism and well-being. J Int Med Res 35(3):277–289

30. Bendich A (1993) Physiological role of antioxidants in the immune system. J Dairy Sci 76(9):2789–2794
31. Slavin JL, Lloyd B (2012) Health benefits of fruits and vegetables. Adv Nutr 3(4):506–516
32. Sarhill N et al (2001) Evaluation and treatment of cancer-related fluid deficits: volume depletion and dehydration. Support Care Cancer 9(6):408–419
33. Cranganu A, Camporeale J (2009) Nutrition aspects of lung cancer. Nutr Clin Pract 24(6):688–700
34. Kanarek N, Petrova B, Sabatini DM (2020) Dietary modifications for enhanced cancer therapy. Nature 579(7800):507–517
35. Hijiya N, Van Der Sluis IM (2016) Asparaginase-associated toxicity in children with acute lymphoblastic leukemia. Leuk Lymphoma 57(4):748–757
36. Krall AS et al (2016) Asparagine promotes cancer cell proliferation through use as an amino acid exchange factor. Nat Commun 7(1):1–13
37. Knott SR et al (2018) Asparagine bioavailability governs metastasis in a model of breast cancer. Nature 554(7692):378–381
38. Dillon BJ et al (2004) Incidence and distribution of argininosuccinate synthetase deficiency in human cancers: a method for identifying cancers sensitive to arginine deprivation. Cancer 100(4):826–833
39. Lind DS (2004) Arginine and cancer. J Nutr 134(10):2837S-2841S
40. Kremer JC et al (2017) Arginine deprivation inhibits the Warburg effect and upregulates glutamine anaplerosis and serine biosynthesis in ASS1-deficient cancers. Cell Rep 18(4):991–1004
41. Ensor CM et al (2002) Pegylated arginine deiminase (ADI-SS PEG20, 000 mw) inhibits human melanomas and hepatocellular carcinomas in vitro and in vivo. Can Res 62(19):5443–5450
42. Poillet-Perez L et al (2018) Autophagy maintains tumour growth through circulating arginine. Nature 563(7732):569–573
43. Palmer RM, Ashton D, Moncada S (1988) Vascular endothelial cells synthesize nitric oxide from L-arginine. Nature 333(6174):664–666
44. Ohshima H, Bartsch H (1994) Chronic infections and inflammatory processes as cancer risk factors: possible role of nitric oxide in carcinogenesis. Mutat Res/Fundam Mol Mech Mutagen 305(2):253–264
45. Poursaitidis I et al (2017) Oncogene-selective sensitivity to synchronous cell death following modulation of the amino acid nutrient cystine. Cell Rep 18(11):2547–2556
46. Cramer SL et al (2017) Systemic depletion of L-cyst(e)ine with cyst(e)inase increases reactive oxygen species and suppresses tumor growth. Nat Med 23(1):120–127
47. Farber S et al (1947) The action of pteroylglutamic conjugates on man. Science 106(2764):619–621
48. Farber S et al (1948) Temporary remissions in acute leukemia in children produced by folic acid antagonist, 4-aminopteroyl-glutamic acid (aminopterin). N Engl J Med 238(23):787–793
49. Wilson PM et al (2014) Standing the test of time: targeting thymidylate biosynthesis in cancer therapy. Nat Rev Clin Oncol 11(5):282–298
50. Shuvalov O et al (2017) One-carbon metabolism and nucleotide biosynthesis as attractive targets for anticancer therapy. Oncotarget 8(14):23955
51. Field MS et al (2018) Dietary uridine decreases tumorigenesis in the $Apc^{Min/+}$ model of intestinal cancer. Curr Dev Nutr 2(5):nzy013
52. DeBerardinis RJ et al (2007) Beyond aerobic glycolysis: transformed cells can engage in glutamine metabolism that exceeds the requirement for protein and nucleotide synthesis. Proc Natl Acad Sci 104(49):19345–19350
53. Cluntun AA et al (2017) Glutamine metabolism in cancer: understanding the heterogeneity. Trends Cancer 3(3):169–180
54. Metallo CM et al (2012) Reductive glutamine metabolism by IDH1 mediates lipogenesis under hypoxia. Nature 481(7381):380–384

55. Biancur DE et al (2017) Compensatory metabolic networks in pancreatic cancers upon perturbation of glutamine metabolism. Nat Commun 8(1):1–15
56. Lacey JM, Wilmore DW (1990) Is glutamine a conditionally essential amino acid? Nutr Rev 48(8):297–309
57. Moloney JN, Cotter TG (2018) ROS signalling in the biology of cancer. In: Seminars in cell & developmental biology. Elsevier
58. Son J et al (2013) Glutamine supports pancreatic cancer growth through a KRAS-regulated metabolic pathway. Nature 496(7443):101–105
59. Momcilovic M et al (2018) The GSK3 signaling axis regulates adaptive glutamine metabolism in lung squamous cell carcinoma. Cancer Cell 33(5):905–921. e5
60. Tardito S et al (2015) Glutamine synthetase activity fuels nucleotide biosynthesis and supports growth of glutamine-restricted glioblastoma. Nat Cell Biol 17(12):1556–1568
61. Niklison-Chirou MV et al (2017) TAp73 is a marker of glutamine addiction in medulloblastoma. Genes Dev 31(17):1738–1753
62. Yang L et al (2016) Targeting stromal glutamine synthetase in tumors disrupts tumor microenvironment-regulated cancer cell growth. Cell Metab 24(5):685–700
63. Sayin VI et al (2017) Activation of the NRF2 antioxidant program generates an imbalance in central carbon metabolism in cancer. Elife 6:e28083
64. Sullivan LB et al (2018) Aspartate is an endogenous metabolic limitation for tumour growth. Nat Cell Biol 20(7):782–788
65. Garcia-Bermudez J et al (2018) Aspartate is a limiting metabolite for cancer cell proliferation under hypoxia and in tumours. Nat Cell Biol 20(7):775–781
66. Birsoy K et al (2015) An essential role of the mitochondrial electron transport chain in cell proliferation is to enable aspartate synthesis. Cell 162(3):540–551
67. Sousa CM et al (2016) Pancreatic stellate cells support tumour metabolism through autophagic alanine secretion. Nature 536(7617):479–483
68. Carracedo A et al (2012) A metabolic prosurvival role for PML in breast cancer. J Clin Investig 122(9):3088–3100
69. Schafer ZT et al (2009) Antioxidant and oncogene rescue of metabolic defects caused by loss of matrix attachment. Nature 461(7260):109–113
70. Camarda R et al (2016) Inhibition of fatty acid oxidation as a therapy for MYC-overexpressing triple-negative breast cancer. Nat Med 22(4):427–432
71. Zaugg K et al (2011) Carnitine palmitoyltransferase 1C promotes cell survival and tumor growth under conditions of metabolic stress. Genes Dev 25(10):1041–1051
72. Caro P et al (2012) Metabolic signatures uncover distinct targets in molecular subsets of diffuse large B cell lymphoma. Cancer Cell 22(4):547–560
73. Tucci J et al (2018) Switch to low-fat diet improves outcome of acute lymphoblastic leukemia in obese mice. Cancer Metab 6(1):1–8
74. Beyaz S et al (2016) High-fat diet enhances stemness and tumorigenicity of intestinal progenitors. Nature 531(7592):53–58
75. Pike LS et al (2011) Inhibition of fatty acid oxidation by etomoxir impairs NADPH production and increases reactive oxygen species resulting in ATP depletion and cell death in human glioblastoma cells. Biochim Biophys Acta (BBA) Bioenerg 1807(6):726–734
76. Jeon S-M, Chandel NS, Hay N (2012) AMPK regulates NADPH homeostasis to promote tumour cell survival during energy stress. Nature 485(7400):661–665
77. Carracedo A, Cantley LC, Pandolfi PP (2013) Cancer metabolism: fatty acid oxidation in the limelight. Nat Rev Cancer 13(4):227–232
78. Lövestam E et al (2019) The international nutrition care process and terminology implementation survey: towards a global evaluation tool to assess individual practitioner implementation in multiple countries and languages. J Acad Nutr Diet 119(2):242–260
79. Lacey K, Pritchett E (2003) Nutrition care process and model: ADA adopts road map to quality care and outcomes management. J Am Diet Assoc 103(8):1061
80. Nuttall FQ (2015) Body mass index: obesity, BMI, and health: a critical review. Nutr Today 50(3):117

81. Cushen S (2015) Nutrition assessment in oncology. Top Clin Nutr 30:103–119
82. Cao DX et al (2010) Resting energy expenditure and body composition in patients with newly detected cancer. Clin Nutr 29(1):72–77
83. Hudson MM et al (2003) Health status of adult long-term survivors of childhood cancer: a report from the childhood cancer survivor study. JAMA 290(12):1583–1592
84. Bourdel-Marchasson I et al (2014) Nutritional advice in older patients at risk of malnutrition during treatment for chemotherapy: a two-year randomized controlled trial. PLoS ONE 9(9):e108687
85. Langius JA et al (2013) Effect of nutritional interventions on nutritional status, quality of life and mortality in patients with head and neck cancer receiving (chemo)radiotherapy: a systematic review. Clin Nutr 32(5):671–678
86. Kang WX et al (2016) Effects of nutritional intervention in head and neck cancer patients undergoing radiotherapy: a prospective randomized clinical trial. Mol Clin Oncol 5(3):279–282
87. Heber D, Li Z (2016) Nutrition intervention in cancer. Med Clin North Am 100(6):1329–1340
88. Gibson RS (2005) Principles of nutritional assessment. Oxford University Press, USA
89. Cena H, Calder PC (2020) Defining a healthy diet: evidence for the role of contemporary dietary patterns in health and disease. Nutrients 12(2)
90. Birla M et al (2022) The advent of nutrigenomics: a narrative review with an emphasis on psychological disorders. Prev Nutr Food Sci 27(2):150–164
91. Mayne ST, Playdon MC, Rock CL (2016) Diet, nutrition, and cancer: past, present and future. Nat Rev Clin Oncol 13(8):504–515
92. Donaldson MS (2004) Nutrition and cancer: a review of the evidence for an anti-cancer diet. Nutr J 3(1):19
93. Speakman JR (2019) Use of high-fat diets to study rodent obesity as a model of human obesity. Nature Publishing Group, pp 1491–1492
94. Xiu L et al (2019) High-fat diets promote colon orthotopic transplantation tumor metastasis in BALB/c mice. Oncol Lett 17(2):1914–1920
95. Zeng H et al (2018) Colonic aberrant crypt formation accompanies an increase of opportunistic pathogenic bacteria in C57BL/6 mice fed a high-fat diet. J Nutr Biochem 54:18–27
96. Cranford TL et al (2019) Effects of high fat diet-induced obesity on mammary tumorigenesis in the PyMT/MMTV murine model. Cancer Biol Ther 20(4):487–496
97. Zhu Y et al (2017) Pubertally initiated high-fat diet promotes mammary tumorigenesis in obesity-prone FVB mice similarly to obesity-resistant BALB/c mice. Transl Oncol 10(6):928–935
98. Yang T et al (2018) Maternal high-fat diet promotes the development and progression of prostate cancer in transgenic adenocarcinoma mouse prostate offspring. Cell Physiol Biochem 47(5):1862–1870
99. Nguyen NM et al (2017) Maternal intake of high n-6 polyunsaturated fatty acid diet during pregnancy causes transgenerational increase in mammary cancer risk in mice. Breast Cancer Res 19(1):1–13
100. Okeyo-Owuor T et al (2017) Exposure to maternal obesogenic diet worsens some but not all pre-cancer phenotypes in a murine genetic model of prostate cancer. PLoS ONE 12(5):e0175764
101. Lambertz IU et al (2017) Early exposure to a high fat/high sugar diet increases the mammary stem cell compartment and mammary tumor risk in female mice. Cancer Prev Res 10(10):553–562
102. Jordan BF, Gourgue F, Cani PD (2017) Adipose tissue metabolism and cancer progression: novel insights from gut microbiota? Curr Pathobiol Rep 5(4):315–322
103. Khadge S et al (2018) Immune regulation and anti-cancer activity by lipid inflammatory mediators. Int Immunopharmacol 65:580–592
104. Steck SE, Murphy EA (2020) Dietary patterns and cancer risk. Nat Rev Cancer 20(2):125–138

105. Klement RJ (2017) Beneficial effects of ketogenic diets for cancer patients: a realist review with focus on evidence and confirmation. Med Oncol 34(8):1–15
106. Weber D (2019) Ketogenic diet in the treatment of cancer—where do we stand? Mol Metab
107. Aminzadeh-Gohari S et al (2017) A ketogenic diet supplemented with medium-chain triglycerides enhances the anti-tumor and anti-angiogenic efficacy of chemotherapy on neuroblastoma xenografts in a CD1-nu mouse model. Oncotarget 8(39):64728
108. Allen BG et al (2013) Ketogenic diets enhance oxidative stress and radio-chemo-therapy responses in lung cancer xenografts. Clin Cancer Res 19(14):3905–3913
109. Morscher RJ et al (2015) Inhibition of neuroblastoma tumor growth by ketogenic diet and/or calorie restriction in a CD1-Nu mouse model. PLoS ONE 10(6):e0129802
110. Nakamura K et al (2018) A ketogenic formula prevents tumor progression and cancer cachexia by attenuating systemic inflammation in colon 26 tumor-bearing mice. Nutrients 10(2):206
111. Weber DD, Aminazdeh-Gohari S, Kofler B (2018) Ketogenic diet in cancer therapy. Aging (Albany NY) 10(2):164
112. Piazzi G et al (2019) A Mediterranean diet mix has chemopreventive effects in a murine model of colorectal cancer modulating apoptosis and the gut microbiota. Front Oncol 9:140
113. Kabata P et al (2015) Preoperative nutritional support in cancer patients with no clinical signs of malnutrition–prospective randomized controlled trial. Support Care Cancer 23(2):365–370
114. Carli F, Gillis C, Scheede-Bergdahl C (2017) Promoting a culture of prehabilitation for the surgical cancer patient. Acta Oncol 56(2):128–133
115. Kim DH (2019) Nutritional issues in patients with cancer. Intest Res 17(4):455–462
116. Müller-Richter U et al (2017) Nutrition management for head and neck cancer patients improves clinical outcome and survival. Nutr Res 48:1–8
117. Einarsson S, Laurell G, Tiblom Ehrsson Y (2019) Experiences and coping strategies related to food and eating up to two years after the termination of treatment in patients with head and neck cancer. Eur J Cancer Care (Engl) 28(2):e12964
118. Steele CM et al (1997) Mealtime difficulties in a home for the aged: not just dysphagia. Dysphagia 12(1):43–50
119. Ackerman D et al (2018) Nutrition management for the head and neck cancer patient. Cancer Treat Res 174:187–208
120. Zoran D (2003) Nutritional management of gastrointestinal disease. Clin Tech Small Anim Pract 18(4):211–217
121. Muszkat Y (2009) Nutritional issues in cancer patients. Med Care Cancer Patients, p.292
122. Furbetta N et al (2021) Perioperative nutritional aspects in total pancreatectomy: a comprehensive review of the literature. Nutrients 13(6)
123. Shadad AK et al (2013) Gastrointestinal radiation injury: symptoms, risk factors and mechanisms. World J Gastroenterol 19(2):185–198
124. Britton B et al (2019) In reply to Lee and Douthit, and Champ and Klement. Int J Radiat Oncol Biol Phys 103(5):1283–1284
125. Wu XS, Miles A, Braakhuis AJ (2021) Texture-modified diets, nutritional status and mealtime satisfaction: a systematic review. Healthcare (Basel) 9(6)
126. López-Jornet P et al (2021) Chemosensory function in burning mouth syndrome a comparative cross-sectional study. Nutrients 13(3):722
127. Jensen SB et al (2019) Salivary gland hypofunction and xerostomia in head and neck radiation patients. J Natl Cancer Inst Monogr 2019(53):lgz016
128. Wang K, Tepper JE (2021) Radiation therapy-associated toxicity: etiology, management, and prevention. CA Cancer J Clin 71(5):437–454
129. Muscaritoli M et al (2021) ESPEN practical guideline: clinical nutrition in cancer. Clin Nutr 40(5):2898–2913
130. Hoption Cann SA (2001) The immune system and breast carcinoma: implications of dietary and other associated factors
131. Aprile G et al (2015) Treatment-related gastrointestinal toxicities and advanced colorectal or pancreatic cancer: a critical update. World J Gastroenterol 21(41):11793

132. Joffe L, Ladas EJ (2020) Nutrition during childhood cancer treatment: current understanding and a path for future research. Lancet Child Adolesc Health 4(6):465–475
133. Duncanson K et al (2021) Mechanisms of food-induced symptom induction and dietary management in functional dyspepsia. Nutrients 13(4)
134. Gangadharan A et al (2017) Protein calorie malnutrition, nutritional intervention and personalized cancer care. Oncotarget 8(14):24009
135. Schiffman S, Graham B (2000) Taste and smell perception affect appetite and immunity in the elderly. Eur J Clin Nutr 54(3):S54–S63
136. Padilla GV (1986) Psychological aspects of nutrition and cancer. Surg Clin North Am 66(6):1121–1135
137. Ackerman D et al (2018) Nutrition management for the head and neck cancer patient. Multidisciplinary care of the head and neck cancer patient. Springer, pp 187–208
138. Galaniha LT, McClements DJ, Nolden A (2020) Opportunities to improve oral nutritional supplements for managing malnutrition in cancer patients: a food design approach. Trends Food Sci Technol 102:254–260
139. Aoyagi T et al (2015) Cancer cachexia, mechanism and treatment. World J Gastrointest Oncol 7(4):17–29
140. Álvaro Sanz E et al (2020) Evaluation of a protocol to detect malnutrition and provide nutritional care for cancer patients undergoing chemotherapy. Sci Rep 10(1):21186
141. Fearon K (2008) Cancer cachexia: Developing multimodal therapy for a multidimensional problem. Eur J Cancer (Oxford, Engl 1990) 44:1124–1132
142. Michels N et al (2021) Eating disorders and the risk of developing cancer: a systematic review. Eat Weight Disord 26(4):1021–1035
143. Engineer DR, Garcia JM (2012) Leptin in anorexia and cachexia syndrome. Int J Pept 2012:287457
144. Bossi P et al (2021) The spectrum of malnutrition/cachexia/sarcopenia in oncology according to different cancer types and settings: a narrative review. Nutrients 13(6)
145. Muscaritoli M, Arends J, Aapro M (2019) From guidelines to clinical practice: a roadmap for oncologists for nutrition therapy for cancer patients. Ther Adv Med Oncol 11:1758835919880084
146. Carruba G et al (2016) Nutrition, aging and cancer: lessons from dietary intervention studies. Immun Ageing 13:13
147. Shen Y et al (2017) The impact of frailty and sarcopenia on postoperative outcomes in older patients undergoing gastrectomy surgery: a systematic review and meta-analysis. BMC Geriatr 17(1):188
148. Maruthappu M et al (2016) Economic downturns, universal health coverage, and cancer mortality in high-income and middle-income countries, 1990–2010: a longitudinal analysis. Lancet 388(10045):684–695
149. Copyright © World Health Organization (2007) Cancer control: knowledge into action: WHO guide for effective programmes: module 3: early detection. World Health Organization, Geneva
150. Lampe JW (2020) Diet and cancer prevention research: from mechanism to implementation. J Cancer Prev 25(2):65–69
151. Caro MMM, Laviano A, Pichard C (2007) Nutritional intervention and quality of life in adult oncology patients. Clin Nutr 26(3):289–301. https://doi.org/10.1016/j.clnu.2007.01.005. Epub 2007 Mar 21. PMID: 17368656

GPSR Compliance

The European Union's (EU) General Product Safety Regulation (GPSR) is a set of rules that requires consumer products to be safe and our obligations to ensure this.

If you have any concerns about our products, you can contact us on ProductSafety@springernature.com

In case Publisher is established outside the EU, the EU authorized representative is:

Springer Nature Customer Service Center GmbH
Europaplatz 3
69115 Heidelberg, Germany

Batch number: 10706310

Printed by Printforce, the Netherlands